Praise for Lose It for Life Institute

"This is a comprehensive approach to victory over weight issues . . . Lose It for Life isn't just about weight; it's about life—the abundant life the Good Shepherd promises to all His sheep."

"I've decided I will not pay the price for the sins of others and that I truly desire the best for me. Thanks for getting me on the path and telling me the truth that I will have to persevere. Mostly thank you for your love and the hope you've given me to create a new life for myself."

"Thank you for helping me find the grace and peace that God has given freely and I never accepted until now. I did not realize until last night that I had not surrendered the pain and anger of my daughter's death. Now I have, and I am free of that hiding in my body."

"LIFL changed my life and my thinking about diets and my weight. I know I am not alone and can now face the future and make some needed changes."

"I *can* keep it off, and I *can* make positive and gradual changes in my life! The biggest change for me has been to my goal—from just losing weight to living a truly healthy life."

LOSE IT FOR LIFE

THE TOTAL SOLUTION—
SPIRITUAL, EMOTIONAL, PHYSICAL—
FOR PERMANENT WEIGHT LOSS

Revised and Updated
with Workbook

Stephen Arterburn, M.Ed.
and Dr. Linda Mintle

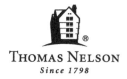

THOMAS NELSON
Since 1798

NASHVILLE   DALLAS   MEXICO CITY   RIO DE JANEIRO

© 2004, 2011 Stephen Arterburn and Linda Mintle

All rights reserved. No portion of this book may be reproduced, stored in a retrieval system, or transmitted in any form or by any means—electronic, mechanical, photocopy, recording, scanning, or any other—except for brief quotations in printed reviews or articles, without the prior written permission of the publisher.

Published in Nashville, Tennessee by Thomas Nelson. Thomas Nelson is a registered trademark of Thomas Nelson, Inc.

Stephen Arterburn published in association with Alive Communications, 7680 Goddard Street, Suite 200, Colorado Springs, Colorado 80920.

Unless otherwise noted, Scripture quotations are taken from the Holy Bible, New International Version®, NIV®. © 1973, 1978, 1984, 2011 by Biblica, Inc.™ Used by permission of Zondervan. All rights reserved worldwide.

Scripture quotations designated MSG are taken from *The Message* by Eugene H. Peterson. © 1993, 1994, 1995, 1996, 2000, 2001, 2002. Used by permission of NavPress Publishing Group. All rights reserved.

Scripture quotations marked NASB are from the New American Standard Bible. © 1960, 1962, 1963, 1968, 1971, 1972, 1973, 1975, 1977, 1995 by the Lockman Foundation. Used by permission. All rights reserved.

Scripture quotations designated NLT are taken from the Holy Bible, New Living Translation. © 1996, 2004, 2007 by Tyndale House Publishers. Wheaton, Illinois, 60189. Used by permission. All rights reserved.

Scripture quotations designated TLB are taken from *The Living Bible* by Kenneth N. Taylor. © 1971. Tyndale House Publishers, Inc. Used by permission. All rights reserved.

Scripture quotations designated NKJV are taken from the Holy Bible, New King James Version. Thomas Nelson Publishers, Nashville, TN. © 1982. Used by permission. All rights reserved.

Scripture quotations designated AMP are taken from THE AMPLIFIED BIBLE, Old Testament, © 1965, 1987 by the Zondervan Corporation and THE AMPLIFIED BIBLE, New Testament, © 1958, 1987 by The Lockman Foundation. Used by permission. All rights reserved.

Scripture quotations designated KJV are taken from the Holy Bible, King James Version.

This book is not intended to provide therapy, counseling, clinical advice or treatment or to take the place of clinical advice and treatment from your personal physician or professional mental health provider. Readers are advised to consult their own qualified health-care physicians regarding mental health or medical issues. Neither the publisher nor the author takes any responsibility for any possible consequences from any treatment, action or application of information in this book to the reader.

Cover Design: Micah Kandros; micahkandrosdesign.com

Interior Design: Walter Petrie

Library of Congress Cataloging-in-Publication Data

ISBN 978-0-8499-4726-1

Printed in the United States of America

11 12 13 14 15 VG 5 4 3 2 1

To the thousands of "losers" who have attended the Lose It for Life Institute. Thank you for helping me shape this material into what it is today. And thanks for staying in touch and connected.

Contents

Getting Started

If you are struggling to lose weight or to keep off pounds already lost, you are in good company. Obesity is a veritable epidemic in our society. Nearly 65 percent of American adults (or more than 120 million people) are considered overweight or obese.[1] And despite billions of dollars spent on countless diet books and health products, we Americans are more overweight than ever.

To be *overweight* or *obese* means to have a medical condition caused by an excess of body fat. By general definition, you are overweight if your body mass index (BMI) is between 25 and 29.9; obese if it is above 30.[2] And while these terms can be easily defined and measured through a number of techniques, most of us need only look in the mirror or stand on the scale to know if we are in trouble.

Samuel Klein, president of the North American Association for the Study of Obesity, notes that technically advanced societies with an abundance of food and sedentary lifestyles are especially at risk for producing overweight people.[3] The speed at which this is happening in America is reason for concern. If you are like most people, you are probably trying to lose weight right now, or you are at least thinking about it. And while losing weight seems like an uphill battle in which the mountain is never fully climbed, it is in truth a battle that can be won.

It is our hope that this book is the last one you'll ever have to read concerning the topic of weight loss. We know most of you have stacks of books you've purchased over the years that detail all sorts of angles and fads for shedding unwanted pounds. Each of those diet books represents your good intentions to conquer that mountain. But for reasons only you know, you haven't won the battle . . . yet.

Perhaps you know someone who is losing weight on the fad diet of the day, or maybe you are trying yourself. After a while, were you right back where you started or in even worse shape than before? It's a familiar story, and it's likely that you are reading this book with a bit of mistrust or skepticism. Let us reassure you that it's okay. We aren't here to help you embark upon another failure. We don't want to promise hope and not deliver. We want you to be successful—to lose weight for life.

Actually, losing weight isn't really the issue. Your closet full of multiple-sized clothing is testimony to the number of times you've lost and gained weight in your lifetime. Some of you are experts at weight loss and could write your own books about your experiences: eating grapefruits, downing vats of "fat burning" cabbage soup, consuming liquid shakes, protein bars, low-fat brownies, and low-carb ice cream. Our personal favorite is the diet in which you lose weight by breathing differently. It's enough to make us all crazy!

We Americans are tempted by quick fixes. The problem with quick weight-loss ideas is that they don't work for very long and require drastic changes in the way we eat—changes that are impossible to maintain over time. Some fad diets are even dangerous and can lead to serious health problems. Recently, I (Steve) was sitting in an airport with executives from my publisher. We were reviewing the cover for this book when the woman at the table next to us overheard our conversation. She wanted to know which diet we thought was the best and asked if Lose It for Life was a healthy plan. She explained that she had just quit a diet because of her health. Though she had lost weight, her cholesterol was at 148 and manageable when she started the diet. However, after only a short time she was forced to take medication to get her cholesterol under control and had to stop using that particular diet. She is only one of many who have hurt their health while trying to lose weight the wrong way.

The real issue isn't *if* you can lose weight. You can. But can you lose weight sensibly and keep it off? Can you Lose It for Life? The answer to both questions is yes.

There is no foolproof diet. Look around. For all our obsession with weight-loss gimmicks, we continue to experience record rates of obesity. We must change our lifestyles, learn to eat sensibly, and exercise. This doesn't sound exciting or terribly new, but it is a long-term strategy that works. And this book can help you make change happen. We encourage you to try again if you have struggled or failed with other methods of weight loss. And if this is your first time trying to lose weight, welcome! We'll share what we know from both personal and clinical experience.

I, Steve, used to weigh sixty pounds more than I do today. I know the heartache of losing the weight, feeling great, and then losing control and gaining it all back. I know how it feels to essentially carry around the equivalent of a third grader on my person. And I know the horror of another approaching summer when everyone will be in a swimsuit and I will have no place to hide.

For years I felt like a second-class citizen because I was fatter than any of my friends. But I was more than that. I was unhealthy. My blood pressure was so high that I was on medication while I was still in my early twenties. I was out of breath and out of energy most of the time. I couldn't run around the block, even at a slow jog! I was facing an early death. And just like you, I had a brain that functioned . . . my weight problem was not a result of lacking IQ points. The problem went deeper; it was emotional and it was spiritual. There was within me a stubborn resistance to do what would eventually change my life.

For a long time, I counted on my troubled mind that had gotten me into trouble to get me out of trouble. I tried the same old tactics over and over again, only to fail over and over again. But fortunately, I awoke one day sick and tired of being sick and tired. My life was never to be the same again. I had experienced a spiritual awakening that led to a new willingness to change. Based on those changes, I developed the Lose It for Life plan—not a diet, but a plan that can work with any diet. Not a behavioral plan that leads to a temporary change in the way you look, but a healthy plan to address spiritual and emotional needs at the core of your being.

The Lose It for Life plan is really a strategy for a healthy life. I have been living by it for years, and the results in my own life have been profound. I have seen what poor eating habits can do to a person. My father was a great man, but he didn't know how to eat. His cholesterol was horrible, and he was on blood-pressure medication, just as I was in my early twenties. He died at sixty-eight of a massive heart attack. It broke my heart because I had so many plans for us over the years that would have followed. Because I was a sitting duck for the same health problems, I gave up some old family eating patterns and adopted the Lose It for Life plan.

So far so good. I just had an annual checkup and my blood work was fantastic. Not one indicator was above or below normal. And the indicators for heart disease showed that I was at one-fourth the risk for heart disease compared to other males my age. I look forward to a long future, and I hope to hear one day that you have experienced the same results.

These radical life changes began from a spiritual place within me—a place of surrender that led me to a new willingness to do whatever it took to get the weight off. I began to lose the weight and have kept it off for more than twenty years. That same willingness to learn and heal and change is the same willingness I try to instill in the hearts of those people who attend the Lose It for Life Institute I have conducted biannually for the past few years. People have paid $1,600 to attend the conference and often had to buy two airline seats to come (that was just for one person!). Many have tried everything; some are on their third gastric bypass surgery. But even after having paid all of that money and going to all the trouble to attend, they often come with little willingness to change.

By the end of the five-day experience, there is real change and they are on a different path. We have followed up with attendants to discover that many do lose weight. I have learned much from those who attend these institutes. Others haven't lost weight but have changed their lives and are actually living for the first time. And sadly, there are also those who make no changes and continue down the same path as before.

Lose It for Life is the culmination of a lifelong journey of first having a weight problem, then finding a way to be free of it for life, and sharing the method of that victory with others. I also bring with me thirty years of experience of working with fellow strugglers of all types of addiction and dependency.

And I, Dr. Linda, bring more than twenty years of personal experience working with clients' eating disorders and food and weight problems. Over the years, I've worked with hundreds of people who have tried all kinds of diets, felt the agony of defeat, been stigmatized because of their weight, endured shame and humiliation due to their size, and felt hopeless in terms of overcoming the compulsion to overeat.

I've consulted with low-calorie diet programs, completed presurgical evaluations for patients considering surgical treatment for obesity, and been instrumental in reviewing medication options for patients. I have spent countless hours with patients in individual, marital, family, and group therapy sessions for eating disorders, including those struggling with compulsive overeating and binge eating. All that to say, I've heard your stories and witnessed the tremendous effort you have put forth to lose weight.

Personally, I struggled with my own weight during a traumatic time in my life. Following the death of my oldest brother, I unconsciously used food to soothe my cycling emotional state and deal with his passing. At the time, I had no idea that my eating was connected to my emotional pain. My training as a therapist and faith in God helped me make this connection and gradually lose the excess thirty pounds. I have maintained that weight loss for twenty years.

We intend to be practical, helpful, insightful, and spiritually alert. We want you to be successful, and we want to help you lose weight without feeling shame, guilt, pressure, or condemnation. Though the weight-loss journey isn't easy, it is possible to lose weight and keep it off. You *can* lose weight for life.

Lose It for Life (LIFL) is not about dieting. It's not about exercising, although exercise does play a part. There is no quick fix, magical diet, or even the promise of a thin body. Losing weight and keeping it off has more to do with changing how you think, feel, and act at any given moment rather than what you eat or whether you take part in a regular exercise program. Lose It for Life is about creating a *lifestyle* of permanent weight management that emphasizes the whole you: your spirit, mind, body, and emotions. It is about discovering meaningful connections with others, support, and community.

Spiritual renewal and transformation, an important part of LIFL, are not typically part of weight-loss programs. Yet without both, you will struggle to keep weight off. It is through a deeper relationship with God and others that hope and encouragement will flood your soul.

When you read the word *spiritual,* what do you picture? Do you envision an angry fundamentalist who throws rules and regulations at you while grinning insincerely? Or perhaps you think of some esoteric experience that no one ever really "gets." If you can relate to either of these scenarios, you're in for a pleasant surprise. We want to help you understand authentic spirituality, and also to examine why the counterfeit of that very thing may be keeping you fat. You are a physical being, and a diet may help you address that. But you are also a spiritual person from the inside out, and it is in that core of you that the battle is fought and then won or lost. We are going to help you with that spiritual battle.

Have you ever found yourself saying, "All I have to do to lose weight is . . ."? It's a common lie that most of us who have struggled with weight have told ourselves—that if we change just one thing, the weight will go away. We want to believe that there is a simple solution to our very complex problem, but there isn't. Instead, there are many variables within your own personal equation to consider. With the help of this book, and by combining the necessary components to maintain your weight-management lifestyle, you will form a personal plan for living a healthier life.

Be encouraged, because you can Lose It for Life! There are so many positive reasons to go forward. Losing it for life is exciting and completely possible. Commit to these ten positive reasons to begin this journey as you:

1. Improve your health. As you gain a proper view of food and nutrition and become more active, you will lose excess pounds. Research shows that even losing a small amount of weight can bring physical benefit!

2. Accept God's free gift of grace and become less judgmental as you are freed of your own guilt and shame.

3. Become defined by who you are, not what you weigh.

4. Gain an awareness of the difference between physical, emotional, and spiritual hunger—and learn ways to satisfy all three.

5. Find yourself more in tune with your body as you accept God's design for you as good.

6. Take your negative thoughts captive, renew your mind, and think in more positive ways.

7. Assume responsibility for your behavior and lose the victim position.

8. Practice managing your emotions instead of allowing them to manage you. Emotions won't be frightening as you learn to confront them head-on and work through the pain.

9. Make new and healthy connections with others—an important part of your recovery.

10. Learn how to preserve spiritual gains and persevere to the finish.

Introduction to the Workbook Sections

These Lose It for Life workbook sections have been designed as a companion to the book *Lose It for Life*. The two are designed to work together. The book offers you the information and tools you will need to understand what's lacking in your current approach to eating and how to begin the process of restoring balance in that area of your life. The workbook sections give you a tool for completing a wide variety of exercises and activities that are crucial to the process. It's an eleven-week (five days per week) program to help you reclaim the power to control your life in the area of food. To prepare for each week, you will be asked to read the appropriate chapter in the book. Then you should use the workbook to help you wrestle with the issues raised in the book.

While not required for you to complete the program, the LIFL family of products has additional resources that you might find helpful, including an interactive journal planner and a day-by-day devotional. There is also a teen version of the book *Lose It for Life*.

The workbook has been developed to urge you to reflect more deeply. It will prod you to examine your thoughts and habits. It will ask you to remember past events—both pleasurable and painful. Mostly, it will push you to take all the facts and wise principles presented in the *LIFL* book and put them into practice. The workbook is your private place to scribble notes, to jot questions, to record feelings and thoughts. The only rule? Be honest. Pretending never got anybody anywhere. Only the truth can set us free.

At times this workbook will likely tick you off. You may feel like hurling it across the room. Please understand our goal isn't to elicit sharp anger or sadness. Rather, through pointed questions and practical exercises, we simply want to lead you to a deeper, richer understanding of why you do what you do and show you how you can shed bad habits for good and how, with the help of God and others, you can develop a whole new approach to life, to eating, to living healthy and free.

So read thoughtfully. Answer honestly. Work through the workbook diligently. Pursue God desperately. Pursue connection with others relentlessly. And, lastly, expect realistically.

Do these things faithfully, and over the long haul, you will succeed. A healthier soul will lead to a healthier mind-set. That will lead to healthier habits. That in turn, will result in a healthier body. Food will lose its powerful hold on you. You will shed unwanted pounds. Can you really do it? Absolutely! God has promised to help, and you have what it takes. Faith in a good and powerful God, together with personal commitment, is an unbeatable combination.

A final warning: If your goal is simply to drop fifty pounds as fast as possible, to get skinny so you'll look better in a bathing suit, LIFL is probably not what you're looking for. But if, at long last, you want to go beneath the surface—if you're finally ready to identify and grapple with all the underlying, unaddressed thoughts and feelings that have been driving your unhealthy eating and exercise habits—then we're ready to begin.

Buckle up. Let's get started. Let's begin to Lose It for Life.

Part One

SEVEN KEYS TO LOSE IT FOR LIFE

Surrender

Acceptance

Confession

Responsibility

Forgiveness

Transformation

Preservation

*At one time we too were foolish, disobedient, deceived
and enslaved by all kinds of passions and pleasures. . . .
But when the kindness and love of God our Savior
appeared, he saved us, not because of righteous
things we had done, but because of his mercy.*

—Titus 3:3–5

1

What Do You Have to Lose?

Food is everywhere! Enticing ads fill the pages of magazines. Billboards loaded with images of pizzas and burgers grab our attention. Television commercials lure us to the refrigerator in search of late-night, feel-good snacks. And if we really want to be scintillated, we can tune in to an entire television network dedicated to scrumptious food preparation, as well as experiencing (however vicariously) the ecstasy associated with eating those specialties. Anyone who is triggered to eat by the mere mention of food or easy access to it is in big trouble in our snack-infested, food-congested society.

Hurried schedules give way to too many fast-food meals eaten on the go. And fast food almost always means fat food. Portions are supersized and a bargain to boot. Some authorities insist that much of our society's obesity comes from one source: carbonated soft drinks—a fancy name for flavored sugar water—consumed in vat-like 32- to 64-ounce containers called "Big Gulps." High prices discourage the purchase of organic and whole foods, fresh fruits, and vegetables. Public high schools subsidize their funding by placing soda and snack machines in their halls of learning. And school lunches are filled with nutritionally bankrupt food.

The food industry isn't solely to blame for amplifying our problem with food. The multibillion-dollar fashion industry promotes an ideal body image that is nearly impossible to replicate, so we give up and collapse into the extreme opposite of the ideal. Guilt and shame glare back from the mirror as we camouflage our thighs and secretly purchase cellulite-reducing creams. Thanks to the media, any chance for a healthy body image is gone before puberty hits. Food becomes our enemy and our lover, truly a relationship as complicated as any other.

When it comes to eating, American culture is toxic. As consumers, we are encouraged to ignore the consequences of overindulgence and our mentality of always needing more. Among the "You deserve a break today" mantras, the messages are consistent: you are entitled to what you want, and you should be immediately gratified (whenever you wish!). However, giving in to these hedonistic messages has led to a serious fallout. As a country, we are fatter than ever and playing roulette with our physical health, mental health, and spiritual health. Our sedentary lifestyles, combined with a poor diet, have led to an obesity epidemic.

American culture promises satisfaction from the pursuit of pleasure. Yet one of the richest and wisest kings of all time (Solomon) concluded that chasing pleasure as an end unto itself only leads to despair. When we lose sight of the Giver of all pleasure (food, taste, and eating included), we carry a burden of excess, both physically and spiritually.

Even the church culture can add to our difficulties. So much of what goes on outside of a Sunday service—most of the social opportunities of the church, in fact—revolve around food. Surely the potluck was invented in a church somewhere in the Midwest. It is almost as if we look for occasions to get together and eat. Additionally, we hear sermons about the evils of alcohol, drugs, and sex outside of marriage, but we seldom hear the Word on gluttony. In fact, some of the best Christian speakers have not resolved their own food issues, so they do not address them with their followers. They would be fired if they entered the pulpit drunk, drugged, or holding a pornographic magazine, but they are excused from taking an extra two hundred pounds up onto the platform. They send an unspoken message that food is the one acceptable addiction of the church.

In society at large, there is a strange dichotomy surrounding food and weight. Our culture simultaneously encourages gorging at the fast-food trough and the all-you-can-stuff buffets, while also frowning deeply on those who pack on extra pounds and look anything less than walking advertisements for anorexia. It is an unwritten American eleventh commandment: thou shalt not be fat. Yet, like the original Law, we are living evidence that this commandment cannot be carried out in our own power. With more than 120 million overweight people,[1] another 5 to 10 million suffering from eating disorders, and still another 25 million suffering from binge-eating disorders,[2] more than willpower is involved in this battle.

The cultural vilification of overweight people guarantees we will try anything to escape the stigma. The billion-dollar dieting industry plays us like a fine violin. When we aren't feeling momentarily defeated, we will embrace another gimmick and believe in its power even when the claims defy all logic. Our sensibilities are lost on the fact that if any of these dieting schemes actually worked, all serious weight-loss programs would go out of business.

But desperation leads to drastic measures—we will try anything for the promise of becoming the incredible shrinking woman or man. The industry knows this and persuades us to keep trying to be thin. And if we buy into the seduction, we can live our lives chasing false images perpetuated by the media. Witness the horror and fascination on MTV as people spend thousands of dollars and suffer intense pain under the knives of plastic surgeons in order to have their frames and faces remade to look like famous stars they idolize. What isn't often shown to the general public are the horror stories of such procedures. A recent television story shared the despair of a mother whose daughter choked to death on her own blood while she recovered from a liposuction procedure in the office of a local plastic surgeon. Truly, does a sixteen-year-old really need to undergo such a surgery in order to live a happy and fulfilled life?

And we forget, or fail to realize, that our spiritual connection to a loving heavenly Father offers real help and truth without distortion in a way no advertiser or program could ever deliver. Dissatisfied and unhappy with life, the hope is that external beauty will translate into opportunity, acceptance, and new life. But as the book of Ecclesiastes reminds us, this is vanity and only leads to emptiness. Lasting happiness and a rich and fulfilling life will only be found in a right relationship with God and others.

So what's the message? *This culture is not going to endorse your decision to change.* It will neither help you control your eating nor offer friendly support. In fact, it may oppose the very measures that contribute to you successfully losing weight for life. But there is reason to hope. In the midst of all the negative influences of our food-saturated society and weight-conscious culture, there is another message: it is possible to lose weight and keep it off.

Seven Keys[3] to Lose It for Life

1. **Surrender**. "So humble yourselves under the mighty power of God, and at the right time he will lift you up in honor" (1 Peter 5:6 NLT). You must be willing to discover what is driving the hunger and want healing more than you want food. You are unable to accomplish your goals without relinquishing control and surrendering to His way of doing things.

2. **Acceptance**. "O Lord, you have examined my heart and know everything about me" (Psalm 139:1 NLT). You must be determined to face and own the emotional issues, pain, and loss that you uncover behind the hunger. Accept the reality of your weight and the need for help. Stay in the reality of your life, accepting your need for help. God sees your heart. He knows your need and will provide the help you require.

3. **Confession**. "Confess your sins to each other and pray for each other so that you may be healed" (James 5:16 NLT). Come out of hiding. Open up to God and others about the reality of your struggles. While it is often difficult to admit your shortcomings and areas of weakness, it is what keeps us honest and real with each other. Confession truly is good for the soul. You must find people you can trust who can handle your secrets and help you heal.

4. **Responsibility**. "For we are each responsible for our own conduct" (Galatians 6:5 NLT). Taking responsibility for change, moving out of the victim position, and owning up to your mistakes is necessary to Lose It for Life. When you are hurt or experience loss, it's easy to blame others or feel like a victim. However, you must believe that God will bring purpose and meaning out of pain, and then you must move on.

5. **Forgiveness**. "If you forgive those who sin against you, your heavenly Father will forgive you" (Matthew 6:14 NLT). Forgive your own failures and the failures of those who have hurt you. Forgiveness is not optional in the Christian life, yet many of us hold on to bitterness and wonder why we don't experience joy and other benefits of the Christian life. When you give up grudges and make restitution for past wrongs, you experience spiritual blessings.

6. **Transformation**. "All praise to God, the Father of our Lord Jesus Christ. God is our merciful Father and the source of all comfort. He comforts us in all our troubles so that we can comfort others. When they are troubled, we will be able to give them the same comfort God has given us" (2 Corinthians 1:3–4 NLT). Transform your struggle, pain, and loss into a purposeful mission. God's way is to take those things you have suffered and use them for His glory. Out of pain and difficulty come compassion for others and a willingness to reach out because of the grace and mercy shown to you.

7. **Preservation**. "Make every effort to respond to God's promises. Supplement your faith with a generous provision of moral excellence, and moral excellence with knowledge" (2 Peter 1:5 NLT). Perseverance is required to make it through life's inevitable struggles and keep the spiritual gains made. When you discover the signs and phases of relapse, you will learn to maintain your weight loss for life.

CONTROL OR SURRENDER?

Life is difficult. Just when we think we have things under control, something happens to remind us that control is elusive. The children who brought such pleasure early on now bring headaches and heartbreaks with rebellion and even rejection. The promotion at work gives you more money but robs you of valuable time and peace of mind. The truth is, we aren't really in control. And until we come to terms with this reality, our lives are destined to be full of anxiety, fear of the future, guilt over the past, and anger at others. Notice—each of these is an excuse to eat!

We can, however, pretend to be in control, especially when it comes to losing weight. We pretend by lying to ourselves about the quick fix that fixes nothing or the instant solution that only makes matters worse. We delude ourselves with the mantras of all those who have failed before us:

- All I have to do is have more willpower.
- All I have to do is just stop eating so much.
- All I have to do is quit being so lazy and exercise more.
- All I have to do is take more control of my life.
- I can do anything if I try hard enough.

And when I no longer believe the lie that I can do whatever I set my mind to, I succumb to the opposite extreme, believing I can do nothing and all is hopeless. The murmurs of my aching soul are:

- My weight is genetic and there is nothing I can do about it.
- It's a sin to dig up the past—what's done is done.
- If I was supposed to be thin, I would have been born that way.

We beat our heads against that same brick wall many times before we realize that our own power is not getting us very far. Check your head. I bet there are many bruises! If so, it's time for a change.

Rather than fight with the same ineffective weapons that have backfired so many times, why not surrender this battle for weight loss? Pull out the white flag and vigorously wave it. Give yourself over to a higher authority; relinquish control to God. He can be trusted, especially when we feel weak and defeated. As the apostle Paul reminds us, "When I am weak, then I am strong" (2 Corinthians 12:10). In fact, when we come to the end of ourselves, God is waiting to step in and provide rest for the weary, and chances are you could use a little reprieve from this exhausting fight. After all, what do you have to lose?

Why not give up the illusion of control and yield to God's mercy and grace? First Peter 5:6 tells us, "So humble yourselves under the mighty power of God, and at the right time he will lift you up in honor" (NLT). Acknowledge your weakness, and invite God into the process. Accept the radical notion that if you could have fixed your weight problem on your own, under your own power, you would have done it by now and the struggle would be over. You have to make an admission. You have to admit you cannot handle this on your own. You have to admit that God can. And you have to let Him do this work, even if it means working with God's people to accomplish the transformation that is necessary (it will!). When you let go of your life and put it into God's hands, you are in good hands.

God is the Creator of all life and the Lord of the universe. But since the garden of Eden, men and women have continually played God and tried unsuccessfully to rule over their own destinies. From Genesis through Revelation, Scripture reveals humankind's natural incapacity to live healthy, God-pleasing lives. The Old Testament describes a colorful assortment of characters who turned their backs on God's ways and inevitably experienced fear, foolishness, and failure. Fortunately, some of them surrendered to the ultimate power of God, allowing Him to intervene in their lives with divine power and wisdom. In the New Testament, Christ's death on the cross made God's intervention even more accessible—He took upon Himself the willfulness and rebellion of the entire world. His resurrection brought hope for new life.

Through years of failed weight-loss attempts, the road of self-effort and control has not taken you where you wanted to go. Proverbs 14:12 tells us, "Before every man there lies a wide and pleasant road that seems right but ends in death" (TLB). To stay on this road is to choose further heartache and destruction. Consequently, we must be willing to admit that our lives have spun out of control. Self-control and our forms of self-treatment have failed us and must be abandoned.

Although we are limited by our weaknesses, God is not. By acknowledging that He alone has the power to change the courses of our lives, we surrender to Him our powerlessness and begin the process of spiritual renewal. Only when we relinquish our control to God does He release His supernatural power in our lives, and it is only through His power that we can be transformed by the renewing of our minds (Romans 12:2).

Every limitation we have can be seen as an invitation from God to do for us what we cannot do for ourselves. When we surrender, we don't just give up or play dead or wait for God to fix us. Instead, we become active participants with God in making a new path of hope toward healing. We drop our guard and give up our solitary and isolated efforts to heal. We sincerely and humbly reach out to others who can help us restore our lives to spiritual vitality. Surrender is not passivity, nor is it resignation. Its motion requires an active and conscious turning toward God wherein we reflect our willingness to submit to His power by living out our newfound truth and sharing it with others.

Surrender means:

- humbling ourselves before the God of the universe
- admitting that God is all-powerful and releasing our struggles to Him
- refusing to escape into the old patterns, habits, and attitudes that continue to distract us and add to the destruction of our lives
- no longer saying, "I can handle this myself"
- submitting to God's way of doing things even when we don't understand
- getting past our pain and fear and clinging to our hope in God and His love for us
- setting aside our human understanding and becoming childlike, and acknowledging that we have no answers that work

Surrender allows you to grow as you submit to God's authority. In order to submit, you must trust that God has good things for you and that His plans and purposes far outweigh what you bring to the table. There are times in our lives when it is very tough to believe that God has good plans in store. When I (Steve) discovered my marriage would end in divorce, it caused a huge faith crisis for me. Surely God would want to spare me the embarrassment and humiliation of being divorced in front of radio listeners, book readers, friends, and family, wouldn't He? What could ever come out of this that would be good? Though I never doubted Jesus was the only way to heaven, I did start to doubt if God really was involved with my life on this side of heaven. I was in deep pain and didn't know if I could trust God to be personally involved with me.

Daily surrender was a daily battle. I felt the need to control based on the absence of God's "felt" concern for me. So I set out in the beginning to do the best I could under my own power. Fortunately that plan did not last long. I began to see God at work and trusted that His love was still there for me in the midst of my failed marriage. Through this pain I came to realize that much of my life was not surrendered to God. As a result of that crisis, I came to a fresher seeking of the true and living God, complete with a new desire for intimacy with Him. The divorce was just the excuse God used to bring me to my knees and to get to know Him once again.

In my own life, I (Dr. Linda) struggled with this concept after my oldest brother was killed. I falsely believed that God could not be trusted because He didn't protect my family and prevent this tragedy from happening. At a time of great loss, I believed a lie—that God could not be trusted. So why would I submit to such an authority?

The difference between surrender and control looks like this:

Surrender	Control
God is the Master of the universe.	I can master all things.
God's perspective is higher than mine.	What I feel is all that is important.
My circumstances are part of God's eternal perspective.	If God is God, my circumstances must be changed now.
I must allow God's plans to open up before me.	My plans are all that matter. I demand immediate results.
I am not alone and will never be.	If there is a God, He is not a part of my life, and I alone can change my reality.
I accept life knowing that all things will work together for my good.	I blame God when life doesn't go the way I think it should.

The lie became so ingrained that a few years later, I refused to put the words "submit" and "obey" in my wedding vows. I loved my husband-to-be, but would I submit to his authority and trust that he had good things for me? No way. I believed that my husband, like God, could not be trusted; both had the potential to hurt me. My belief wasn't based on any reality—I just wasn't about to give control to anyone for fear of being hurt. Disappointed with God, I thought I could prevent bad things from happening. I figured the more I took charge of my life, the less chance I had to be hurt again. You can guess how well this strategy worked!

The years of heartache this type of thinking caused could have been avoided if I had recognized the lie under which I was operating. I had an inaccurate view of God based on my traumatic experience of loss. As a young adult, this prevented me from submitting my life to God's greater purposes, a step that could have saved me much grief. Be assured that it is never too late to abandon yourself to God's power and authority. He can redeem lost time and work His purposes in your life. This has been true in my own life. And when you release yourself from self-effort and striving, a huge burden is lifted.

Thus, your first step to Lose It for Life is to acknowledge your incredible need for God to take the reins. If you don't do this, you are doomed to continue to try every new diet or scheme that offers you false hope and false security. But if you can grasp this concept of surrender and implement it, you can be free from your obsessions and find a new life you never dreamed could be so great. But understand, before you can have that life, you must surrender the one you have.

Surrender acknowledges God's existence and is the first act of faith that will begin your transformation. If you want to get off the weight-loss roller coaster, then surrender to God's way of doing things. Acknowledge that He is in the driver's seat and you are along for the ride. Your way hasn't worked, and His grace is sufficient. His power will be made perfect in your weakness. Surrender leads to healing and the promise God gave us in Jeremiah 29:14: "'I will be found by you,' declares the LORD, 'and will bring you back from captivity.'"

Dear Lord,

I surrender my life to You. Open my eyes to the truth of who You are and what You desire to do in my life. Show me specific areas of my life that need to be surrendered to You. Help me seek You with my whole heart so that You may reveal yourself to me and I may find You. Lead me to those who will help me on this journey. Fill me with Your love and give me what I need to choose Your way and not mine. I trust You enough to surrender my life to You without condition or demands. I trust You to love me, to take care of me, and to never leave me. Please help me realize whenever I am trying to control You so that I can surrender to You and let You control my life. Amen.

MEET GRACE, A NEEDED FRIEND

Once the decision to surrender all to Christ is made, transformation begins. During the process, you'll be introduced to a friend who can really help. Perhaps you've never met this person, or maybe you have but never took the time to get to know Him.

Lose It for Lifer—meet Grace. Grace is divine, a gift from God to you. He offers new life based on nothing you have to offer. There is no way to earn His affections or coax His love for you. He already delights in you and befriends you. The fact that you are overweight and feel like a failure doesn't impact Him. When you fail, He says, "Not to worry. I am with you, and we can start afresh. Lean on Me, not on your own strength. I am strong when you are weak. I have a plan and purpose for your life that I'm dying to reveal."

This guy seems too good to be true, you think. *Perhaps there is a catch.* But as you become more acquainted with Grace, you see He is authentic. There is no pretending. He is compassionate and He cares deeply. And He has the capacity to be intimately involved in your life. His friendship and promises are mind-boggling. People sing and talk about Him and describe Him as "amazing." Apparently He has quite the reputation for being "The Man," despite His feminine name. One reason relates to His astounding ability to see sin, not excuse it, but love anyway. He hangs out with the failed, the most desperate, and the most defeated. He walks along, holding their hands, and pours out healing salve, mercy, and hope. Grace is shocking in the way He upholds the unlovely.

And He knows your critical thought: *If I really wanted to lose weight, I would!* But He responds with such confidence, "I know what you want . . . but don't worry about your life, what you will eat or what you will drink; or about your body, what you will put on." Grace's passion for you is so powerful that it overcomes your fears.

Grace understands the angst involved in doing what you hate—overeating, dieting, gaining momentary control, and overeating again—and says, "Hey, you can't do this on your own. There are healthy ways to eat, but you won't make it with self-imposed rules. I am here to help you change your life, not just your eating. Without Me, it's pretty hopeless—a sort of grit-your-teeth-and-hang-on existence. You need Me in your life. Take Me on your journey."

According to our reports, Grace was recently spotted having lunch with a bunch of overeaters. Many were downright obese and had given up hope for any future joy. But Grace didn't seem to be embarrassed. His kindness was so refreshing. And His eyes . . . well, all you could see was compassion.

Patiently He listened as the group recited their various individual struggles from a week of dieting. Then He gently spoke. "Wow! All you talk about are standards and rules: Never mess up the diet. Don't touch chocolate again. Condemn yourself if you fall into temptation. And these rules seem to be written in stone! You guys need a break. These laws and rules are *guidelines* for eating, but they are impossible to keep all the time. Aren't you human? It's okay to mess up. Just acknowledge when you do, turn from it, and start over.

"With My help, you can keep moving toward the goal. However, remind yourself about Me. I'm going to be here every day. Without Me, your heart will condemn you. But I won't withhold any good thing from you if you walk uprightly."

Stunned, the group sat in silence. One brave woman spoke. "I've never met anyone like You. My friends and coworkers judge me because of the way I look. They say I am fat and lazy and will never be promoted. You say You have good things for me? By the way, did You notice I weigh 280 pounds?"

"I noticed," Grace replied. "But I fail to see how that relates to My offer. Apparently you don't get it. I'm not basing My care for you on anything you do or on how you appear. I would love your devotion in return, but it isn't contingent on Me loving you."

"Okay!" an angry man yelled back. "How much is this going to cost us? What's the bottom line?"

"The cost has already been paid. You were bought with a price. What I have, I give freely. There is no additional cost. It was a onetime deal. Paid in full. Sealed."

Who is this marvelous friend? John 1:17 reveals Him: "For the law was given through Moses; grace and truth came through Jesus Christ." The grace of God is revealed through the divine person and work of Jesus Christ. He both embodied grace and benefited from God's grace. By His death and resurrection on the cross, Christ brought salvation to each of us and restored our broken relationship with God. The Holy Spirit, called the "Spirit of grace" (Hebrews 10:29 NKJV), is the one who binds Christ to us so that we can receive forgiveness, adoption, and new life.

Grace requires faith. We must trust in the mercy of God and realize His favor on us even though it is undeserved. This unmerited favor is a free gift given by our affectionate heavenly Father. As we Lose It for Life, we must remember that God's grace abounds in our lives. He is for us, not against us. He cheers us on to victory, and He uses others to pour out that grace in our lives as well.

If you find you are beating yourself up all the time, saying to yourself things you would never say to someone else, then you have Grace Deficiency (GD). If you think you are so bad no one can love you, you have GD. If you judge yourself based solely on your weight, you have GD. Thankfully, this misery-inducing disease has a cure! God's extravagant grace is what heals it. Give yourself a Grace transfusion through the reading of God's Word, communing with His people, and utilizing a new vocabulary for your self-talk. It is time you started treating yourself the way God treats you . . . with Grace!

COUNTING THE COSTS

Grace is an amazing gift from God. But it does not entitle us to a free ride with no effort on our part. Losing weight and keeping it off under a shower of God's grace still requires small amounts of sacrifice and pain. It is going to cost you more than just developing some good intentions, which people usually have when they approach weight loss. However, in our experience, few people really think through all the ramifications of their weight-loss decisions up front. We believe this has something to do with why so many people fail to keep weight off and give up the battle so quickly. But we are not interested in witnessing your failure, so read on!

Do you recall the story of Jesus and the rich young ruler found in Matthew 19:16–22? The story illustrates the importance of counting the cost before you make a decision. In the story, a rich young ruler approaches Jesus and says, "Good Teacher, what good thing shall I do that I may have eternal life?" Jesus answers by stating five of the Ten Commandments and adds that the man should love his neighbor as himself. The young man acknowledges having done all these things and further asks, "What do I still lack?" to which Jesus replies, "Sell what you have and give to the poor . . . Come, follow Me" (NKJV). Suddenly, the rich young ruler feels the weight of what he is being asked to do. It's one thing to be good and keep the commandments, another to give up what he already has (or thinks he has). You see, his wealth really wasn't his problem. A divided heart was the issue. He wasn't sure he could give up his security for the promise of eternal life. Sadly, he did not follow Jesus because he concluded that the cost was too great.

Do you see the parallels? Whenever you make a decision to change things about your life, there are costs to consider, and your heart cannot be divided as you decide. Perhaps you are more comfortable with dieting than you even know. You try to be good—you even keep all the dieting commandments (Thou shall eat only low-fat foods; Thou shall have no chocolate, etc.) and also wonder, "What do I still lack?" Notice the specific answer Jesus gives. There is no question what is required—total surrender.

Note that Jesus not only gave a specific answer but also addressed the heart condition of the young man. He was looking for a heart sold out to Him. In order to live a life undefined by your weight, your heart condition is critical. Your weight isn't the root problem. Oh, it's tipping the scales too high or causing you distress; we understand this. But there is more to losing and keeping weight off than meets the eye. The good outcome you desire requires changes of behavior, thinking, and the heart.

Even though this might be difficult to accept, it should be a source of hope for you. Other diet books have not helped you because they have addressed only one aspect of the problem—what is going into your mouth. And you have likely proven that for a specific amount of time you can change what you eat. But it is a change of the heart that sustains change in terms of what you eat and fuels a desire to find the weight that is right for you. Heart change is not easy work, but it is easier than staying where you are and experiencing the same frustrations and failures.

We want to be clear from the start: There are no magic pills to offer you. We have no gimmicks, no quick fixes; there are no melt-away-the-pounds creams or cookies that fuel your metabolism into burning like the blazing sun. But there is a path to follow that will transform your life and bring about a stronger, clearer sense of you, as well as healing, renewed thoughts, and meaningful connections.

So let's begin to identify the possible changes you could encounter. Think about these *before* the going gets tough so you can remain tough and keep going. We believe the benefits of a changed life are worth the costs, but you must decide for yourself by counting the costs before committing.

Overeating serves a purpose. This purpose may not be healthy, desired, or even in your awareness, but it is there. Try to think about what it would mean to lose that extra weight and keep it off for life. It's important to be realistic when seeking answers for why you want to be thin. Think about what your life would be like if you didn't spend so much time and energy with food. For example, you might have extra time to fill. With what would you fill it? Would you feel more anxious if your life didn't revolve around food? Most people do experience anxiety when they stop using food to cope with stress because they have to learn new ways to cope. Change, even when desired and positive, can be stressful.

One important question to ask is this: "Will I be confronted with issues in my life I have worked hard to avoid?" For example, maybe you are secretly angry over your husband's request for a divorce and you have stuffed those feelings away by eating. If you stop using food to dull the pain, those feelings of hurt may surface. And though you can learn to tolerate this, it won't be pleasant. You will have to learn to manage those feelings and deal with them directly.

In Order to Lose Weight and Keep It Off, I Might Be Changing . . .

There are a multitude of changes that occur when people try to give up a lifetime of food and weight problems. Although some of these may apply to you, others will not. And there may be personal changes that will occur that only you know about, so we've left a blank line. Take a moment to read through this list and decide if any of these apply to you. And feel free to jot down others that come to mind.

1. **A comfortable habit and way of life**. Eating is what I do when I am happy, comfortable, and feeling good. It's social and a way of life. Go to a movie without a bucket of popcorn? No way.

2. **My best and most acceptable form of distraction**. For example, it's easier to think about the next meal, binge, or snack than the way my boss just treated me on the phone.

3. **A meaningful expression of love**. Food and love are closely associated. Cooking and eating high-calorie foods may be a way I give and receive love.

4. **A way to satisfy needs**. Do I eat as a response to a felt need? Even though the food doesn't satisfy that need, I eat *as if* it does.

5. **Protection from my own sexual impulses**. To lose weight means feeling more attractive. Can I control those impulses related to feeling more sexual and satisfied with my body when I lose weight?

6. **Protection from the sexual advances of others**. If I was raped or sexually abused when I was thin, I might believe that my weight has served as protection against further abuse. If I lose weight, will I feel more vulnerable? Am I ready and willing to face this?

7. **A strategy to keep an intimate other at bay**. When I feel unattractive and don't like my body, I have an excuse to avoid intimacy (especially with my spouse). Am I ready to confront *all* the issues that come with building intimacy?

8. **A cover-up for fears, including failure**. The reason I'm not married, the reason I lost my job, the reason I can't make friends . . . is because I'm fat. Could there be other reasons?

9. **A way to control my life with false structure**. When I feel out of control, eating can be a way to structure my life.

10. **A major coping mechanism for life's stresses**. A general pattern has developed. When I am stressed, I eat. Yes, *stressed* is *desserts* spelled backward!

11. **My tried-and-true way to deal with boredom**. Boredom can be relieved by adding a little spice to life—with extra pasta, a little more sauce. When I open the refrigerator, I find something interesting.

12. **My best friend**. Food never lets me down. I can always depend on it being there and making me feel good for the moment.

13. **My most dependable way to experience pleasure**. There is pleasure in eating, in taste, in texture. And hey, according to our culture, I deserve to feel pleasure (and lots of it!) whenever I want it.

14. **The best or most acceptable numbing device used for emotional pain and anger**. Eating really works to distract me from emotional pain and anger. I don't have to think or feel—just eat.

15. **Protection from rejection**. My layers of fat protect me from possible rejection. I don't have to date, ski, go to the beach, or assert myself—after all, I am fat.

16. **Fantasy versus reality**. If I were thinner . . . ahhh, let me dream of the good life and fantasize about all my problems melting away with the fat. There's no need for reality to interfere.

17. **A way of thinking that reinforces those feelings of not being good enough**. When I am overweight, I can continue to find reasons that people won't like me. They won't look beyond my weight to really get to know me. Without the weight, well . . . I don't want to think there could be other things about me they might not like.

18. **Waiting for the future to avoid the *now***. When I am down to a size 14, *then* I'll visit my relatives. When I fit into that dress, *then* I'll talk to men. The list for future action just grows with the weight gain.

19. **Pretending I have no problems**. Hey, I'm the life of the party, easygoing, and can get along with anyone. Everyone likes me. It's true. I never assert myself and instead pretend I don't have needs. I use food to cover hurtful feelings. My life is dedicated to helping others. It's selfish to think about me.

20. _____

_____

WHAT WORKS AND WHAT DOESN'T

Finally, you may be wondering if this program will be any different from your past efforts to lose weight. Perhaps you've yo-yo dieted or lost a great deal of weight only to put it all back on with a few additional pounds. If so, consider the following ten pros and cons of why other programs fail, as well as the alternatives offered by Lose It for Life.

Other Diets and Programs	Lose It for Life
Unrealistic expectations. People are often disappointed by the reality that weight loss doesn't fix other problems.	**Realistic expectations**. This especially applies to losing weight slowly and sensibly. Other areas of your life may require examination.
Weight loss motivated by appearance. Improving health is less important than becoming thin.	**Changing the focus to health and lifestyle**. This is a lifelong journey with a focus away from weight to that of improved health.
Eating low-fat but still gaining weight. We've developed a diet mentality in which we think low-fat means weight loss. Actually you can eat low-fat food in large quantities and still gain weight.	**Cutting back on high-glycemic foods (sugar and refined carbohydrates)**. For long-term success, feeling more energetic, and eating healthier, this helps.
Physical activity was not increased. Long term, you won't maintain weight loss if you don't increase your physical movement.	**Increased exercise and movement**. In most cases, thirty to sixty minutes of exercise, five to seven days a week keeps the weight off. The more active you are, the better.
All the issues involved in overeating are not addressed. Too many programs focus only on weight loss. Weight loss must address all aspects of your life.	**Resolving emotional issues**. Filling emotional and relational needs with food doesn't work.
Health issues that contributed to weight gain were ignored. You need to know what is causing your weight gain.	**Encouraging self-monitoring**. This means weighing regularly, being aware of how your clothes fit, and looking at your body. In addition, medical monitoring may be necessary if you have health issues.
Disconnecting the spiritual and the body. Your spiritual life is directly related to your physical life. Your body is the temple of the Holy Spirit. Both need to be fed.	**Support a vibrant spiritual life**. We are all in desperate need of mind renewal and allowing God to give us hearts of flesh in exchange for our hearts of stone.

Other Diets and Programs	Lose It for Life
Nutritional plan didn't work. In the world of food and eating, one size does not fit all. You have to develop eating habits that work for you, are balanced, and provide proper nutrition.	**Eating at regular times in order to maximize your body's metabolism.** The idea of skipping meals doesn't work. It sets you up to overeat and to crave foods, and it slows down your metabolism.
Lack of support. Research shows that social support helps sustain weight-loss efforts and maintenance. Spouses are especially important because they can unknowingly sabotage your efforts.	**Connection and support.** Research is clear that support is needed. You will need to build community with people who will support and help you.
Not patient enough. Any lifestyle change takes time to incorporate. Remember, slow and steady wins the race. Quick weight-loss methods usually fail long term.	**Balance and moderation**. It will become your mantra: "There are no forbidden foods." By not feeling deprived, you will stick with the plan and Lose It for Life!

When making any decision, weigh the pros and cons related to change. If you desire in your heart to do this, God will empower you to deal with the hurdles along the way—that is His promise. Through His Spirit, as you surrender to Him and accept His grace, He will transform you to His image. He is your help and source of strength. Invite Him to walk alongside you. His desire is to change your entire life, both physically and spiritually.

Surrender is one of the transforming keys that begins the process of losing the weight for life. In order to give up control and trust God, get to know Him better. Read what the Word says about who He is and what He promises He will do for you. "Taste and see that the LORD is good; blessed is the one who takes refuge in him" (Psalm 34:8). Around the corner is true freedom—much more than just weight loss! The decision is yours.

Workbook Week 1

WHAT DO YOU HAVE TO LOSE?

DAY 1

Losing It for Life

Despite all our diet books, health products, and billions of dollars spent on weight-loss efforts, Americans are more overweight than ever. Obesity is a growing epidemic with 64.5 percent of American adults, or more than 120 million people, overweight or obese.[4]

LOOKING AT YOUR *LIFE*

List the various diet plans you've tried over the course of your life.

_____

_____

How would you rank those diets, best to worst, in terms of long-term effectiveness?

_____

_____

_____

What words or phrases describe your experiences with the assorted weight-loss programs and plans you listed above (for example: "frustration," "the yo-yo syndrome," and so forth)?

_____

_____

_____

List the exercise regimens you've followed and/or the fitness equipment you've purchased in your attempts to control your weight. What were your favorite(s) and least favorite(s)?

_____

_____

_____

_____

How do you feel—at the core of your soul—when you see an infomercial full of hard bodies hawking some new weight-loss or fitness system?

_____

_____

_____

What words best describe your feelings as you begin this _Lose It for Life_ workbook?

_____

_____

_____

LEARNING A NEW WAY OF _LIFE_

Losing weight isn't really the issue. We all know people with closets full of multisized clothing—testimony to the number of times they've lost and gained weight in their lifetimes. Many of us are experts at weight loss. The real issue is, can we lose weight and keep it off?

Why do you think our culture is so enamored with new diet fads and so susceptible to the promise of a quick, easy fix?

_____

_____

_____

_____

> **We don't want to promise hope and not deliver. We want you to be successful— to lose weight for life.**

What feelings stir in you when you see a magazine headline that promises "Lose 10 pounds in one week" or when you see an ad for an exercise gizmo that promises "six-pack abs" in just three minutes a day, three days a week?

_____

_____

_____

_____

Someone has observed, "It's not so hard to change; what's really difficult is maintaining change." Do you agree? Why or why not? In what areas of your life have you experienced lasting change?

_____

_____

_____

_____

The authors assert, "There is no foolproof diet. Look around. For all our obsession with weight-loss gimmicks, we continue to experience record rates of obesity. We must change our lifestyles, learn to eat sensibly, and exercise. This doesn't sound exciting or terribly new, but it is a long-term strategy that works."

What do you think about this statement? Does it encourage or discourage you? Fill you with hope or dread? Why?

_____

_____

_____

LOSING IT FOR *LIFE*

Whether you have long struggled with weight-loss efforts or this is your first time trying to lose unwanted, unhealthy pounds, welcome. We want you to be successful, without feeling shame, guilt, pressure, or condemnation. We know the weight-loss journey isn't easy. But we also know it is possible to shed excess weight and keep it off. You *can* lose weight for life.

The real issue isn't if we can lose weight; rather, can we lose weight sensibly and keep it off?

Dream a little bit. How do you imagine your life would be different if you were able to reach and maintain your ideal weight?

_____

_____

_____

The authors state, "Lose It for Life (LIFL) is not about dieting. It's not about exercising, although exercise does play a part. There is no quick fix, magical diet, or even the promise of a thin body. Losing weight and keeping it off has more to do with changing how you think, feel, and act at any given moment rather than what you eat or whether you take part in a regular exercise program."

Does this explanation surprise you? How does the LIFL approach seem different from other weight-loss plans you've attempted in the past?

_____

_____

_____

The LIFL plan speaks overtly and unashamedly about the central role that spiritual renewal and transformation play in one's long-term success. Spend a few minutes reflecting and writing about your own faith journey. How would you describe your own relationship with God? When did God become more than an idea or concept to you?

_____

_____

_____

In LIFL you will discover what essential ingredients are missing in your quest to be healthy in all aspects of your life. Look at the list below. Rank from 1 to 10 the current "health status" of the various components of your life (1 = "on life support" and 10 = "fit as a fiddle").

_____ My general emotional condition

_____ My family life

_____ My friendships and connections with others

_____ My work or school relationships

_____ My optimism about the future

_____ My ability to handle difficulties and setbacks

_____ My overall view of things

Compose a short prayer that expresses your hopes as you begin this workbook. Tell God what is on your heart. Ask Him to do great things. Trust that He will.

_____

_____

_____

Lose It for Life is about creating a lifestyle of permanent weight management that emphasizes the whole you: your spirit, mind, body, and emotions.

The Culture of Eating

Food is everywhere we look. Enticing ads fill the pages of magazines. Highway billboards loaded with pizzas and burgers grab our attention. Television commercials lure us to the refrigerator in search of late-night feel-good snacks. And if we really want to be tantalized, we can tune in to an entire television network dedicated to scrumptious food preparation and vicariously experience the ecstasy associated with eating it.

LOOKING AT YOUR *LIFE*

If alien creatures visited and studied American culture for a week, what conclusions do you think they would draw about us and food? About us and fitness?

_____

_____

To what degree do you order your days around food—lunch plans, dinner preparation, seeking out your next snack, and so forth? Why do you think you do this? Have you always been this way?

_____

_____

Would you say you live to eat or eat to live? Why?

_____

_____

How often do you eat out? On average, in a typical week, how many fast-food meals do you grab and consume? How many all-you-can-eat buffets do you visit?

_____

_____

The same media that bombard us with around-the-clock temptations to consume fattening foods also broadcast a steady stream of images that convey the necessity of being thin and fit. What is the wide-scale cultural impact of this mixed message? How does this food frenzy—versus—fashion/fitness craze play out in your own life?

_____

_____

_____

LEARNING A NEW WAY OF _LIFE_

American culture is toxic in terms of eating. We are encouraged to pursue the pleasure of eating—whenever we feel like it. When it comes to food, we can never get enough; however, giving in to these hedonistic messages has serious fallout. We are fatter than ever. Our sedentary lifestyles combined with poor diet have led to an obesity epidemic.

Meanwhile, the cultural vilification of overweight people guarantees we will try anything to escape the stigma. The billion-dollar dieting industry plays us like a fine violin. When we aren't feeling momentarily defeated, we will embrace another gimmick and believe its claims even though those claims defy all logic. Our sensibilities are lost on the fact that if any of these dieting schemes actually worked, all serious weight-loss programs would go out of business.

Read Ecclesiastes 2. What did wise King Solomon conclude after his extensive experiment in pursuing pleasure as an end in itself? What is the lesson for us? Is food really able to satisfy the deep longings of our souls?

_____

_____

_____

Thanks to media images, any chance for a healthy body image is gone before puberty hits.

Jesus stated, "Therefore I tell you, do not worry about your life, what you will eat or drink. . . . Is not life more than food?" (Matthew 6:25). What do you think He meant?

_____

_____

_____

Most of us understand that you don't get something for nothing and that anything worth having requires effort. Why, then, do you think many people fall prey to "breakthrough" diet pills or natural supplements that promise miraculous results without a serious change in lifestyle? How susceptible are you to this kind of thinking?

_____

_____

_____

What are your current exercise habits? Have you always followed this regimen?

_____

_____

_____

The Bible makes it clear that God is the generous supplier of all the food we enjoy. For example:

He makes grass grow for the cattle, and plants for people to cultivate—bringing forth food from the earth. (Psalm 104:14)

Give thanks to the LORD. . . . He gives food to every creature. (Psalm 136:1, 25)

He has shown kindness by giving you rain from heaven and crops in their seasons; he provides you with plenty of food and fills your hearts with joy. (Acts 14:17)

God . . . richly provides us with everything for our enjoyment. (1 Timothy 6:17)

American culture has adopted an eleventh commandment— thou shalt not be fat.

Why does our focus so easily shift away from the great Giver of food to the good gift of food? How can we reverse this tendency?

_____

_____

_____

_____

Based on the verses cited above, is it wrong or sinful for us to enjoy a delicious dinner? Why?

_____

_____

_____

_____

In your opinion, where is the fine line between appreciating food and idolizing food? (Be specific.)

_____

_____

_____

_____

LOSING IT FOR _LIFE_

When we lose sight of the Giver of all pleasure (food, taste, and eating included) and pursue pleasure as an end in itself, we carry a burden of excess, both physically and spiritually. We forget that our spiritual connection to a loving heavenly Father is where we find liberating truth, guidance for everyday living, and powerful help of the sort no advertiser or program could ever deliver. Lasting happiness will only be found in a right relationship with God and others.

Our culture will neither help you control your eating nor offer friendly support. In fact, it may oppose the very things that contribute to you losing weight for life.

Is this a new thought to you—that your physical health is tied intrinsically to your spiritual condition? Do you agree with this premise? Why or why not? Record your thoughts, observations, or objections.

_____

_____

_____

_____

In a few sentences, describe your own willpower. How effective are you at setting and reaching goals? At summoning the strength to fight long-term battles?

_____

_____

_____

Many people who struggle with addictive or obsessive behaviors have found great help in the twelve-step programs. One common feature of these programs is an admission of one's powerlessness to change and of one's need for outside help. How might such a confession help a person with a lifelong struggle against overeating?

_____

_____

_____

God doesn't magically change us by "zapping" us. He doesn't routinely take away our desires for certain foods. Instantaneous, once-for-all life change is a pipe dream, not a reality. Given those facts, what are some realistic expectations for any weight-management plan you embark upon?

_____

_____

_____

DAY 3
Control or Surrender?

Life is often difficult and uncertain. Just when we think we have things under control, something happens to remind us that control is elusive. The truth is we don't have control over much of anything. And until we come to terms with this reality, our lives will be full of anxiety, fear of the future, guilt over the past, and anger at others.

The key is surrender—surrender of our entire lives to God's higher perspective and power. Once you've made the decision to surrender all to Christ, true transformation begins. During the process, you'll meet (and need!) a "friend" who can really help. That friend is grace. Let's look closer at the struggle of surrender and this mysterious miracle called grace.

LOOKING AT YOUR *LIFE*

Do you consider yourself a "control freak"? How much and in what specific ways do you try to orchestrate and direct the events and people in your life?

_____

_____

When have you felt the most out of control? What finally happened?

_____

_____

When it comes to weight loss/weight management, check off the following statements you find yourself saying (either internally or externally).

___ "I need to stop eating so much. I need to just say no."

___ "Quit being so lazy and exercise!"

___ "As soon as _____, I will get my weight under control."

___ "I can do this if I try harder."

___ "I wish I had his/her willpower."

___ "If I can just hit upon the right diet, I'd lose weight."

For most people, the word *surrender* brings to mind images of losing, giving up, being defeated and humiliated. But the key to victory in weight control is surrender. One key concept to grasp is grace.

How would you define *grace*? Give it a shot in the space below. (Note: Try to avoid religious lingo.)

_____

_____

_____

Grace is divine, an undeserved gift from God. There is no way to earn God's affections or coax Him to love you. He already delights in you.

What is the opposite of grace? Or, what would a world be like that was devoid of grace? Describe it.

_____

_____

At what time in your life did someone—perhaps even God—treat you in an especially gracious manner? What happened?

_____

_____

LEARNING A NEW WAY OF *LIFE*

Through years of failed weight-loss attempts, the road of self-effort and control has not taken us where we wanted to go. Proverbs 14:12 says, "Before every man there lies a wide and pleasant road that seems right but ends in death" (TLB). To stay on this road is to choose further heartache and destruction. Self-control and our various forms of self-help have failed us and must be abandoned.

What do you think the apostle Paul meant when he said, "When I am weak, then I am strong" (2 Corinthians 12:10)? How can acknowledged weakness lead to strength? How does this truth apply to those who are facing "the battle of the bulge"?

_____

_____

The Bible urges, "So humble yourselves under the mighty power of God, and at the right time he will lift you up in honor" (1 Peter 5:6 NLT). What does humbling ourselves before God look like in practical, everyday terms? What might this look like when dieting? Give some specific examples.

_____

_____

The authors say, "By acknowledging that [God] alone has the power to change the course of our lives, we surrender to Him our powerlessness and begin the process of spiritual renewal. Only when we relinquish our control to God does He release His supernatural power in our lives."

What do you have to lose (other than stress and heartache and excess weight!)? Why not acknowledge your weakness and invite God into the process? What is stopping you?

_____

_____

Grace may seem too good to be true. _There's gotta be a catch,_ you may think. But God's grace is authentic, compassionate, and has the capacity to transform your life. Consider these Bible passages that speak of God's grace:

> [Jesus Christ] became flesh and made his dwelling among us. We have seen his glory, the glory of the one and only Son, who came from the Father, full of grace and truth. . . . Out of his fullness we have all received grace in place of grace already given. (John 1:14, 16)

> [God] has saved us and called us to a holy life—not because of anything we have done but because of his own purpose and grace. (2 Timothy 1:9)

What new insights do they shed on this subject of grace? According to John 1:14, who is the personification of grace?

_____

_____

LOSING IT FOR *LIFE*

Surrender is not passivity, nor is it resignation. It is an active, conscious turning toward God, reflecting our willingness to submit to His power and to share our truth with others. Surrender means:

- admitting that God is all-powerful and releasing our struggles to Him
- refusing to escape into the old patterns, habits, and attitudes that continue to distract us from destructive direction of our lives
- no longer saying, "I can handle this myself"
- humbling ourselves and submitting to God's way of doing things, even though we don't understand them

Every wound and weakness is an invitation to God: "Please do for us what we cannot do for ourselves."

Does the thought of surrendering in this manner excite you or terrify you? Why?

_____

_____

The authors compare and contrast a surrendered mind-set with the person who is determined to remain in control:

Surrender	Control
God is the Master of the universe.	I can master all things.
God's perspective is higher than mine.	What I feel is all that is important.
My circumstances are part of God's eternal perspective.	If God is God, my circumstances must be changed now.

Surrender	Control
I must allow God's plans to open up before me.	My plans are all that matter. I demand immediate results.
I am not alone and will never be.	If there is a God, He is not a part of my life, and I alone can change my reality.
I accept life knowing that all things will work together for my good.	I blame God when life doesn't go the way I think it should.

Which column best describes the way you typically approach life?

_____

In order to submit to God, we must trust that God has good things for us. Why is this kind of submission such a difficult thing for so many people?

_____

_____

Do you typically trust God or mistrust Him? Why?

_____

_____

As we Lose It for Life, remember that God's grace abounds in your life. He is for you, not against you.

Grace understands the angst involved in doing what you hate—overeating, dieting, gaining momentary control, and overeating again—and says, "Hey, you can't do this on your own. There are healthy ways to eat, but you won't make it with self-imposed rules. I am here to help you change your whole life, not just your eating habits. You need me in your life." Will we trust in God's mercy and rely on His favor, even though it is totally undeserved?

Meditate on the jaw-dropping promise of Ephesians 1:7–8: "In him we have redemption through his blood, the forgiveness of sins, in accordance with the riches of God's grace that he lavished on us." The verb _lavish_ means "to overflow, to have an excess or superabundance." No matter how much we've screwed up or failed, God's grace is _way_ more than sufficient.

The authors suggest a prayer of surrender. If this prayer expresses the desire of your heart, take the time to say it now.

Dear Lord,

I surrender my life to You. Open my eyes to the truth of who You are and what You desire to do in my life. Show me specific areas of my life that need to be surrendered to You. Help me seek You with my whole heart so that You may reveal Yourself to me and I may find You. Lead me to those who will help me on this journey. Fill me with Your love and give me what I need to choose Your way and not mine. I trust You enough to surrender my life to You without conditions or demands. I trust You to love me, to take care of me, and to never leave me. Please help me realize whenever I am trying to control You so that I can surrender to You and let You control my life. Amen.

— DAY 4 —

What Works, What Doesn't

You may be wondering, *Is the LIFL program any different from my past efforts to lose weight?* Perhaps you've yo-yo dieted, or lost a great deal of weight only to put it all back on with additional pounds. People approach weight loss with good intentions. In this lesson, let's explore the reasons some diets work and some don't.

LOOKING AT YOUR *LIFE*

Based on your own experience with various diet programs, what are the ingredients of a good weight-loss plan? What are the marks of a diet that is destined to fail?

_____

_____

What is the most weight you've ever lost on a single diet? How long did that take?

_____

_____

If you gained the weight back, how quickly did you gain it? Why? Describe your experience. How did your weight gain affect you?

_____

_____

What has been the most significant *lasting* change in your life? To what do you attribute your long-term success?

_____

_____

_____

> Whenever you make a decision to change things about your life, there are costs to consider, and your heart cannot be divided.

LEARNING A NEW WAY OF *LIFE*

Here are the most common reasons the average diet fails. Check the ones that you've encountered in your own experience.

_____ **Unrealistic expectations.** We often fantasize wildly about how different our lives will be when we reach our thin ideal. In dieting, if we begin with foolish assumptions, we are destined to become disillusioned and discouraged.

_____ **Overeating issues are not addressed.** Too many programs focus solely on how much we've lost rather than exploring the underlying issue of *why* we eat so much—especially when we're not physically hungry. A good diet plan will address these factors.

_____ **The diet is never personalized.** In the world of food and eating, one size does *not* fit all. You have to develop eating habits that are balanced, that provide proper nutrition, and that are tailored for you.

_____ **Too much of a good thing.** Many think low-fat equals guaranteed weight loss. Actually one can eat too much low-fat food and gain weight! Bottom line, we have to decrease amount and increase activity.

_____ **Medical factors ignored.** Certain medical conditions or prescriptions can contribute to weight gain. Before dieting, you need to know what is causing your weight gain.

_____ **Lack of support.** Research shows that social support helps sustain weight loss efforts and maintenance. Make sure you have supportive people to pray, encourage, and be available when you need that extra push.

_____ **Superficial motives.** It is important that we are motivated by a desire for all-around *health* rather than a mere longing for a thin appearance.

_____ **Inadequate exercise.** We cannot maintain weight loss unless we increase our physical movement.

_____ **Separating the soul and the body.** We are spiritual and physical creatures, comprised of body *and* soul. A diet that does not take into account both aspects of our human nature is deficient.

_____ **Results were slow in coming.** Any lifestyle change takes time to incorporate. Remember, slow and steady wins the race. Quick weight-loss methods usually fail long term.

LIFL involves no gimmicks, no quick fixes, no melt-away-the-pounds creams or cookies that burn your metabolism. But there is a path to follow that will transform you. Healing, renewed thoughts, and meaningful connections will emerge if you commit to the process.

If a person wants only to be thin (and couldn't care less about being emotionally/spiritually whole), what are his or her quickest options to a skinny body? Why is this a less-than-desirable outcome?

_____

_____

_____

_____

Why is the support of others so important in an endeavor like LIFL?

_____

_____

_____

Read and ponder the story of Jesus and the rich young ruler in Matthew 19:16–24. What was the man's root problem? Materialism? A lack of spiritual desire? What do you think Jesus really wanted from this moral young man?

_____

_____

_____

What does this story illustrate about counting the costs before making a decision, and the dangers of a divided heart?

_____

_____

_____

The authors observe from this story: "Perhaps you are more comfortable with dieting than you even know. You try to be good—you even keep all the dieting commandments (Thou shall eat only low-fat foods; Thou shall have no chocolate, etc.) and also wonder, 'What do I still lack?' Notice the specific answer Jesus gives. There is no question what is required—total surrender."

What do you think of this notion—that far more important than fat grams is *faith*, and more significant than calories is one's commitment to Christ?

_____

_____

Is your heart fully God's? If you are holding back, why are you? What keeps you from giving yourself in total surrender to God?

_____

_____

Sometimes people eat for emotional reasons and because they are spiritually hungry. Weight loss must address all aspects of your life.

LOSING IT FOR *LIFE*

Let's identify the possible changes you may encounter if you lose weight for life. It is important to think about these possibilities up front. Some may apply to you; others will not. The last line is blank for you to fill in your own reasons. Take a moment and read through this abbreviated list (also found in the book). Check any and all that might apply to you.

In order to lose weight and keep it off, I might be changing . . .

☐ **A comfortable habit and way of life**. Eating is what I do when I am happy, comfortable, and feeling good. It's social and a way of life. Go to a movie without a bucket of popcorn? No way.

☐ **My best and most acceptable form of distraction**. For example, it's easier to think about the next meal, binge, or snack than the way my boss just treated me on the phone.

☐ **A meaningful expression of love**. Food and love are closely associated. Cooking and eating high-calorie foods may be a way I give and receive love.

☐ **A way to satisfy needs**. Do I eat as a response to a felt need? Even though the food doesn't satisfy that need, I eat *as if* it does.

☐ **Protection from the sexual advances of others**. If I was raped or sexually abused when I was thin, I might believe that my weight has served as protection against further abuse. If I lose weight, will I feel more vulnerable? Am I ready and willing to face this?

☐ **A strategy to keep an intimate other at bay.** When I feel unattractive and don't like my body, I have an excuse to avoid intimacy (especially with my spouse). Am I ready to confront *all* the issues that come with building intimacy?

☐ **A cover-up for fears, including failure.** The reason I'm not married, the reason I lost my job, the reason I can't make friends . . . is because I'm fat. Could there be other reasons?

☐ **A way to control my life with false structure.** When I feel out of control, eating can be a way to structure my life.

☐ **A major coping mechanism for life's stresses.** A general pattern has developed. When I am stressed, I eat. Yes, *stressed* is *desserts* spelled backward!

☐ **My tried-and-true way to deal with boredom.** Boredom can be relieved by adding a little spice to life—with extra pasta, a little more sauce. When I open the refrigerator, I find something interesting.

☐ **My best friend.** Food never lets me down. I can always depend on it being there and making me feel good for the moment.

☐ **My most dependable way to experience pleasure.** There is pleasure in eating, in taste, in texture. And hey, according to our culture, I deserve to feel pleasure (and lots of it!) whenever I want it.

☐ **The best or most acceptable numbing device used for emotional pain and anger.** Eating really works to distract me from emotional pain and anger. I don't have to think or feel—just eat.

☐ **Protection from rejection.** My layers of fat protect me from possible rejection. I don't have to date, ski, go to the beach, or assert myself—after all, I am fat.

☐ **Fantasy versus reality.** If I were thinner . . . ahhh, let me dream of the good life and fantasize about all my problems melting away with the fat. There's no need for reality to interfere.

☐ **A way of thinking that reinforces those feelings of not being good enough.** When I am overweight, I can continue to find reasons why people won't like me. They won't look beyond my weight to really get to know me. Without the weight, well . . . I don't want to think there could be other things about me they might not like.

☐ **Waiting for the future to avoid the *now*.** When I am down to a size 14, *then* I'll visit my relatives. When I fit into that dress, *then* I'll talk to men. The list for future action just grows with the weight gain.

☐ **Pretending I have no problems.** Hey, I'm the life of the party, easygoing, and can get along with anyone. Everyone likes me. It's true. I never assert myself and instead pretend I don't have needs. I use food to cover hurtful feelings. My life is dedicated to helping others. It's selfish to think about me.

☐ **Other:** _____

Ask yourself: If I embark on this LIFL program, will I be confronted with issues in my life I have worked hard to avoid? What issues?

_____

_____

Any lifestyle change takes time to incorporate. Remember, slow and steady wins the race.

Here are just some of the positive reasons listed in the book for deciding to Lose It for Life. You will:

- Improve your health. As you gain a proper view of food and nutrition and become more active, you will lose excess pounds. Research shows that even losing a small amount of weight can bring physical benefit!
- Accept God's free gift of grace and become less judgmental as you are freed of your own guilt and shame.
- Become defined by who you are, not what you weigh.
- Gain an awareness of the difference between physical, emotional, and spiritual hunger and learn ways to satisfy all three.
- Find yourself more in tune with your body as you accept God's design for you as good.
- Take your negative thoughts captive, renew your mind, and think in more positive ways.
- Assume responsibility for your behavior and lose the victim position.

- Practice managing your emotions instead of allowing them to manage you. Emotions won't be frightening as you learn to confront them head-on and work through the pain.
- Make new and healthy connections with others—an important part of your recovery.
- Learn how to preserve spiritual gains and persevere to the finish.

Which of these positive benefits excites you most? Why?

_____

_____

Who are the people you can depend upon to surround you with support and encouragement in your LIFL endeavor?

_____

_____

Ten Elements of Success

Congratulations! In a few minutes you will have completed the first week of lessons in the Lose It for Life workbook. Hopefully, you are sensing a powerful new hope rising within. You are catching a glimpse that substantive change really *is* possible—not just another short-term spin on the old diet yo-yo, but real and lasting transformation, a brand-new way of living.

LOOKING AT YOUR *LIFE*

What are your biggest fears or concerns as you embark on this life-altering adventure?

_____

_____

Imagine being free from any and every sort of unhealthy preoccupation with food. Imagine being truly satisfied with smaller amounts of healthier foods. Imagine getting to the place that your body is toned and fit. Imagine enjoying dinners with friends and the taste of certain dishes without being obsessed. Imagine not lugging around all those excess pounds. Imagine instead feeling energetic. In the space below, write about some of your hopes and dreams.

_____

_____

LEARNING A NEW WAY OF *LIFE*

Romans 8:31 says that God is "for us." Spend a few minutes pondering that phrase. What does it do to your heart to realize that God is pulling for you, that He's in your corner, that He wants you to succeed?

_____

_____

A big part of the LIFL philosophy is recognizing that our beliefs determine our behaviors. When we engage in wrong behaviors, including unhealthy eating habits, it's because we've embraced wrong beliefs (Romans 12:1–2). Therefore the deepest and surest way to change how we live is to change the way we think.

Can you begin to identify certain beliefs (about food, about dieting, about thinness) or wrong ways of thinking (about yourself, about how to handle struggles) that need to be changed? Write your observations here:

_____

_____

LOSING IT FOR _LIFE_

If you truly desire to embark wholeheartedly on the LIFL plan, God will empower you to deal with the hurdles along the way. That is His promise. Through His Spirit, as you surrender to Him and accept His grace, He will transform you to His image. He is your help and source of strength. Invite Him to walk alongside you. His desire is to change your life—not just your body.

In the prior session (Day 4) we looked at the typical reasons most diet plans fail. This time, let's look at those factors that contribute to losing and keeping weight off long term. These are the principles upon which the Lose It for Life system is based.

Ponder each statement below. In the space that follows, jot down your thoughts, questions, or responses.

1. **You will set realistic expectations**. This is how we lose weight, slowly and sensibly. (Other areas of your life may also require examination.) Develop goals, but make them realistic and reachable.

_____

_____

2. **You will eat at regular times in order to maximize your body's metabolism**. The idea of "skipping meals" doesn't work. It sets us up to overeat, crave foods, and slows down our metabolism.

_____

_____

The more active you are, the better.

3. **You will begin to exercise and move your body**. In most cases, thirty to sixty minutes of exercise, five to seven days a week, keeps the weight off.

_____

_____

4. **You will monitor your progress**. This means weighing on a regular basis and being aware of how your clothes fit. If you have a history of eating disorders, you may not want to weigh daily, but you will want to establish some accountability. In addition, medical monitoring may be necessary if you have health issues.

_____

_____

5. **You will strive, by God's grace, for balance and moderation**. This will become your mantra: "There are no forbidden foods." However, you have to exercise God-aided self-restraint for the sake of your health. It's the amount we eat and the reasons we eat it that matter most.

_____

_____

6. **You must cut back on high-glycemic foods (sugar and refined carbohydrates)**. For long-term success, feeling more energetic, and eating healthier, this is mandatory.

_____

_____

7. **You will begin addressing emotional issues related to personal and interpersonal relationships.** Filling emotional and relational needs with food doesn't work and isn't healthy.

_____

_____

8. **You will cultivate a vibrant spiritual life.** We are all in desperate need of a rich walk with God. We need to work actively to change how we think (Romans 12:1–2) so that our actions and habits also change.

_____

_____

9. **You will enlist support.** Research and experience are clear that we cannot find victory alone. We need to build community with people who will support and help us (and who we can support and help).

_____

_____

10. **You will develop a more holistic focus.** Lifelong weight control is an ongoing process, that requires much more than a mere focus on body shape/size. Our emphasis must be on total emotional/ spiritual/physical health.

_____

_____

Remember, surrender is the step that begins the process of losing it for life. Give up control. Trust God. Get to know Him better. Read what the Bible says about who He is, what He promises, and what He will do in you and for you. "Taste and see that the LORD is good; blessed is the one who takes refuge in him" (Psalm 34:8).

2

Take the Red Pill

O Lord, you have examined my heart
and know everything about me.

—Psalm 139:1 NLT

If you saw *The Matrix*, you'll understand this next challenge. It involves just one question: Will you take the red pill? For those of you who didn't see the movie or prefer not to, here's the context. In *The Matrix*, a computer hacker named Neo lives a rather ordinary life in what he thinks is the year 1999. Morpheus, a rebel warrior, contacts Neo and explains to him that his reality is in fact false. The truth is that it is two hundred years later, artificial intelligence runs the world, and humans are living in a complex system in which they are placated and used for fuel to run the machines that have very nearly taken over the world. Neo, fresh with this revelation, is confronted with a life-altering choice: he can take the blue pill, wake up the next morning remembering nothing of this meeting, and go on living in his false world, or he can take the red pill. If he swallows the red pill, he'll see life as it really is (and save the world, of course!).

Think of yourself as Neo. We (Morpheus) are confronting you with a life-altering choice. Do you want to continue to live in the false world of dieting, where emotional pain is numbed, health risks are ignored, and false promises are made? Or do you want to take the red pill, as it were, and see the reality of a world in which food and eating don't dominate or take over your life? If you accept this challenge, you will have to face moments of pain from the past you might prefer be left alone, deal with relationship difficulties, and make changes in possibly all aspects of your lifestyle. As you consider, ask yourself what would happen if your body were how you wanted it to be and food no longer ruled your day.

Lose It for Life is a program that can make this happen. Change is possible, and the support and insight in this book can help you be successful as you commit to getting healthy and staying on track. One step at a time, through making decisions and evaluating your needs, you will find the answers you need.

If you do choose the red pill, you won't be saving the whole world, but your whole world will change as you reclaim your sanity and health!

ACCEPTING REALITY

Once you fully surrender the weight-loss battle to God, you must open your eyes to reality and stop lying to yourself or making excuses. This is a vital step in the process. Incredible insight concerning truth is offered by Dostoevsky in his novel *The Brothers Karamazov*:

> The important thing is to stop lying to yourself. A man who lies to himself, and believes his lies, becomes unable to recognize the truth, either in himself or anyone else, and he ends up losing respect for himself as well as others. When he has no respect for anyone, he can no longer love and, in order to divert himself, having no love in him, he yields to his impulses, indulges in the lowest forms of pleasure, and behaves in the end like an animal, in satisfying his vices. And it all comes from lying—lying to others and to yourself.[1]

In order to lose weight for life, you have to face reality or you end up lying to yourself and others. Tough questions must be asked and answered:

- What is my part in gaining this weight?
- How do I respond to difficulty?
- What unmet needs do I have that I try to meet through food?
- When life gets tough, do I get going or start eating?
- Am I hung up on "why" my life feels so out of control?
- Am I disconnected from others?
- Do I live in denial, refusing to acknowledge my weight problem and the impact it has on my life?

The words of Jesus in John 16:33 provide truth and hope. Jesus tells His disciples, "These things I have spoken to you, that in Me you may have peace. In the world you will have tribulation; but be of good cheer, I have overcome the world" (NKJV).

Jesus doesn't lie to us. As the Son of God, He is incapable of lying. He tells us that difficulty and suffering will be part of life—He wants us to know reality. And this is the reason we can trust Christ: He is the Truth and He speaks truth. Jesus offers hope. He has overcome the world! During His life on earth, He overcame Satan's temptation. On the cross, He overcame the power of sin by becoming sin. And through His death and resurrection, He broke the power of death. He is our hope no matter what difficulty we face. "I am the way, the truth, and the life. No one comes to the Father except through me," He declares (John 14:6 NKJV). "And you shall know the truth, and the truth shall make you free" (John 8:32 NKJV). Acceptance involves first realizing the full depth of your problem . . . which means taking the red pill and seeing life as it really is.

So often it is easier to replace these realities with lies of our own making. We tell ourselves there really is nothing we can do; that it isn't our fault we got so heavy; or that to face the reality will mean facing pain, which is potentially worse than letting ourselves go and merely surviving through life. Or we assume that if God wanted to, He would take this burden from us. He would take away this pain if it were His will. All are very tempting lies to hold on to, but when we reach that point of acceptance, the lies start to peel away. Reality is no longer denied, and the truth comes out: being over-weight is not about the past, or food, or even the temporary relief and comfort found in food. *It is about right now and what you choose to do about it.* A weight problem either continues to get worse or gets better with the next choice made. Take note—no matter what path was chosen before, choosing differently *now* is the key to where this program begins.

- Your overweight body is a symptom of an underdeveloped soul.
- No one else caused your problem, and no one else is going to fix it for you.
- When you decide to change, it is going to be painful.
- No one can walk through that pain but you, and you must walk through it.

BREAK THROUGH YOUR DENIAL

All of us struggle with blind spots in our lives, and to some degree we all live in the company of denial and self-deception. But rather than confront our area(s) of struggle and pain, we often point to others and focus on them or find alternatives to distract and anesthetize ourselves from what really needs to be faced.

Acceptance is being willing to lift the curtain of denial and look at the big lie of your life. Breaking through denial means being aware of your struggle and pain and consciously confronting the behaviors and patterns that have deterred you from God's best. Only with God's help and a supportive, healing community can the blinders be removed.

Deception and denial give way to seeing yourself as you really are—trapped in your patterns, paralyzed by fear, and making choices that produce short-term results rather than long-term change. God is patient, loving, and able "to do far more than we would ever dare to ask or even dream of—infinitely beyond our highest prayers, desires, thoughts, or hopes" (Ephesians 3:20 TLB). Take a moment and examine your heart. How have you avoided reality? See if any of these actions play a role in how you avoid the truth:

- You avoid prayer, times of silence and looking at your situation, honest conversations that touch a sensitive area of your life, or people who can speak into your life and encourage you on your journey.
- You minimize or rationalize your behavior.
- You constantly criticize others.
- You are confused as to why others react to you and what you say or do.
- You find yourself lying repeatedly.

If you are willing to confront the reality of your overeating, these positive signs will be evident:

- You focus on what you can do to change rather than on what you want others to do to make you feel better.
- You humble yourself in order to confront who you really are.
- You look for what really causes the conflicts you experience.
- You honestly face your past pain and failures head on.
- You stop blaming others for your difficulties.
- You seek, receive, and apply God's wisdom to your situation.

- You look at what you've done in the light of God's mercy and grace—not judgment or condemnation.
- You accept that you are unable to help yourself without God's help.
- You can name your character defects and mistakes rather than deny them.

By being honest you can move out of the past and into the reality of the present. Only when you face the truth can God teach you to resolve your problems rather than reproduce them within relationships with family and close friends. Are you ready to take the red pill? It's a big dose of reality, but with God's help and the help of others, you can take it.

Dear Lord,

Open my eyes to see the truth about You and myself. Show me the things that need to be changed. Put me on the right path that I may walk in Your truth. Amen.

LETTING GO OF EXCUSES

Making excuses is perhaps the most common way to justify overeating—and deal with failure. With a good excuse, guilt and anxiety about overeating dissipate. But the sad reality is that making excuses to feel better about overeating actually fosters continued overeating by simply lessening the momentary anxiety—which means making excuses becomes part of a vicious cycle of overeating again and again.

For example, it's late at night. You are watching TV and you start thinking about ice cream because you've just seen a tantalizing commercial. Anxiety begins to mount as you try to decide if you should eat the ice cream sitting in your freezer . . . or say no. You aren't thinking about the fact that you are *not* hungry. The ice cream just looks so good—it would be a terrific treat right now . . . and it's calling to you from the freezer . . . and you've had a long and exhausting day. All of these are excuses that hide the truth: *you are not hungry*. But the excuses come so easily, so smoothly, it has become your habit to just ignore the truth when it comes to overeating. Excuses take the focus off of the long-term consequences.

Certainly you don't want to think about the long-term effects of overeating right now. And the longer you postpone eating the ice cream, the greater your anxiety becomes. *Should I eat or shouldn't I?* Eventually you become so uncomfortable over this dilemma that you get up, walk to the kitchen, and serve yourself a scoop of ice cream.

Then you think, *There isn't that much ice cream left in the carton. I'll finish it off and won't buy any more. I'll start dieting tomorrow when it's all gone.* As you begin to overeat, the momentary anxiety disappears. The ice cream tasted great, or at least you think it did—you ate it so fast, you really didn't taste it. Now it's late, and now you are really tired. Feeling uncomfortably full, you go to bed.

Excuses prompted you to avoid the reality that you weren't hungry. Sound familiar? Happily, there is an alternative, but the first step is to see excuses for what they really are.

Think It Through—Delay Gratification

When you ate the ice cream, you gave in—you bowed under pressure to the moment (and the anxiety) without thinking about the long-term consequences. You are an advertiser's dream TV viewer! Immediate gratification is the message advertisers sell. Their job is to persuade you to be impulsive, to give in to temptation.

To lose weight and keep it off requires you to delay momentary gratification and think with a long-term perspective—to engage in the reality of your decisions. Advertisers hope you won't think that hard. They would prefer that you live in the moment and give in to the immediate pleasures they are selling. However, when you are tempted, think about the impact of this one choice on your life. Taking the earlier example, ask yourself questions like these:

- How will I feel after I eat this?
- How will I feel in thirty minutes?
- How will I feel about this tomorrow morning?
- Will I beat myself up over this choice?

You get the idea. To delay an urge to overeat, don't rationalize what you are doing. Think about the long-term consequences and learn to tolerate your anxious feelings, which generally will pass after only a short time. Tell yourself it's normal to feel anxious when making a decision. Take a few deep breaths and relax your body; the urge will likely subside within twenty minutes or so.

Or wait for that anxious feeling to go away by distracting yourself with something else. Turn off the TV, pull out a book, call a friend, take a walk, go to the bathroom (people tend not to eat in the bathroom), get in the car and go for a drive, attend a meeting, or just go to bed. Whatever you do, don't stare at the refrigerator and try to exercise willpower.

These strategies work for overeating and other impulsive behavior as well. And sometimes the best strategy is to avoid any tempting situation altogether. Late-night TV viewing may be a trigger for you to overeat. If so, don't watch late-night TV! Instead, do something different: play a game, read, pray for your family, or do a Bible study.

If you do decide to give in to the immediate pleasure of eating, take *one* scoop of ice cream and no more. Eat it slowly and enjoy every bite. You won't gain a pound from one small scoop, but eating the entire carton will certainly do some damage. The next day, be sure that you go to the store and replace that high-fat, high-carb, high-sugar ice cream with a no-sugar-added substitute. Make your freezer safe for the next time you just can't resist or are unwilling to delay gratification.

Delaying gratification is a process that involves self-control, an area we often feel we lack in. According to Galatians 5:22–23, self-control is a fruit of the Spirit. This fruit is an attribute of those who walk in the Spirit. As we grow in the Lord, we become more like Him.

Just as fruit begins with a seed, so, too, does a fruitful spiritual life. Both need nourishment to thrive. We need to read the Word of God and let it soak very deep in our hearts. The more we desire to please God in all we do, the more obedient we become. Obedience produces self-discipline, which gives way to self-control. We are not talking about control born of self-effort, but self-control born of the Spirit working in us.

The enemy of our souls wants to discourage us from ever thinking we could have a supernatural self-control. Satan even tested Jesus in the wilderness. This fallen angel came to Jesus when He was physically weak, hungry, and tired from fasting. Just think: the first wilderness temptation involved food, as did the original temptation with Adam and Eve!

Satan, knowing the toll of hunger on Jesus' earthly body, suggested a shortcut—an immediate gratification. However, the biblical account begins with an important fact. *The Spirit* led Jesus into the wilderness. Don't miss the importance of this—being led by the Spirit is what we all need in order to overcome our weaknesses.

And Jesus' defense against succumbing to immediate gratification was to quote the Word to His enemy. The Living Word quoted the Word. This is your model for overcoming. As you soak yourself in the Word, you nourish your spiritual life. The seed bears fruit—in this case, self-control. Be ready for times of testing. Nourish yourself with plenty of time in the Word and allow your life to bear the fruit of the Spirit.

RESPONSIBILITY—THE BALANCE TO SURRENDER

Another key element of a life no longer controlled by appetite or weight is a newfound sense of responsibility. We must refuse to blame anyone else for the extra weight and acknowledge that we are responsible, yet we can't fix this on our own power. This is the balance of surrendering to God: we allow God to do what we cannot do, but we do what we can.

Responsibility involves the treatment of old wounds that may be triggering your overeating. It also requires making strong decisions and changes in your life. Hurts that drive you to inappropriate behaviors and destructive habits are hurts that you may not have fully worked through. Diverting yourself from problems or anesthetizing your emotions with food, hurtful people, or activities may be a common pattern in your life.

The Steps of Accepting Responsibility

1. Facing problems rather than escaping them, including bearing the full responsibility of misconduct.
2. Taking time to grieve the loss and experience pain—"Blessed are those who mourn, for they will be comforted" (Matthew 5:4).
3. Reaching out to Christ, who suffered Himself and understands our hurt.
4. Accepting the hope that God's plans for us are good and loving—we must purposefully look beyond the loss to God's deeper purposes.
5. Refusing to allow anything from the past to serve as an excuse for lack of growth, character, or development, including living in the role of victim.

In our world, it's easy to take on the role of victim and live a life of victimization. Yet, as horrendous as your past problems and abuse may have been, when you own them as part of you, you learn to see them as purposeful, deepening, and integral to your development of godly character. It takes courage to walk through this pain, but God can provide the strength and support to truly overcome past hurts and, ultimately, to use them for His glory. As the psalmist David wrote, "It was good for me to be afflicted so that I might learn your decrees" (Psalm 119:71).

Avoiding pain and problems is a natural human response. Most people feel they have "suffered enough" and have no desire to feel overwhelmed by sorrowful emotions. But grief is a necessary process of this earthly life, because we all fail, suffer, and deal with loss. It is important to note that experiencing grief over our failures and losses connects us to God's grace. Saint Augustine affirmed this when he said, "In my deepest wound I saw your glory and it dazzled me." It is not pleasant, but it is necessary. We must experience (or grieve) the pain we feel today so we will not be driven by it in the future. Too often we point to our past pain as an excuse and miss the fact that it very definitely *is* part of God's plan for us. It is so easy to blame others for everything that has gone wrong. When we don't accept responsibility, we live in a victimized state and blame others for our problems. For the overeater, food will continue to be used to deaden pain and numb reality.

Prayer for Accepting Responsibility

Dear Lord,

    I realize that You have given me life and that living is my responsibility. Lord, I want to accept responsibility for my whole life. I know You want my life to be fruitful, but sin and tragedy have infected my life—both by my hand and the hands of others. Help me to accept responsibility to remove these weeds that have been sown in me. Lord, I confess that sometimes I blame others for my own disobedience to You. I now accept responsibility for these things. Please forgive me and fully restore the relationship between us. Amen.

EXAMINE YOUR MOTIVATION

When you give up your excuses, pray a prayer of acceptance and responsibility, and then examine your motivation for wanting to lose weight. If your main motivation is to be thin so you can do all the things you never could do before, or to be the person you were never allowed to be and have all your dreams come true, it's time to reevaluate (definitely take the red pill!).

    Research tells us that people become more successful at long-term weight loss when their motivation is to become *healthier,* not thinner. This change in attitude or motivation is essential. Improving your health involves lifestyle changes that we will delineate in this book. To be thin, you have to lose the weight. And we know you can do that. Many of you have done so, *over and over.* To Lose It for Life, you have to take a more comprehensive approach. All the areas involved with overeating must be addressed.

WRITE IT DOWN

Perhaps you are frustrated because it seems as if you've been dieting forever and haven't lost a pound. We can relate. My college "cottage cheese diet" caused me (Dr. Linda) to gain fifteen pounds my freshman year. Here's what I did. I skipped breakfast every day (and slept instead), ate cottage cheese and fruit for lunch, and then ate a regular dinner. As I stared at my little bowl of white mealy curds every lunchtime, I believed I was making the ultimate sacrifice to lose weight. For the record, I don't believe cottage cheese is real food! But I ate it religiously and sincerely thought the pounds would fall off.

What I failed to take into account was a small but important fact. Snack machines were placed in the dorms and right next to the room where I studied. In addition to my meals, I was also ingesting late-night fruit pies from those machines. Oh yes, and those cinnamon buns . . . and maybe a few Doritos too. And when the chocolate was passed around the study room, I broke off my share of the bar. All those extra calories that didn't "count" because they weren't part of my meals added up to quite a shocking number! No wonder I didn't lose weight.

Maybe it seems as if you eat very little. Or you think you can't lose weight on a 1,200-calorie diet because of metabolic problems or heredity issues. Yet in truth, very few people have metabolic disorders or genetic factors that cause them to be overweight. Because so many people reported eating small amounts of food and gaining weight, researchers studied this. What they found was that people grossly underestimated what they ate in a day, and they also exercised less than they thought.[2] It wasn't that people were intentionally lying about what they ate. They just forgot about moments in the day when they grabbed a handful of M&Ms or tasted spoonfuls of chili while preparing dinner. A little here and a little there really adds up.

Perhaps the largest number of "hidden" calories and carbs are consumed in the most unnoticed way—in what you drink. Soft drinks and hard liquor and everything in between fill us up with calories that often go unaccounted. Consider this reality: if in a single day you consumed a twelve-ounce mocha, two glasses of orange juice, two glasses of milk, a can of regular soda, and a twelve-ounce bottle of beer, you added nearly a thousand calories to the total number of calories you consumed in actual food!

Studies show that people who record what they eat lose more weight and keep it off compared to those who don't. In fact, the more days a person keeps a food journal, the greater the weight loss.[3] So, based on studies and our personal experience, keeping a food journal is important. Begin by writing down everything you eat in a day for a week or two. It sounds tedious, but recording this data will provide you with a greater awareness of what you are eating. A food journal will also pinpoint eating patterns—when you eat, how much, how often, the amount of what you eat, etc. This information will later be used to make changes. Here is a sample of a simple food journal. (See Appendix A for a blank copy. The *Lose It for Life Interactive Journal Planner* is another resource and is available from LoseItForLife.com.)

It was eye-opening for Jane to track her food intake every day for two weeks. You can see just by glancing at this first day of Jane's food journal, as she did, how the calories added up and how many empty-calorie, nonnutritive foods she consumed. Fruits, vegetables, and protein were lacking in her food choices. In addition, she often ate on the run while doing errands in her car, with only one meal being eaten at her kitchen table. There were times she ate when she wasn't even hungry, as well as instances where the meal included multiple servings or large-size items. Without the help of a dietitian, Jane could see she had to make changes—thanks to the food journal, which provided her an objective view of her eating patterns.

FOOD JOURNAL

Name: Jane Doe

Date: Wednesday, May 18

When I ate	Where I ate	What I ate	How much I ate	Was I hungry?
Breakfast (8 a.m.)	Kitchen table	Jelly donuts	3	Yes
		Coffee with cream and sugar	3 cups, 3 tbsp., 2 tbsp.	Yes
		Orange juice	1 cup	Yes
10 a.m.	Desk at work	Pop Tart	2	Yes
11 a.m.	Car	Bag of chips	12 oz.	No
Lunch (12 p.m.)	Mall Plaza	Pizza	3 slices	Yes
		Coke	1 24-oz. cup	Yes

When I ate	Where I ate	What I ate	How much I ate	Was I hungry?
	Car	Heath ice cream	1 Klondike bar	No
2 p.m.	Desk	Cupcakes	2	No
4 p.m.	Car	French fries	1 large	No
		Coke	12 oz.	No
		Burger	1 regular	No
Dinner (6 p.m.)	In front of TV	Lasagna	2 large helpings	Yes
		Salad with dressing	1 bowl with 1/4 cup blue cheese	Yes
		Bread sticks	3	No
		Dr. Pepper	2 8-oz. cans	Yes
		Cheesecake	1 large slice	No
		Coffee with cream and sugar	2 cups, 3 tbsp., 2 tbsp.	No
8:30 p.m.	Movie	Buttered popcorn	Large bag	No
		Sprite	2 8-oz. glasses	No

IDENTIFY YOUR EATING PATTERNS

There are basically three eating patterns to look for when you keep a food journal. The first is called *grazing.* Picture a cow grazing . . . all day she is chewing grass. We know it's not a flattering visual, but that picture is similar to what some overeaters do! They eat all day, with a little here and a little more there—never really eating huge amounts at once, but continuously eating, all day long. Physical hunger is not what motivates grazing. This type of eating happens because food is available or it sounds good at the time.

A second pattern is to overeat during any particular eating episode. According to Jane's journal, she ate two helpings of lasagna instead of one. At the end of the second helping, she felt uncomfortable, but she continued to eat. *Overeating* is when you eat past a feeling of being full or to the point of feeling uncomfortable. A third pattern is *binge eating,* which involves uncontrolled eating episodes in which a person consumes a large number of calories in a short amount of time. Usually bingeing is secretive and occurs when the person is alone; often this type of eating ends with feelings of disgust and a very uncomfortable physical feeling. Bingeing obviously results in weight gain and, in many cases, weight fluctuations. Emotionally, this type of eating leads to depression, anxiety, low self-esteem, powerlessness, anger, fear, and numbness. Social withdrawal and isolation, as well as a social preoccupation with food, are also common. The secrecy involved produces additional guilt and shame.

Use your food journal as an objective information source to help you identify your overeating habits. At this point in the weight-loss journey, it's best not to judge your eating by subjective feelings—you simply can't trust them to be accurate. And remember, people who consistently record food intake lose weight!

WEIGHT LOSS DOES NOT EQUAL HAPPINESS

One of the greatest myths people hold is that losing weight will make them happy. Granted, it is true that shedding extra pounds does make a person feel better on the outside. However, losing weight uncovers more than we sometimes imagine. And it isn't always happiness, as Cathy describes in her journal:

> This week has been a rough one. Lately I've been thinking about the past through rose-colored glasses. Somehow, I remember being happier and more jovial at 350 pounds. I remember being a social butterfly—loud, crazy, and extremely talkative— always looking for spontaneous fun! Sort of like a female John Candy. Boy, have I

changed! Without the white stuff (sugar), my personality now is nothing like the one I describe.

Bottom line: I have somehow manipulated my memories into believing that being fat was fun, and I know this isn't true. I guess I'm looking for a good reason to sabotage my new healthy lifestyle. I need help on this one!

What Cathy is experiencing happens to most people who lose as much weight as she has—other issues begin to surface. Cathy is making significant changes and finding out why permanent weight loss is so difficult. Keeping the weight off requires changes in thinking and doing. Once she stopped using food to numb her feelings, past memories began to creep in, memories she had previously avoided. Happily, she was able to analyze what was happening.

Past hurts are usually the root reasons that a person begins to overeat in the first place. The good news is that the root reasons can be healed. Cathy is at a crossroads. If she chooses to confront the reality of her life, she won't feel happy all the time. But if she will learn to deal with those past hurts (and eventually move on), she will no longer need food as a cover-up and she will maintain a healthy weight.

It's easy to be a social butterfly when you are overweight because being fun and jovial is an acceptable way to cover negative feelings. In the same way, it's often easier to laugh and be the life of the party and avoid the reality of hurts and bruised feelings. If you see yourself doing this, you haven't yet taken the red pill. In Cathy's case, as she peels away the excess weight, she is peeling away her old defenses. What's left is the reality . . . the pain she has feared facing. For some overweight people, the past is full of hurtful experiences that were never resolved.

One woman struggles with her weight because her past includes sexual abuse. As she gains control of her compulsive overeating, sexual abuse memories surface. The feelings are intense; she is angry, hurt, and anxious. All kinds of emotions are flooding her as she faces the reality of a past she didn't want to face. Like Cathy, she is at a crossroads. She must face the emotional pain or go back to old habits. The amazing thing is that if she faces those wounds, they can be healed. The woman she was created to be can and will surface. She is living proof of the grace of God demonstrated in Isaiah 61:2–3:

> GOD sent me to announce the year of his grace—
>   a celebration of GOD's destruction of our enemies—
>   and to comfort all who mourn,

To care for the needs of all who mourn in Zion,
   give them bouquets of roses instead of ashes,
Messages of joy instead of news of doom,
   a praising heart instead of a languid spirit.
Rename them "Oaks of Righteousness"
   planted by GOD to display his glory. (MSG)

HAPPY ALL THE TIME

In my (Steve's) book *Toxic Faith*, I address a faith issue that is actually a fat issue for many. One problem people have with Christianity is that they are offered some false promises if they surrender their lives to Jesus. They are told that everything changes and happiness is the result, but this is simply not true. Becoming a Christian does not mean everything will immediately change. Real-life residue is present that must be processed out of our lives. And there are some realities like loss, struggle, temptation, and betrayal that cause us to be anything but happy.

I (Dr. Linda) remember singing a song in Sunday school when I was very young. The boys would karate chop their way through the action motions and the girls would watch and sigh because those young males weren't doing it right! But the lyrics are a little disturbing when I think about them now. Go ahead and do the motions as you sing with me:

I'm in-right, out-right, up-right, down-right happy all the time.[4]

Now, don't misunderstand, I am *thrilled* that Jesus came into my life. But the idea of being happy all the time leads me to believe it's time for the red pill! We are *not* happy all the time. We have to learn to deal with difficulty and affliction. We may have to grieve the losses of a less-than-perfect family, or a disappointing marriage, or children making bad choices, or critical and controlling bosses. The important thing to remember is this: You can learn to tolerate bad feelings, to walk through them and let go of them. Or you can overeat and numb out those feelings while gaining weight. And you may need counseling to walk you through those difficult times. That's okay. Walking through the pain is better than avoiding it.

Many new Christians are disappointed, broken by the falsehoods of faith not coming through what they heard about or were promised. They eat to comfort and soothe their loss of heart. Fulfillment, purpose, meaning, and security—this is what we have in our relationship with Christ. We do not and should not expect to have happiness for every moment of the rest of our lives.

LOSE THE UNREALISTIC EXPECTATIONS

Thinking your life will be happy if you lose weight is only one of many unrealistic expectations concerning weight loss. Reevaluating your expectations is both necessary and an important part of accepting reality. Here are seven general expectations to reconsider:

1. **All I have to do is lose weight. Nothing more will be required.** This isn't true in most cases. Usually there are reasons you've gained weight unrelated to hunger. Uncovering the reasons you overeat and then making changes will be required for most people to be successful on a long-term basis.

2. **All kinds of opportunities will come to me when I lose weight.** We can't tell you how many times this thought sets up disappointment. We've worked with people who believed that, after losing the weight, their dating lives would explode. They were so disappointed when this didn't happen. Other potential opportunities that might be expected include new job opportunities, healed marriages, and blossoming friendships. It's not that these things can't happen, but they have less to do with losing weight and more to do with how you act and feel about yourself.

3. **I will like myself better when I'm thinner.** Reality check! Red pill time! You may like yourself less for a short time as you confront things about you that need changing! As Cathy reminded us, losing weight can mean letting go of a significant way to cope with stress and painful memories. And it can also take away your excuse not to work on you. You can hide behind the weight and blame your life on being "fat," or you can face the not-so-nice parts of yourself and make changes. For example, your office worker may pass you up for a party invitation because you are insensitive, not because you are overweight. Ouch! But as you make necessary changes, you will really like who emerges.

4. **I'll be giving up a good thing.** Food is a poor substitute for community and connection. In the end, it brings neither and leaves you more disconnected than ever. We long to be a part of something bigger than ourselves, to have people who love and care for us, as well as find the one thing that truly

feeds us emotionally and spiritually. We won't find these things in food. They can only be found through connection with God and others.

5. **I must be perfect for God to work in me.** Holding this thought, we tend to cover up problems and be dishonest about our struggles because we think God is looking for perfection in order to work. But the reality is that He invites you to be His with every cellulite wrinkle and flaw. One of the problems of the modern church is that we are often taught to cognitively fix things by declaring a Scripture like John 8:32, "Then you will know the truth, and the truth will set you free." This scripture is absolutely right on! But we need to read the one before it as well (v. 31): "To the Jews who had believed him, Jesus said, 'If you hold to my teaching, you are really my disciples.'" Jesus is telling us that the truth cannot just be read; it must be lived out in our lives—following His commands, loving one another, seeing ourselves as He says we are, picking up our daily cross and following Him, crucifying the flesh, etc. Do you see the difference?

The living truth says no to self and selfish desires and requires an authentic life lived out with others and before the Lord. The truth transforms us, but we have to cooperate during the process in order to look like the Christ who does the transforming. Sadly, we see little of this transformation in our churches because the church often penalizes us for being honest. Problems are hidden as we are encouraged to hang on to Jesus and put on a happy face (and sing that song!).

Interestingly, God didn't hide truth in His Word. For instance, even though it wasn't pretty, the story of the first biblical family (the one with the original problem with choosing the wrong food to eat) involved murder. Throughout the Bible there are unflattering details of sins committed by biblical characters, yet God so loved the world that He gave His only begotten Son (John 3:16). This is powerful. God sees our imperfections and is able to transform us anyway! But we have to let Him do His work.

6. **I've screwed up so many times, it's just too late.** It's never too late with God. Repeat this twenty times until it sinks into your thick skull! God doesn't hold grudges and He certainly doesn't keep on punishing you for sins already confessed. He forgives and calls you to Him. When you accept guilt and shame from your past, you basically tell God that His sacrifice didn't matter. Jesus Christ has taken all your guilt and shame to the cross

and doesn't want you holding on to it. He says, "I'll take your failures and build your future." And He has a great one planned for you.

Witness the life of Peter. Jesus knew Peter would deny Him and lie about being one of His disciples when the going got tough. And when it did, Peter failed miserably. Yet Peter was the man upon whom Jesus chose to build His church. If that doesn't get you excited, we don't know what will!

And we love the fact that, later, Jesus gave Peter three chances to redeem himself personally to the Lord:

> When they had finished eating, Jesus said to Simon Peter, "Simon son of John, do you love me more than these?" "Yes, Lord," he said, "you know that I love you." Jesus said, "Feed my lambs." Again Jesus said, "Simon son of John, do you love me?" He answered, "Yes, Lord, you know that I love you." Jesus said, "Take care of my sheep." The third time he said to him, "Simon son of John, do you love me?" Peter was hurt because Jesus asked him the third time, "Do you love me?" He said, "Lord, you know all things; you know that I love you." (John 21:15–17)

We have to believe that Jesus asked him three times just to correct those earlier three denials. He wanted Peter restored, not punished. That's our God—using our failures and redeeming our losses. But we've got to be honest and not hide our faults and struggles.

7. **I can do this alone**. Perhaps this is the mother of all unrealistic expectations. If you could do it alone, you would have by now. Going it alone feeds your appetite. God uses connections to heal us. Going it alone is just a very long and painful path to going right back to where you were before.

JUDGED BY OTHERS BUT NOT BY GOD

Unfortunately, you are judged by your weight. People will think you lack willpower and self-discipline. Have you ever heard, "Just stop putting the food in your mouth"? And don't you want to scream back, "If it were that easy, I'd be at my ideal weight right now!"? So what's the lesson? You won't always find the acceptance you desire from other people. Because they are human, they have the potential to fail you. And you can't control what people think or say. Therefore, it's important to find a few people who do understand the battle you are in and who won't judge you but will pray and encourage you. We'll talk more about this later. But for now, we want you to begin this journey with people who will encourage, love, and accept you.

If you are having trouble finding those people, join our online community at LoseItForLife.com. This website is a wonderful resource for weight loss. And remember, God is always with you. His Word is a great source of encouragement. In prayer, say, "God, I refuse to accept words such as *lazy, ugly, out of control,* or [fill in the blank] as definitions of who I am. With Your help, I will discover the true me. You created me and declared Your creation good."

Scriptures that declare who you are in Christ are a wonderful source of comfort and support. Put them on index cards or do whatever you need to do to be reminded of your true worth—whatever gets it in your head. You are not what you weigh. You have worth just because God created you. He esteems you already. He's not waiting for you to lose ten pounds. He values you now! He chose you, and He loves you unconditionally. Nothing you do impresses Him. He looks at your heart, not your outward appearance (1 Samuel 16:7).

Losing weight doesn't make you more acceptable to God, but unfortunately it influences the judgment of other people. However, don't make the opinions of others a motivation to lose weight. Anytime you try to lose weight for other people, it's a setup for failure.

We are fans of fantasy, but not when it's used for your body and health. Save it for the movies, a great novel, or some other outlet! A good, hard-hitting look at reality isn't as scary as you might imagine. We are going to walk you through it so you face life with your eyes wide open. You can make good decisions when you become aware of what you are doing and then stay aware. If you are used to answering questions about why you overeat with answers like, "I don't know" or "I just wasn't thinking," prepare to have better answers after reading this book. The choice to overeat will still be yours, but it won't be an unconscious choice!

With each Lose It for Life Institute, I (Steve) begin the sessions with a reality check for those present. Living between expectations and reality brings misery. We must alter our expectations to coincide with reality, a step that will remove misery from our lives. Understand, we can't live every moment without pain, as difficulties do happen, but we can live without misery. Personal desires to be healed by a quick fix or instant solution, or by working harder or just praying more, only give us more misery and more excuses when we fail yet again and reach for food to comfort us. Instead, we need to walk in reality.

Walk in the reality of your needs and expect God to act on your behalf. His way may not always be what you expect, but He can be trusted to intervene. The assurance we have that nothing could ever separate us from God's love is based on His past and present actions on our behalf. Christ sits and pleads our case to the Father; He is always interceding for us on our behalf. "What then shall we say to these things [the reality of our life]? If God is for us, who can be against us?" (Romans 8:31 NKJV).

There are no shortcuts. Body weight is controlled by the number of calories you eat and the number of calories you use each day; that is the reality of taking the red pill. To lose weight, you need to take in fewer calories than you consume. The bottom line is that simple. This happens by becoming more physically active and eating less. Lose It for Life will help you lose the weight and keep it off by sharing suggestions for change in your physical activity and eating habits that will stay with you the rest of your life. Along the way may come changes to your lifestyle, a new awareness of your body, and counsel to deal with potential issues that might keep you from losing the weight permanently.

If you're ready, the time is now. Will you take the red pill? If so, welcome to a new Matrix—Lose It for Life!

Workbook Week 2

TAKE THE RED PILL

DAY 1
The Matrix . . . or Reality?

The film *The Matrix* tells the story of a computer hacker named Neo who lives a rather ordinary life in what he thinks is the year 1999. Then he meets a man named Morpheus, who explains to Neo that his reality is false. It is actually two hundred years later, artificial intelligence runs the world, and all humans are trapped in a complex computer "matrix" in which they are used for fuel to run the machines. Morpheus gives Neo a life-altering choice. He can go on living in his false world or he can take the red pill. Once he swallows the red pill, he'll see life as it really is!

LIFL confronts you with a similar life-altering choice. Do you want to continue to live in the false world of dieting, where emotional pain is numbed, health risks are ignored, and false promises are made? Or do you want to "take the red pill" and see the reality of a world in which food and eating don't dominate your life or take over? If you take the challenge, you will have to face things you have avoided, deal with relationship difficulties, and make changes in your lifestyle.

LOOKING AT YOUR *LIFE*

How we spend our hours is how we spend our days, and how we spend our days is how we spend our lives. All of us are headed in a certain trajectory; unless we do something to alter our direction, we will end up where we are headed.

How are you spending your days? Where are you headed?

_____

_____

If you don't change some things about how you think about and deal with food, about how you take care (or don't take care) of your body and soul, where do you think you will you end up? (Try to project ten, twenty, or thirty years into the future.)

_____

_____

Would the people who know you best and love you most say that you are a wide-eyed realist or someone who easily falls prey to deceptive ideas? Would they say you more readily take responsibility for your life situation or that you are prone to make excuses, justify, rationalize, and blame others?

_____

_____

Dostoevsky's novel _The Brothers Karamazov_ is a classic. One of the main characters observed, "The important thing is to stop lying to yourself. A man who lies to himself, and believes his lies, becomes unable to recognize the truth, either in himself or anyone else, and he ends up losing respect for himself as well as others. When he has no respect for anyone, he can no longer love and . . . behaves in the end like an animal, in satisfying his vices."[5]

When it comes to your relationship with food, are you lying to yourself? (Be honest!)

_____

_____

LEARNING A NEW WAY OF _LIFE_

In order to lose weight for life, we have to face reality or we end up lying to ourselves and to others. We must ask (and answer) tough, uncomfortable questions such as:

- What is _my_ part in gaining weight?
- How do I respond to difficulty?
- What unmet needs do I have that I try to meet through food?
- When life gets tough, do I get going or start eating?
- Am I hung up on _why_ my life feels so out of control?

We can facilitate change . . . But you will have to make some hard decisions and re-evaluate your motivations for wanting to lose weight.

- Am I disconnected from others?
- Am I in denial?

What are your first-blush reactions to these probing queries?

_____

_____

Read John 16:33 in your Bible. "In this world you will have trouble," Jesus said. Difficulty and suffering will be part of life. How does that reality make you feel?

_____

_____

In the same breath, Jesus offered hope. "Take heart! I have overcome the world." During His life on earth, He overcame temptation from Satan. Through His death on the cross and the power of His resurrection, He destroyed the power of sin and death. Now He is able to offer otherworldly peace and freedom—a whole new way of living.

When it comes to food and weight and dieting, are you more often "at war" within or flooded with God's peace? Why?

_____

_____

_____

When is the last time you felt truly at peace, relaxed to the depths of your soul? What were the circumstances? What would it be like to experience a whole life of such rest?

_____

_____

As the perfect Son of God, Jesus is incapable of lying. He can only tell the truth. What does John 14:6 reveal about the character of Christ?

_____

_____

The psalmist prayed, "LORD, you have examined my heart and know everything about me" (Psalm 139:1 NLT). How can this fact free us up to be honest with God, others, and ourselves?

LOSING IT FOR *LIFE*

We take steps toward true freedom and true peace when we soberly and realistically decide to "take the red pill." We choose to give up our false and foolish ways of thinking and living, and accept certain truths:

"You will know the truth, and the truth will set you free" (John 8:32).

- My overweight body is a symptom of an underdeveloped soul.
- No one else caused my problem and no one else is going to fix it for me.
- When I decide to change, it is going to be painful.
- No one can walk through that pain but me, and I must walk through it.

Record your true thoughts about these statements.

In the *LIFL* book, the authors state, "All of us struggle with blind spots in our lives, and to some degree we all live in the company of denial and self-deception. But rather than confront our area(s) of struggle and pain, we often point to others and focus on them or find alternatives to distract and anesthetize ourselves from what really needs to be faced."

Do you agree? Why or why not?

Acceptance is being willing to see, to lift the curtain of denial and look unblinkingly at the "big lie" of your life. Breaking through denial means being aware of your struggle and pain and consciously confronting the behaviors and patterns that have detoured you from God's best.

Take a moment and rigorously examine your heart. Ask God for the courage to be brutally honest. How have you avoided reality? How many (if any) of these truth-avoiding "symptoms" are a regular part of your life? Check all that apply.

___ I avoid honest prayer.

___ I avoid times of silence.

___ I avoid discussions that focus on my life situation.

___ I avoid honest conversations that touch on sensitive or painful areas of my life.

___ I avoid people who can (and would) speak into my life and encourage me on the journey.

___ I minimize or rationalize my behavior and its effect on others.

___ I find myself constantly criticizing or pointing the finger at others—either outwardly or inwardly.

___ I am confused as to why others react the way they do to me and what I say or do.

___ I catch myself lying repeatedly—or stretching and twisting the truth.

With God's help, remove the blinders of deception and denial. Begin to see yourself as you really are. Then see God as He is: patient and loving.

Here's how you'll have to change if you want to leave behind a life of delusion and excuse-making. Here are the positive signs that will mark your life:

- You will focus on what *you* can do to change rather than on what you want others to do to make you feel better.
- You will humble yourself in order to see and confront who you really are.
- You will look hard for what really causes the conflicts you experience.
- You will honestly face your past, pain, and failures head on.
- You will stop blaming others for your difficulties.
- You will actively seek, receive, and apply God's wisdom to your situation.
- You will look at what you've done in the light of God's mercy and grace—not judgment or condemnation.
- You will accept that you are unable to change without God's help.
- You will name your character defects and mistakes rather than deny them.

What's your gut-level reaction to this list? What hopes or fears are stirred in you as you contemplate it?

_____

_____

By being humble, courageous, and honest, we can move out of the past and into the reality of the present where God can teach us to resolve our problems rather than reproduce them in family and close friends. Are you ready to take the red pill?

Letting Go of Excuses

Are you ready to be completely honest with yourself and others and stop making excuses for why your life is the way it is?

LOOKING AT YOUR *LIFE*

What are your five best qualities?

_____

_____

What are your three worst habits?

_____

_____

How about "making excuses" for your eating/exercise habits? Are you guilty? On a scale of 1 to 10, with 1 being "I'm afraid I do it all the time!" and 10 being "I never make excuses!" how would you rank yourself?

_____

_____

Remember the following example from the book portion:

It's late at night. You are watching TV and you start thinking about ice cream because you've just seen a tantalizing commercial. Anxiety begins to mount as you try to decide if you should eat the ice cream sitting in your freezer . . . or say no. You aren't thinking about the fact that you are *not* hungry. The ice cream just looks so good—it would be a terrific treat right now . . . and it's calling to you from the freezer . . . and you've had a long and exhausting day. All of these are excuses that hide the truth: *you are not hungry*. But the excuses come so easily, so smoothly, it has become your habit to just ignore the truth when it comes to overeating. Excuses take the focus off of the long-term consequences.

Certainly you don't want to think about the long-term effects of overeating right now. And the longer you postpone eating the ice cream, the greater your anxiety becomes. *Should I eat or shouldn't I?* Eventually you become so uncomfortable over this dilemma that you get up, walk to the kitchen, and serve yourself a scoop of ice cream.

Then you think, *There isn't that much ice cream left in the carton. I'll finish it off and won't buy any more. I'll start dieting tomorrow when it's all gone.* As you begin to overeat, the momentary anxiety disappears. The ice cream tasted great, or at least you think it did—you ate it so fast, you really didn't taste it. Now it's late, and now you are really tired. Feeling uncomfortably full, you go to bed.

When do you most often catch yourself in similar situations as the ice cream example?

_____

_____

_____

LEARNING A NEW WAY OF *LIFE*

Giving in to strong, momentary urges (in order to ward off anxious feelings) is a dangerous habit. By refusing to think about long-term consequences, we become pawns or puppets in the hands of advertisers. Think about it—immediate gratification is the strong, underlying message of every ad or commercial. The whole marketing industry is designed to persuade us to think and act impulsively. If we're ever going to find true freedom and peace and victory, we must learn a new way of thinking and living.

Excuses are simply ways we lessen momentary anxiety so we can overeat.

Are you a short-term thinker or a long-term thinker? Why do you say that? What would your friends and family say?

_____

_____

Circle the statement in either column that best describes how you usually react.

I react impulsively.	**I respond thoughtfully.**
1. $100! Let's go to the mall!	$100! Maybe I should save this?
2. I do things spur of the moment.	I like to plan things out in advance.
3. I'm blunt. I say what's on my mind.	I'm tactful. I fret over how to say hard things.
4. I don't know what I'm doing next week.	I have a life plan or personal mission statement.
5. I buy my Christmas gifts at the last minute.	I Christmas shop far in advance.
6. Retirement? 401K? IRA? Ha!	I just got back from an appointment with my financial planner.
7. My kids? Hmm. I guess they're okay.	I'm deeply concerned about my kids' futures.
8. Sounds good to me! Let's do it.	How could this decision affect others?
9. What would feel good now?	What is God calling me to be and do?
10. You only go around once in life.	One day I will stand before God.

How common is it for you to stop (before eating) and ask questions such as these?

- How will I feel after I eat this?
- How will I feel in thirty minutes?
- How will I feel about this tomorrow morning?
- Will I beat myself up over this?

_____

_____

_____

If you're not in that habit, what would it take for you to develop this habit—thinking through the ramifications of your decisions?

_____

_____

Read Galatians 5:22–23. This passage depicts the character qualities of a person who is surrendered to God's Spirit and living under His control. Notice the last fruit of the Spirit listed. What does this suggest to you? What hope does this give in the whole weight-loss/weight-control battle?

_____

_____

_____

Fruit always comes from a seed. Interestingly, Jesus spoke of the Word of God as being like seed (Luke 8:1–15). What are the implications of this? What role does the Bible play in learning to Lose It for Life?

_____

_____

How—realistically and practically—do we plant the seed of God's Word deeply in our lives so that it bears fruit over time?

_____

_____

The original temptation to sin involved food (Genesis 3), as did Christ's temptation in the wilderness. Read Luke 4:1–13. How did Jesus fight the lure of immediate gratification?

_____

_____

_____

Here are some practical, tried-and-true suggestions for battling the anxious temptations to overeat (or to eat when you're not really physically hungry):

- Tell yourself, "It's normal to feel anxious when making a change. This feeling will pass shortly."

- Breathe deeply and relax your body. Usually the urge subsides within twenty minutes or so.
- Distract yourself with something else. Turn off the TV, pull out a book, go to the bathroom (people tend not to eat in the bathroom), take a walk, chew some sugar-free gum, or go to bed. Don't stare at the refrigerator and try to exercise willpower.
- Try to avoid tempting situations altogether. If you are realizing that late-night TV viewing is a trigger for you to overeat, don't watch late-night TV! Do something different—play a game, read a good book, pray for your family, work on a Bible study, and so forth.
- If you do decide to eat, eat a piece of fruit, chewing it slowly. Or go ahead and take one small scoop of ice cream and no more. Eat it slowly and enjoy every bite. You won't gain a pound from one small scoop, but eating the entire carton will do some damage.

Which of these suggestions do you think will work best for you? Why?

_____

_____

Jesus' defense against succumbing to immediate gratification was to quote God's Word to His enemy. That's our model for overcoming.

LOSING IT FOR *LIFE*

A big part of the LIFL approach is taking responsibility. We stop blaming others for our situation. We surrender to God, trusting Him to do what we cannot do, and we take responsibility for doing all that we can. Responsibility also means confronting old wounds that can trigger our overeating. We could fill volumes with the stories of people who have used overeating as a way of numbing emotional hurts. Perhaps you, too, have spent your life anesthetizing your emotions with food rather than addressing your disappointments and grief. LIFL wants to provide you with the truth and encouragement to face your pain and grieve your losses, so that you find deep healing.

There is much psychological talk about our "victim" culture. What does this mean? Why are so many so quick to take on the role of victim and live a life of victimization?

_____

_____

King David wrote, "It was good for me to be afflicted so that I might learn your decrees" (Psalm 119:71). How can affliction and pain end up serving God's good purposes for our lives?

_____

_____

The authors state, "Avoiding pain and problems is a natural human response. Most people feel they have 'suffered enough' and have no desire to feel overwhelmed by sorrowful emotions. But grief is a necessary process of this earthly life. . . . Grief over our failures and losses connects us to God's grace. Saint Augustine affirmed this when he said, 'In my deepest wound I saw your glory and it dazzled me.'"

How do you respond to that thought? Is this a new perspective for you?

_____

_____

It would be easy to use your past pain as a lifelong excuse for not changing (but you'd miss God's best). Many people choose to live this way. It would also be easy to blame others for everything that has gone wrong in your life. Accepting responsibility is a bold step, and a better way.

Are you willing to . . .

- ☐ face your problems rather than run from them?
- ☐ take the time now to finally grieve your losses?
- ☐ believe Jesus' words, "Blessed are those who mourn, for they will be comforted" (Matthew 5:4)?
- ☐ stop playing the role of victim?
- ☐ bear the full responsibility of your own misconduct?

- ☐ reach out to Christ, who is fully capable of understanding your emotional pain because He suffered abuse and rejection Himself?
- ☐ look beyond your loss to God's deeper purposes?
- ☐ accept the hope that God's plans for you are good and loving?
- ☐ refuse to allow anything from your past to be an excuse for lack of growth or character development?

If you checked any boxes, you have taken a wise and courageous step! We applaud your brave heart. With God's truth, God's power, God's indwelling Spirit, and God's people, you can Lose It for Life—by appropriating fully the new life that Christ gives.

The book offers a prayer for accepting responsibility. If you wish, pray it silently right now.

Dear Lord,

I realize that You have given me life and that living is my responsibility. Lord, I want to accept responsibility for my whole life. I know You want my life to be fruitful, but sin and tragedy have infected my life—both by my hand and the hands of others. Help me to accept responsibility to remove these weeds that have been sown in me. Lord, I confess that sometimes I blame others for my own disobedience to You. I now accept responsibility for these things. Please forgive me and fully restore the relationship between us. Amen.

DAY 3
New Motives and Methods

Once you have decided to give up a lifestyle of making excuses, and after you have prayed through your acceptance and responsibility, then it's time to examine your motivation for wanting to lose weight.

LOOKING AT YOUR *LIFE*

If you had a magic wand and could wave it over your life, what three big changes would you most like to see and why?

_____

_____

_____

_____

Our emotions are the warning lights on the dashboard of our lives. When we find ourselves flashing with a strong emotion—fear, anger, worry, sadness—it's time to "pull over," so to speak, and "look under the hood" at what's really going on inside us. Does the idea of self-examination trouble you or excite you? Why?

_____

_____

_____

_____

Research tells us that people become more successful at long-term weight loss when their motivation is to become healthier, not thinner.

Be honest—which of the following options might you choose? Why?

- Living another *thirty* years, while enjoying an absolutely flawless physique—a body off the cover of some magazine.
- Living another *fifty* years, in a reasonably fit and healthy body— though not necessarily a body that would cause people to stop and stare in envy.

_____

_____

_____

_____

_____

LEARNING A NEW WAY OF *LIFE*

As you learn more about making good food choices and self-care, your focus should be on becoming a healthier, not just thinner, you. This change in attitude and motivation is essential.

If one's goal is merely to look more attractive, rank the following ways to do that, from 1 to 10 (1=most effective; 10=least effective):

"I am the
Lord, the
God of all
mankind.
Is anything
too hard
for me?"
(Jeremiah
32:27).

____ liposuction and other forms of plastic surgery

____ gastric bypass surgery

____ vegetarian diet

____ low-fat diet

____ low-carb diet

____ aerobics classes

____ new wardrobe

____ cosmetic dental surgery

____ tanning booth sessions

____ weight/strength-training

If one's goal is to become an overall healthier, happier person, what activities might need to be added to the above list and why?

Healthy Habit or Practice	Why and How This Contributes to Overall Health

Read 1 Timothy 4:7–8. What does this passage suggest is important in achieving overall health?

_____

_____

_____

In Philippians 4:13, the apostle Paul exclaims, "I can do all this through him who gives me strength." What is the significance of this statement to those who are opting for the long-term view of lifelong weight loss/management?

_____

_____

LOSING IT FOR *LIFE*

Perhaps you are frustrated because it seems as though you've been dieting forever and haven't lost a pound. We know the drill!

In the *LIFL* book, Dr. Linda tells of her college "cottage cheese diet" that helped her gain fifteen pounds her freshman year. She reports how she skipped breakfast every day (food or sleep was her option), ate cottage cheese and fruit for lunch, and ate a regular dinner. Staring daily at her little bowl of white mealy curd lunch, she believed she was making the ultimate sacrifice to lose weight. She ate it religiously and thought the pounds would fall off.

What she forgot to add to the equation were her nightly visits to the dormitory snack machines. In addition to her 7 a.m. to 7 p.m. dietary discipline, Dr. Linda was also ingesting late-night fruit pies and cinnamon buns and chips and chocolate. Add up all those extra study snack calories that didn't "count" because they weren't part of her "healthy" meals, and it's no wonder she didn't lose weight.

Studies also show that people who record what they eat lose more weight and keep it off compared to those who don't.[6]

What are your snack habits?

_____

_____

_____

When do you find yourself most susceptible to nibbling and grazing?

_____

_____

_____

Research shows that very few people have metabolic disorders or genetic factors that cause obesity. The truth is that most people grossly underestimate what they eat in a day and they exercise far less than they think.[7] It's not that people intentionally lie about what they eat. They just forget all those random moments in the day when they grab a handful of chocolates or taste a few spoonfuls of chili while preparing dinner. A little here, a little there adds up.

Get a small blank tablet that you can carry with you. Begin right now writing down everything you eat in a day for a week or two. This may sound tedious, but it will provide you with a greater awareness of what you are eating. The food journal will also pinpoint eating patterns—when you eat, how much, how often, what you eat, etc. This information will later be used to make changes.

Find a companion who will do this with you. Having a partner to remind you and encourage you is a great way to develop this new, important habit. Use the following format (also provided in Appendix A) to help monitor your progress.

Food Journal				
Name: Jane Doe **Date**: Wednesday, May 18				
When I ate	**Where**	**What I ate**	**How much**	**Was I hungry?**
Breakfast (8:00 a.m.)	Kitchen table	Jelly donuts	3	Yes
		Coffee	3 cups, 3 tbsp. cream, 2 tbsp. sugar	
		Orange Juice	8 oz glass	Yes
Snack (10:00 a.m.)	Desk at work	Pop Tart	2	Yes

After you have set up your food journal, commit this exercise to God with this prayer:

Father,

I have begun this new adventure that I hope and pray will become a new way of life. I do not want to be controlled by food or by unhealthy emotions. Give me the grace to lean on You at all times. Help me change my mind-set so that I am motivated by a deep desire to be healthy. And grant that I might attain that goal, to Your glory and my own good. In Jesus' name, amen.

Looking Below the Surface

When you keep a journal, you should look for these three eating patterns: grazing, overeating, and binge eating.

Keeping a food journal provides you with an objective view of your eating patterns.

LOOKING AT YOUR *LIFE*

What adjectives would you use to describe your current eating habits (for example, "unpredictable," "insatiable," and so forth)?

_____

_____

_____

When during the day or week was your appetite biggest? When was it smaller? Why?

_____

_____

_____

Picture a cow grazing all day, chewing grass. We know that's not a flattering visual, but that picture is similar to what some overeaters do. They graze all day on food, a little here and there—never really eating huge amounts at once, but continuously eating thoughout the day. How much a part of your daily routine is grazing?

_____

_____

_____

Overeating is when you eat past a feeling of being full or to the point of feeling uncomfortable. Maybe you wolf down three servings quickly, or you keep going back to the buffet.

What's behind this habit? When do you see this tendency in yourself?

_____

_____

_____

Binge eating involves uncontrolled eating episodes in which you consume a large number of calories in a short amount of time. Usually bingeing is done in secret. It happens when you are alone, and it ends in disgust and a very uncomfortable physical feeling.

If you are a binger, describe how it makes you feel. (If you are not, speculate on why this habit has so many in its grip.)

_____

_____

Physical hunger is not what motivates grazing. You eat because food is available or because it sounds good at the time.

   Use your food journal as an objective information source for the purpose of helping you identify your overeating habits. At this point in the weight-loss journey, it's best not to judge your eating by subjective feelings. You simply can't trust them to be accurate. Remember, *those who consistently record food intake lose weight.*

LEARNING A NEW WAY OF *LIFE*

One of the greatest myths people believe is that losing weight guarantees happiness. It's true that shedding extra pounds does make people feel better on the outside. But losing weight can also uncover more than we sometimes imagine.

   The authors cite the following letter from a woman named Cathy:

This week has been a rough one. Lately I've been thinking about the past through rose-colored glasses. Somehow, I remember being happier and more jovial at 350 pounds. I remember being a social butterfly—loud, crazy, and

Emotionally, binge eating leads to depression, anxiety, low self-esteem, powerlessness, anger, fear, numbness, social withdrawal, and isolation.

extremely talkative—always looking for spontaneous fun! Sort of like a female John Candy. Boy, have I changed! Without the white stuff (sugar), my personality now is nothing like the one I describe.

Bottom line: I have somehow manipulated my memories into believing that being fat was fun, and I know this isn't true. I guess I'm looking for a good reason to sabotage my new healthy lifestyle. I need help on this one!

What examples can you think of in your life of a good thing resulting in consequences that were different from what you expected?

_____

_____

When people shed weight—especially a lot of weight—other issues begin to surface. Keeping the weight off requires changes in thinking and doing. For example, speculate on the experience of the person who has always used food to numb unpleasant feelings from the past, but who now refuses to use food as a crutch.

How might such a person be tempted to sabotage his or her success?

_____

_____

What is the best solution to overcoming such inner tension?

_____

_____

Our food-obsessed lifestyles may not be healthy, but they surely are familiar and comfortable. As we peel away the weight, we also peel away our old defenses. What's left is the reality we have feared facing. For many overweight people, the past is full of hurtful experiences that were never resolved.

The authors argue that unresolved hurts are usually the root reasons that people begin to overeat in the first place, and that they can be healed. What do you think of this argument?

_____

_____

What have been the great wounding incidents in your life? Be honest. Remember, Jesus said the truth would set us free.

_____

_____

_____

Read Isaiah 61:2–3. This great passage shows God's desire to send a Savior who will heal His defeated, disillusioned people and fill them with hope:

GOD sent me to announce the year of his grace—a celebration of GOD's destruction of our enemies—and to comfort all who mourn, to care for the needs of all who mourn in Zion, give them bouquets of roses instead of ashes, messages of joy instead of news of doom, a praising heart instead of a languid spirit. Rename them "Oaks of Righteousness" planted by GOD to display his glory. (MSG)

Listen. Be still before the Lord. What is God saying to you in this passage?

_____

_____

_____

LOSING IT FOR _LIFE_

Cathy's choices may be yours as well.

- Am I going to push ahead, despite the pain that will surface as I remember the past—without using food to cover it up?
- Will I seek other God-honoring ways to cope with my present stress?
- Will I go back to my old habit of numbing out bad feelings?

What kinds of feelings, questions, and concerns do those choices stir in you?

_____

_____

_____

You can learn to tolerate bad feelings, walk through them, and let go of them. Walk through the pain; don't avoid it.

Dr. Linda remembers being in church as a child and singing a chorus that went: "I'm in-right, out-right, up-right, down-right, happy all the time."[8]

How accurately does that picture life as a Christian? Explain.

_____

_____

_____

If we choose to confront the reality of our lives, we won't feel happy all the time. We will have to learn to deal with difficulty and affliction. We may have to grieve losses of not having the perfect family, of a disappointing marriage, of children making bad choices, of critical and controlling bosses, and so forth. But we will learn to move past those hurts, no longer needing food as a cover-up.

Hebrews 12:2 says, "[Let us fix] our eyes on Jesus, the pioneer and perfecter of faith. For the joy set before him he endured the cross, scorning its shame, and sat down at the right hand of the throne of God." In the short term, what was Jesus called by God to experience?

_____

_____

_____

Because He was willing to endure short-term pain, what did Jesus ultimately receive?

_____

_____

_____

What does Jesus' example suggest with regard to your own experience and path? Why is embarking on the LIFL plan worth it long term?

_____

_____

DAY 5
Lose the Unrealistic Expectations

Thinking your life will be totally happy if you lose weight is only one of many unrealistic expectations concerning weight loss. Reevaluating your expectations is necessary. It's part of accepting reality. Our goal in this workbook session is to uncover other wrong ways of thinking. Are you ready?

LOOKING AT YOUR LIFE

Belief #1: All I have to do is lose weight. Nothing more will be required.

What is fallacious or dangerous about this kind of thinking?

_____

_____

In addition to the "what" of weight gain, why must we also focus on the "why"?

_____

_____

Belief #2: All kinds of opportunities will come to me when I lose weight.

When have you ever fallen victim to thinking that your life would be awash with good if you lost weight, only to be disappointed when it didn't turn out that way?

_____

_____

What do you think about the idea that blossoming friendships, a better marriage, a more active dating life, and so forth have less to do with losing weight and more to do with how you act and feel about yourself?

_____

_____

Belief #3: I will like myself better when I'm thinner.

To this idea, the authors cry, "Reality check! Red pill time! You may like yourself less for a short time as you confront things about yourself that need changing!" Do you agree? Why or why not?

_____

_____

Remember, being thin can take away a very comfortable excuse: "People don't like me because I'm fat." In actuality, they may avoid you because you are insensitive or something else. What concerns you as you realize that LIFL, in addition to being a weight-loss program, is also a call to confront the not-so-nice parts of yourself and make changes?

_____

_____

Belief #4: I'll be giving up a good thing.

In what specific ways is food a poor substitute for community and connection?

_____

_____

Describe a time in your life when a great meal deeply satisfied your innermost longings to be cared for emotionally and spiritually. Did it work? Did it last?

_____

_____

Belief #5: I must be perfect for God to work in me.

How does holding on to this belief cause us to cover up problems and be dishonest about our struggles?

_____

_____

Belief #6: I've screwed up so many times, it's just too late.

How does Jesus release us from this kind of thinking?

_____

_____

Belief #7: I can do this alone.

What is the danger in holding on to this belief?

_____

_____

It's never too late with God. God doesn't hold grudges. He forgives you and invites you to be His, with every cellulite wrinkle and flaw.

LEARNING A NEW WAY OF *LIFE*

Our souls have a great enemy called Satan, or the devil. He is described in the Bible as a liar and a murderer (John 8:44), as the ruler of this age who blinds people to truth (2 Corinthians 4:4), as an accuser of God's people (Revelation 12:10), and as one who is like a roaring lion, intent on destroying lives (1 Peter 5:8). Ephesians 6 speaks of the reality of spiritual warfare against this brutal adversary and of the importance of taking up the armor of God to fend off the evil one's diabolical attacks.

How would you say Satan most effectively wars against you—using food and eating?

_____

_____

Where are the chinks in your armor? Where are his fiery arrows landing in your life?

_____

_____

The truth transforms us, but we have to cooperate in the process in order to look like the Christ, who does the transforming.

When we wallow in guilt and shame from our past, we basically tell God that His Son's sacrifice didn't matter. He's taken all your guilt and shame to the cross, where Jesus died for our sin, and He doesn't want you holding on to it. He says, "I'll take your failures and build your future." And He has a great one planned for you. Do you dare believe this? Respond honestly.

_____

_____

Before His death, Jesus knew that Peter would deny him three times. He knew Peter would fail miserably. Read John 21. What do you see there? How does Jesus use Peter's failures and redeem his losses? How do you think Peter felt before, during, and after this encounter?

_____

_____

Read John 8:31–32. Before the truth can set us free, what must we be willing to do? (See also James 1:22.)

_____

_____

The authors argue that we see so little genuine transformation in our churches because the church often penalizes us for being honest. We hide our problems, as we are encouraged to put on a happy face.

Do you agree with that assessment? What do you think would happen if the people in your church knew all your stuff—your past, your hurts, your wrong choices, your failures?

_____

_____

In the Bible, we find unflattering details of all kinds of biblical characters. What does this suggest about God, His power, His grace, and our future?

_____

_____

LOSING IT FOR _LIFE_

Unfortunately, often we are judged by our weight. If we are heavy, many people will conclude we lack willpower and self-discipline. Haven't you heard,

"Well, just stop putting the food in your mouth!"? And don't you always want to scream back, "If it were that easy, I'd be at my ideal weight right now!"? The lesson? We won't always find the acceptance we desire from others. We can't control what people think or say.

Given this harsh reality, how can we go on? Where do we find acceptance and support?

_____

_____

In light of all the insensitive, impatient people, how can we trust that a few people will prove to be faithful friends and comrades on the LIFL journey?

_____

_____

How do we guard against the ever-present temptation of letting the opinions of others be our motivation for losing weight?

_____

_____

The authors recommend a prayer along these lines:

> God, I refuse to accept such words as *lazy, ugly, out of control,* or [fill in the blank] as definitions of who I am. With Your help, I will discover the true me. You created me and declared Your creation good. Amen.

Why is it important to know who we are in Christ? How does someone develop a biblical self-image?

You are not what you weigh. You have worth just because God created you.

_____

_____

_____

Based on what you've read here so far, how does this weight-loss/weight-management plan differ from others that you have tried?

_____

_____

What would you like to see God do in your life—not just in your body, but also in your heart in the months and years to come?

_____

_____

_____

Remembering that there are no quick fixes or instant solutions, what is your plan for when you encounter hard times on this journey?

_____

_____

3
Lose Dieting (for Life!)

Help! I could write a book on dieting. I don't know if there is one I haven't tried. I could fill a garage sale with all the books I've purchased. Maybe I should stack them up and use them for shelves or plant stands and find some real use for them. All kidding aside, I'm tired, broke, and still overweight. For some reason, I keep trying to lose weight. Do you think I've just missed the diet that will really work for me? Which diet do you recommend?

—Desperate Rita

Desperate Rita,

There is only one word to answer your question: NONE!

We can't think of anything more depressing than dieting. Who wants to willingly embark on a life of deprivation and eating food you don't enjoy? Just mentioning the word is depressing. We can almost hear your groans and moans: "Not another diet!" Any word that contains this three-letter word—*die*—can't be good.

DIETING MEANS DEPRIVATION

See if this self-dialogue doesn't ring some familiar bells:

"It's 7:00 a.m. and I'm going to be really good today. I won't eat one piece of candy or one french fry. I will be perfect starting today and get that thin body that will change my life."

By 8:30 a.m. you are hungry and eat two hardboiled eggs (leftovers from Easter Sunday) out of the refrigerator. Right after you've consumed them, you say, "What is wrong with me!? I already blew my diet. I shouldn't have eaten those eggs! I can't believe I did this. Eggs were not on my list of acceptable foods. I can't even control myself for one day . . . I don't care anymore." Enter [stage left] shame and despair.

By 9:00 a.m. you stare at the candy in the Easter basket and say, "I might as well eat it, too, since I already blew it." You overeat and actually binge on the candy, thereafter becoming disgusted again. "I need a diet that will make me stop eating so much! Okay, here is my plan. I'm going to eat grapefruit every day for two weeks. I'm ready. I'm psyched."

Weight loss (mostly water) begins quickly but then slows down after several days. You now add paper-thin crackers and low-fat bars to the grapefruit diet. Both taste like cardboard. And all you can think about is what you can't eat because what you are eating isn't satisfying at all. Then, you remember. There is Ben & Jerry's cookie dough ice cream in the freezer. *It definitely doesn't taste like cardboard.* You dive into the pint and quickly inhale all of it. The eating binge has begun.

"I am really bad. I have no willpower or self-control. Who am I kidding? I really need to get a serious diet. I can't make food choices. Maybe I should try liquids for a week. There has to be something more drastic out there to help me. I've got to get this weight off fast."

A liquids-only diet for one week really does the trick. You lose ten pounds. The weight is dropped! You go off the liquids. Gradually, over a few weeks, all the weight is regained, with five extra pounds being added to the ten that were lost and then gained. It's a vicious cycle. Your life feels out of control, hopeless, and depressing.

Dieting sets up most people to fail. It is not the solution to losing weight and keeping it off. The cycle of depriving yourself, then giving in, then feeling guilty, which leads to more overeating, is classic. The feelings of failure and shame are inevitable. Beating yourself up for not being able to fix the problem leads to a negative self-obsession mode. You are powerless to do what needs to be done—to address *why* you overeat in the first place.

We should make dieting a disorder and call it what it is—Dieting Disorder! Don't keep doing this to yourself. Food is not your enemy. Diets, however, make food your enemy. And the dietitians' mantra continues to sound: "There are no forbidden foods." Anything in moderation will not make you fat! Sensible choices combine with practicing moderation in all things while eating foods that have good nutritional content. It should be added that balance and moderation are keys not only to healthy eating but to good living. Both are biblical principles.

Moderation is better than muscle, self-control better than political power. (Proverbs 16:32 MSG)

Let your moderation be known unto all men. The Lord is at hand. (Philippians 4:5 KJV)

We must think differently when it comes to choosing food that makes us feel good and is good for us. We need to consider the whole picture. Here's an example from Dr. Linda's life: My children just had their week of SAT testing in school. I made sure they had some protein each morning to feed their brains—they needed foods that would stay with them for a few hours while they concentrated. Though they would have eaten sugary cereal given that option, they needed nutritious food that would sustain them and help them test well. I reminded them there was no good nutrition in sugary cereal and that they would be asleep at their desks in two hours if they made that choice. They agreed and wisely decided to eat a balanced breakfast—proving that even kids can be sensible when it comes to choosing healthy foods.

DIETING DOESN'T FILL THE EMPTY PLACE

Another problem with dieting is that it usually doesn't accomplish what we really need it to do. One of the biggest disappointments is that overeating doesn't fill the emotional needs we have. Yet how many of us overeat because we have emotional needs or want something? As much as we try, food doesn't fill those empty spaces.

When I (Steve) lost weight in my college days (the most at one time), I did it on a low-carb plan. The weight came off quickly, but it also went back on quickly. It was more of a roller coaster than a yo-yo as there were many twists and turns. But the weight always came back because of two disconnection factors: disconnection from God and disconnection from others. I was an independent loner, and rather than work through this chronic problem, I prided myself on my identity. The emptiness of my life drove me back to food over and over again.

So, yes, the low-carb diet worked to get the weight off, but *it didn't keep it off*. It failed to deliver me from a life of obesity and poor health. That state of being only came when I put into place the other factors that would fill the emptiness and heal the emotional conflicts I was experiencing.

To keep the weight off, eventually you have to fill the emptiness with something other than food and start to resolve the emotions. Here's an example: You overeat because you were rejected for a job. As you stuff down the food, your emotions slide right down with it. At the end of this small binge, the rejection is still with you. All that's been accomplished is you have overeaten and numbed out the problem temporarily with food. What really needed to be done was to deal with the rejection. Not getting the job was a loss that must be contended with; it hurt not to be picked.

Perhaps there were things you did in the interview that ruined your chances. Or the interviewer discriminated against you because you were overweight. Or you were under- or overqualified and weren't a viable option. Or perhaps this was not the job for you and God has something better waiting! Whatever the reason, overeating doesn't make the problem go away. At the end of the day, you are still jobless and have overeaten. Overeating actually may compound your bad feelings and make the situation even more painful as feelings of guilt, shame, and failure follow.

Sometimes overeating is triggered because we feel empty. We can feel empty because of unmet emotional needs. Another reason is that we have no active, living relationship with God. We don't go to God with our hurts as He instructs us to do. We don't call on Him for help when we feel helpless. Or we don't trust Him to help us handle our difficult feelings, so we indulge in an activity that covers the pain. We eat to fill the void, cover the void, or pretend it isn't really there.

Our culture rarely suggests God as an answer to combating feelings of emptiness. Instead, it promotes materialism and false solutions. It tells us we need more—more food, more sex, more cars, bigger homes—more and more stuff, and supersized! The message is shouted, advertised, sold, and publicized again and again: *More stuff is the answer to your longings.* Empty? Get more!

The truth is that only a personal, intimate relationship with God can satisfy the emptiness we feel. We were created to want more of God. Apart from God, we won't find satisfaction. And He doesn't leave us without a way to satisfy that longing. In addition, the emptiness must be filled with caring people who can love and support us through difficulty. Filling up with things is a poor substitute for relationships and intimacy. Through community and relationships we meet our needs for love and intimacy. This is a point we will make throughout LIFL because it is so important. You cannot be alone and isolated as you take this road to losing it for life.

DIETING MEANS MISSING SOMETHING

Diets promote us to miss something based on the premise that we may never be able to eat it again. Sound familiar? Let's say it's Christmas and you pass the buffet table at the office Christmas party. It's loaded with your favorite chocolate éclairs. Usually the thinking goes like this: *It's Christmas. I only get these once a year. I'll need to eat one, no . . . two, or three! After all, it'll be an entire year before I see these again. I can't let this chance pass.* Two weeks later you are at a baby shower. The cake has your favorite frosting, rich cream cheese. *Oh, can you believe this? I'm on a diet and I can't eat that cake.*

It's right in front of me and I can't have it. Everyone will enjoy the taste but me. I will miss out . . . I better grab it while I can. One month later, you are in Chicago for business. You pass by Giordano's Pizza, home of the best stuffed pizza you've ever tasted. *I can't be in Chicago and not eat Giordano's pizza. That would be a crime! But I'm dieting. Even though I could order a small single pizza, I would miss eating all I wanted this one time. I'll get the big stuffed pizza and take the rest back to my hotel for later.* Of course, none of the pizza makes it back to the hotel!

Lose this mentality and Lose It for Life! When you diet, you keep restricting yourself in ways that set you up to fail. Dieting means you'll be missing the good stuff, when in fact you could have just a taste, or just one piece, or just one slice of the good stuff. You wouldn't gain ten pounds. But thinking you are going to miss out on something sets you up to overeat. What you can't have, you want. This idea goes all the way back to the garden of Eden. Adam and Eve were given the freedom to eat from any tree in Paradise, except the Tree of Knowledge of Good and Evil. That was the one tree Adam was told to avoid. When the serpent came to tempt Eve, he began by questioning what God had instructed. He sowed doubt in Eve's mind. The very tree Adam and Eve were to avoid, they ultimately ate from! Think about it. They could have eaten from any tree but one! Eve was deceived and thought she was missing out on something, and Adam disobeyed with her. From the beginning, dealing with restriction has been a problem.

There is always a choice: to eat a food, eat less of it, or skip eating it entirely. A little of something may satisfy our want. The problem is we eat without thinking and focus on what we might be missing. Again, like sin, a little of something forbidden usually ends up being highly desirable. Rather than being self-governed, we give in to the temptation.

Please remember there are no "bad foods" (well, perhaps there are no bad foods other than the deep-fried Twinkies at your local fair), but there are wise choices. Actually this is a grown-up idea. Most people over twenty-one can have anything they want, but this doesn't mean they should indulge in everything just because they can. There are activities we should choose to do in moderate amounts, like watching TV or sports, and others we should do more often, like playing with our children. Finally, there are other things we shouldn't do at all, like viewing pornography. In every case, we have a choice. Though we don't have to miss a thing if we don't want to, it is very important to note that though everything may be available to us, it is definitely not all good for us. This is especially true of food.

Let's study this example: A mother complained that she couldn't give up eating ice cream. The reason was that her family stopped regularly at an ice cream parlor after each of her children's soccer games. She would sit at the table, drinking her diet drink and pretending she was having fun. But the more she thought about the taste and what she was missing, the more she wanted ice cream. After the kids were delivered home, she returned to the ice cream parlor, alone, and ordered a big hot fudge sundae. She ate it quickly so no one would see her. Feeling slightly sick to her stomach afterward, she rode home and lied about her absence. Then guilt set in as she felt terrible for lying and being so secretive.

Her mistake in choosing not to eat any ice cream is the reason she ended up at the ice cream parlor by herself. It would have been better for her to order a moderate treat with her family present, or divide a sundae with another person, or take a few bites from her husband's ice cream and not feel as if she were left out of the fun and celebration. Using moderation, she could have participated. Life isn't usually about all-or-nothing choices. There is a lot of gray area in between. In this case, her choices weren't limited to eating an entire supersized hot fudge sundae (black) or drinking a diet drink (white). The "gray" included options to divide a sundae, take a few bites, order a small sundae, or cut back on a dessert later. Or she could say to herself, *I could have a hot fudge sundae, but I choose not to. Later I'll be upset adding those extra calories. It's not worth it to me now.* Thus her decision to not have ice cream would not be made based on feelings of deprivation but feelings of certainty that she would regret her choice.

I (Steve) get kidded often about my ice cream and frozen yogurt strategy. People have told me they just could not do it, but they could if they practiced. The strategy is to always order a child's cone. I will even say to the person making a cone, "Not too much." Then, once I have paid for the treat, I ask anyone if they would like any of it. If the answer is yes, I spoon off the top and give it to them. If I have no takers, I walk over to the nearest trash can and spoon half of it into the trash.

That might seem wasteful to you, but it isn't. I own the cone. It is mine and I am free to do whatever I want with it. If I eat more than I need or want, it does not help one hungry person in Ethiopia. My throwing away a portion of it rather than eating it does not hurt people who are starving either. Each time I do this, I make an adult decision that I do not need the whole cone to feel satisfied. But I know that if I start eating right away (before getting rid of half the ice cream), it will be difficult to stop at the halfway point, or at any point. So I lessen the damage right up front, enjoy the half that I eat, and don't feel deprived at all. In fact, I walk away having had something I really enjoyed while also being proud that I implemented a strategy that worked. It may seem strange, but it's a pretty easy way to save yourself a lot of calories and carbs over a year's time while still enjoying ice cream now and again.

*DIETING GIVES THE CONTROL TO
OTHERS INSTEAD OF YOU

Another problem with dieting is that you constantly give the control of your food over to others. The diet is like Big Brother watching your every move. Imagine him saying, "Ah, Sally, you can't have that! No, those chips are not on my plan. Stop eating that pasta—do you see it written on our plan?" Sally, feeling deprived and frustrated by the diet, tells the voice to be quiet and to stop telling her what to do!

Add this internal voice to the myriad expert voices telling you to eat only low fat . . . *no*, high protein . . . *no*, low carbs . . . *no*, high carbs . . . *no*, only vegetables . . . *no!* It's enough to make any of us throw in the towel and say, "Forget it! I'll do what I want to do!"

Chapter 6 will help you learn to eat what's right for you, to pay attention to your body and how you feel when you eat certain foods, and to make your own choices. Whole 30 Eating is something you do for life. Thus, you need to be in charge of it and not dependent on what others tell you to do. This doesn't mean you can't learn more about nutrition and healthy eating, as it's important to be well informed. But you must learn to make your own decisions and not be so dependent. If you need to enlist the help of a dietitian or nutritionist for a while, that's fine. He or she can instruct you as to how to eat healthy and sensible meals. Or you can follow our guidelines. But ultimately, you need to feel in control of your choices and be a grown-up who makes your own choices.

DIETING SETS YOU UP FOR BINGEING

A serious concern with dieting is that it sets you up to binge, which involves uncontrolled eating episodes in which you consume a large number of calories in a short amount of time, and usually in secrecy.

You may relate to Jim's story. Jim was a rather successful salesman who spent a great deal of time on the road, traveling for his job. He decided to diet after gaining a substantial amount of weight. He was motivated by his desperation to meet someone and settle down.

Because Jim traveled so much, most evenings were spent in a hotel room, preparing his sales pitches for the next day. The evenings were boring and Jim was anxious. He knew the dangers of pornography and avoided porn movies and videos he could view in his room. His father was an alcoholic, so Jim stayed clear of the hotel bars. But when he was bored and needed a break from the monotony and loneliness of his weeknights, he'd make runs to local grocery stores. There he'd load up on goodies—mostly sweets and desserts.

Night after night, he binged and watched his weight steadily climb. For Jim, bingeing became habitual and was always accompanied by self-loathing. No woman would want him, he reckoned. He was obese and out of control. The key issue, however, was that Jim struggled with loneliness and didn't know how to deal with it. Dieting was his solution. The binges followed. He felt powerless over the food, but the truth is that his powerlessness was directly related to his perceived inability to find a wife and have the life he desired.

A PROPER VIEW OF EATING

Since there is so much distortion in our culture concerning food, it's best to look at God's original intention for eating. Obviously, He created us with a physical need to eat and provided food as a way to satisfy that need. So what does the Bible say about diets, eating, drinking, overeating, and indulgence in general?

Eating and drinking were common points of fellowship in biblical days. People held feasts, celebrated weddings, invited guests for meals, and used food to nourish, strengthen, and celebrate. The Gospels record Jesus eating meals with His disciples (including the Last Supper), sharing a meal with Lazarus, and being fed by Martha. There is nothing sinful about eating. In fact, eating is often associated with celebration.

Food and drink were used for miracles—Jesus turned water into wine at a wedding and fed thousands of hungry people with loaves and fishes. In Mark, Jesus likened the coming of His kingdom to a wedding feast. In the Old Testament, several feasts are recorded to commemorate Israel's deliverance from Egypt as well as from the wilderness. These occasions symbolized consecration and devotion to God. The firstfruits of harvest were dedicated to make atonement for sins and to rejoice and give thanks with the completion of another harvest.

Throughout the Bible, food is discussed symbolically as well as literally and is enjoyed and celebrated. However, like most things, eating and drinking can be excessive. When appetite is ravenous and unrestrained, the Bible calls it *gluttony*. A glutton, according to *Webster's Dictionary*, is described as someone who eats excessively and is greedy or excessively indulgent. So what can we learn from Scripture about gluttony, a topic that is rarely discussed in the modern American church?

Let's face the reality. How many sermons have you heard on this topic? I have counted three in my lifetime. All three were from one series on the Seven Deadly Sins (preached in a Protestant church). Most of you know that the list (as it is) originated in the Catholic Church with Pope St. Gregory the Great. The sins are called "deadly" because they wound love and are considered harmful to one's relationship with God and others. Gluttony is often contrasted with the spiritual virtues of faith and temperance.

The point of understanding gluttony in this context is that it can impede one's spiritual progress or hinder a victorious spiritual life. The Seven Deadly Sins are not a formal list in the Bible, but each one is referenced within the Bible between the books of Genesis and Revelation.

Gluttony Brings Poverty

One of the direct references to gluttony is found in Proverbs 23, a chapter about the importance of exercising restraint. In Proverbs 23:2–3, Solomon instructs, "Don't gobble your food, don't talk with your mouth full. And don't stuff yourself; bridle your appetite" (MSG). In verse 21 of that same chapter, he goes on to say, "Drunks and gluttons will end up on skid row, in a stupor and dressed in rags" (MSG). In other words, when you don't exercise restraint over eating, the outcome is negative! The message here is don't overindulge. It's true—too much of a good thing is too much!

Gluttony Is a Negative Behavioral Characteristic

Note the reference to gluttony in Matthew 11:19. Jesus is talking about how the people tried to discredit Him as Messiah by calling Him a glutton: "I came feasting and they called me a lush, a friend of the riffraff. Opinion polls don't count for much, do they? The proof of the pudding is in the eating" (MSG). In this case, gluttony was referred to as a negative behavioral trait. Though feasting was not a problem, becoming a lush was. The intent was to criticize Jesus by calling Him a glutton, someone who couldn't bridle His appetite or exercise control over His life. It's ironic that the Pharisees applied this label to Christ, who is God. He is in total control. There is nothing "excessive" about Him! Those Pharisees didn't like that and so resorted to name-calling, a rather childish maneuver.

Gluttony Is Rebellion

A warning against rebellion is found in Deuteronomy 21:18–21, which speaks to the fallout of a rebellious son in a family. "When a man has a stubborn son, a real rebel who won't do a thing his mother and father tell him, and even though they discipline him he still won't obey, his father and mother shall forcibly bring him before the leaders at the city gate and say to the city fathers, 'This son of ours is a stubborn rebel; he won't listen to a thing we say. He's a glutton and a drunk'" (MSG). Amazingly, the punishment for this was to be stoned to death! Go ahead and thank God for His grace and mercy right now! There are no recorded instances of parents having done this in the

Old Testament. The consequence was meant to deter rebellion. Apparently it worked well. It surely would have made us obedient!

The point of this biblical chapter isn't to provide an extreme model for solving rebellion today. We live under the new covenant in which mercy and grace are freely extended. (Breathe a sigh of relief with us!) We believe, however, that this chapter underscores an important truth—rebellion to family, to proper authority, and to God ultimately leads to destruction and negative consequences—consequences God wanted the children of Israel to avoid for their own good. This is wisdom from which to benefit.

Have you ever thought about your eating as rebellion? In some cases, this is a motive for excessive eating. Do you eat when you want to rebel? Are you compliant on the outside but secretly rebelling on the inside? These are important questions to ask yourself, as it is possible to be eating out of a feeling of rebellion. For example, a man who needed to confront his wife for a hurtful remark she made reported eating to "show her." "She wasn't about to control me by what she said," he angrily cried out. When we got down to the motive for his overeating, which was to rebel against what he thought his wife wanted him to be, we made progress. In his heart, he felt rebellious, even though it wasn't apparent from his physical outlook. Later he realized that he was angry with God too. In fact, he blamed God for his unhappy life. His response was to rebel against his wife, body, and God, and to harbor anger and resentment.

OUR BODIES ARE FOR THE GLORY OF GOD

As you read through these biblical references to gluttony, it's easy to see why more ministers don't preach on this topic! It seems negative and depressing. Yet God created your body. He chose you as His. His spirit lives in you. Read 1 Corinthians 6:19: "Or didn't you realize that your body is a sacred place, the place of the Holy Spirit? Don't you see that you can't live however you please, squandering what God paid such a high price for? The physical part of you is not some piece of property belonging to the spiritual part of you" (MSG). What Paul is saying is that our bodies are sacred and what we do with them affects all parts of us. Our bodies are the dwelling places of the Most High God. We need to take care of them and allow them to be used for God's glory. If gluttony is the sin that is preventing us from being used for God's glory, we need to admit it and repent from it, however painful that act may be.

Lose It for Life is not about wishing for a more sensitive world so our lives would be better. It is about transformation. And transformation will only occur when we face the reality of what we are involved in. Not all who have a weight problem are gluttons, so if you aren't, don't feel falsely accused. But if you are struggling with gluttony, admitting it to God and another person could be the first step toward freedom. If God has been replaced with the food idol and you gluttonously worship that idol with all the devotion you can muster, accepting the true nature, degree, and description of the problem is the way to begin transforming.

Anyone's obsession with food can take on an idol worship–like proportion. When we worry, think, and obsess about what we will eat, or look forward to meals more than our time with God, we are out of balance. Worry is a distracting trait. If we worry about what we eat, how much we'll be able to have, and how often we can get it, we are not following Christ's directive in Matthew 6:25, "If you decide for God, living a life of God-worship, it follows that you don't fuss about what's on the table at mealtimes or whether the clothes in your closet are in fashion. There is far more to your life than the food you put in your stomach, more to your outer appearance than the clothes you hang on your body" (MSG).

A life decided for God has the promise that God will meet your physical needs as well as your emotional and spiritual ones. Accept the promises. God wants you to enjoy eating yet not become a glutton. These words are not meant to be harsh but to help you understand that anything taken to excess can block a vibrant relationship with God. *Moderation is key.*

You are not condemned by God or us for overeating. God wants to bring you to improved health, to remove your obsession with food, to prevent negative consequences related to your overeating, and to help you enjoy meals and fellowship with others. He wants you to experience the enjoyment of food, the pleasure of taste, and the sensation of a full stomach rather than be bound by guilt, physical discomfort, or negative health consequences related to obesity and bingeing.

The Bible also tells us to get out of spiritual poverty by developing self-control, a fruit of the Spirit (Galatians 5:22), and to submit our entire lives to God as living sacrifices (Romans 12:1). Allow Him to use you for His glory—it is a primary reason that you were created!

DISTINGUISHING BETWEEN THE HUNGERS

I eat but I'm not really hungry. At least, I don't think I am. I'm not really sure. Sometimes I feel like I could eat everything in the cupboards, like I'm ravenous. So I just do. I never really think about if I'm hungry or not. I think I just really like food, lots of food. And lots of times, I crave things—like cookies. I'll go to the bakery and pretend to be buying a dozen cookies for my kids at school, but really, I plan on eating them all.

What is hunger? What motivates it? Is the need physical, emotional, or spiritual? The three faces of hunger are very different and often confused, as many of us have discovered. The need for deeper emotional and spiritual fulfillment can be viewed instead as physical hunger. And though there may be immediate gratification when we eat, we will not be truly satisfied unless we are eating to fill a physical hunger.

Physical Hunger

Physical hunger is a normal body sensation, a cue that the body needs refueling. Physical hunger goes away when there is food to satisfy it. Hunger is part of God's creative design. To identify physical hunger, you must learn to recognize the physical sensations that accompany it. Usually hunger builds because you haven't eaten in a while. Your body signals its need for food—whether it is a rumbling, growling, or emptiness in the pit of your stomach. You may also experience low energy or even light-headedness. Eating even a small amount of food usually stops these sensations.

We have other needs apart from our physical bodies. There are the needs to be safe, to belong, to be loved, to be esteemed, and to grow. Emotional hunger relates to an unmet emotional need. Even though emotional needs can't be satisfied by food, that doesn't stop us from trying. Yet as most of us know, this doesn't work. Food is used like a drug to distract, numb, and help us avoid the reality of hurt and pain or the emptiness of an unmet need.

The following table will help you distinguish differences between physical and emotional hunger:[1]

Physical Hunger	Emotional Hunger
Builds gradually	Hits suddenly, "starving"
Stomach starts to rumble and growl	Anxiety; but there is no real physical symptom of feeling hungry
Feel full and stop eating	Overeat even if feeling full
Different foods will satisfy	Crave very specific food; nothing else satisfies
Physically feel empty in pit of stomach	Mouth and mind are tasting the food

Need to eat but can wait	Eat now to ease whatever is happening
Eat and feel fine	Eat and feel guilt and shame
Four to five hours since last meal; feel light-headed, low energy	Upset and want to eat now
Choose foods purposefully	Automatic or absentminded eating

If you had difficulty on your food journal deciding whether or not you were physically hungry each time you ate, this exercise may help. The next time you eat, make a guess as to which type of hunger you are experiencing. List the three columns in the following chart. In the first column, check which hunger you think you are having. In the second column, write down your feelings, physical sensations, emotions, and thoughts right before you wanted to eat. In the third column, write down how you felt after you ate. Read what you listed and decide if you checked the correct type of hunger. A blank copy of this chart is provided in Appendix B. Your chart might resemble this one:

Physical or Emotional Hunger?	**Before I ate, I felt:** *(Feelings and thoughts)*	**After I ate, I felt:** *(Feelings and thoughts)*
Emotional	Upset and mad, wanted to eat, stomach tense from anger	Tired, immediately uncomfortable
Physical	Ate four hours ago, light-headed, stomach growling	Satisfied, energized

Each time you eat, something precedes the eating. We call these "triggers" or "cues." A trigger or cue signals that something is about to begin. A physical trigger involves a physical symptom—something like feeling short of energy, light-headedness, a growling stomach, headache, or dizziness.

Emotional Hunger

Emotional triggers involve feelings: feeling upset, bored, hurt, angry, disappointed, lonely, happy, and so on. If you notice that all your checks are in the emotional column, then we have work to do. The goal is to eat more often in response to physical cues than emotional ones.

If you aren't sure what you are feeling or thinking, here's an additional exercise. Next time you eat, focus on the *experience* of eating and become very aware of your physical and emotional state. The goal is to stay in the moment of eating and avoid eating without thinking.

Sixty seconds before you eat, sit quietly (with no distractions) and think, *What do I feel and what am I thinking about right now?* Record this. Then look at what you are about to eat. Notice how it tastes. Do you like what you are eating? Do you like the feel of it in your mouth? How does it feel in your stomach? After you finish, take another sixty seconds and write down how you feel—energized, tired, unsatisfied, content, and so forth.

This short exercise will put you in touch with the experience of eating. It will slow you down and help you pay attention to all the sensations involved in eating. After emotional eating, you'll often feel tired and sluggish or won't feel satisfied because eating wasn't what you needed to do. In addition, when you choose sugary foods, your blood sugar rises and falls quickly, which makes you feel tired. The goal is to find out why you are eating in the first place and to stop eating when you aren't physically hungry.

Why do we eat when we aren't hungry? Sometimes this behavior happens out of habit—such as when food is treated as a reward or involves a celebration. It also serves as a numbing device or plan of avoidance when we feel unpleasant. Often people eat because they feel impulsive and want to gratify those impulses quickly. Other people eat to indulge in something good because they are feeling deprived by other things in life. Whatever the reason, finding out why you are eating is paramount to losing weight and keeping it off. Once you get a handle on why you eat, you can make changes.

At this point, begin to tune in to your physical, mental, and emotional state. Pay attention to the cues that lead to overeating. Write them down and study them. Stay aware and "in the moment" while eating. Soon you'll know the difference between real hunger and emotional hunger.

Spiritual Hunger

During the Sermon on the Mount, Jesus said, "Blessed are you who hunger now, for you will be satisfied" (Luke 6:21). The Greek word for "hunger" is *peinas*, meaning to be hungry, to be famished, to be starved. Jesus tells us to hunger after Him and we will be satisfied. What we think is hunger for food or even emotional hunger may be a hunger for more of God. We were created with a space for God to live in us, not to be empty. His desire is for us to have life and have it more abundantly. Yet how many of us are satisfied with the scraps from the table when He promises us a feast? We are spiritually starving and don't feed our hunger the right way. We become distracted with other things that won't fill that spiritual void.

Beth Moore says, "Victory is not determined as much by what we've been delivered *from* as by what we've been delivered *to*."[2] She is so right. You won't be victorious over food and overeating unless you look to God to satisfy you. Nothing else will really do. God wants to deliver you from the need to overeat. He wants you to find your purpose, move in His power, and live a life of overcoming. He offers Himself to you. He is your deliverer. With God there is relationship, intimacy, and abundant life, not to mention peace, joy, and so much more! He offers that which will satisfy. Heed His promise! He wants you, chose you, and is waiting to fill your mouth with good things.

When you feel depressed by a gnawing emptiness in your soul, focus on your hope in Christ. God's promises are many, and they are meant to be read and treasured and cried over and praised over. Let these scriptures encourage you and fill that empty space within you:

> For everything that was written in the past was written to teach us, so that through the endurance taught in the Scriptures and the encouragement they provide we might have hope. (Romans 15:4)

> May the God of hope fill you with all joy and peace as you trust in him, so that you may overflow with hope by the power of the Holy Spirit. (Romans 15:13)

> I pray that the eyes of your heart may be enlightened in order that you may know the hope to which he has called you, the riches of his glorious inheritance in his holy people. (Ephesians 1:18)

God has so much more for you. He doesn't want you dragging through life being defeated by your weight. He wants to give you good things—more of His power, more of His Spirit, more of His love and compassion. The urgency you feel to fill up with food, to overeat, could be the Holy Spirit urging you to satisfy your spiritual hunger through God. Are you afraid you won't get what you need? Not to worry. God has enough to go around for all of us. His resources are limitless. He is the Living Water that never runs dry. He is the Bread of Life who promises eternal life. The fullness He has for you cannot be found in the temporal things of this world. And once you experience His fullness, you'll never hunger in the same way again!

So why don't we hunger and thirst after righteousness? Too often it is because we listen to the voice of the accuser. The Bible tells us the accuser is the devil and that he accuses us day and night (Revelation 12:10). Think about it. Satan can't undo our salvation, so he has to have other tricks to trip us up. One of his best schemes is to accuse us with claims that we aren't worthy, we can't lose weight, or that we are all losers. His accusations are constantly ringing in our ears. But we cannot listen to him or believe his lies because we have been cleared of all accusations, as Hebrews 10:19–23 tells us:

> So, friends, we can now—without hesitation—walk right up to God, into "the Holy Place." Jesus has cleared the way by the blood of his sacrifice, acting as our priest before God. The "curtain" into God's presence is his body. So let's do it—full of belief, confident that we're presentable inside and out. Let's keep a firm grip on the promises that keep us going. He always keeps his word. (MSG)

Did you grasp that truth? You are cleansed by the blood of Christ's sacrifice. Once you confess sin, there is nothing Satan can do about it because it's no longer there. So he can accuse all he wants. You just tell him to go take a hike because there is nothing left for Satan to accuse. You have to believe this truth and stop letting the devil take your past and hold it up like an autobiography. Yes, you have sinned, but once confessed, the book's pages are blank. There is no record of those wrongs anymore, because the sin has been cleared.

You've got to get this into your spirit and not allow the enemy to steal your joy. Hunger for more of God. God holds all satisfaction. Perhaps you've tried to find satisfaction in many other ways. Rest in the assurance that nothing completely satisfies except more of God. God wants to fill your hungry, empty life with the bread that truly satisfies, and He will—when you sit down for the meal and open your heart and life to His will and His voice.

Workbook Week 3

LOSE DIETING (FOR LIFE!)

Why Dieting Doesn't Work

We can't think of anything more depressing than dieting. Who wants to willingly embark on a life of deprivation and eating foods you don't enjoy? Just mentioning the word *diet* is depressing. We can almost hear your groans and moans: "Not another diet!"

LOOKING AT YOUR *LIFE*

What was your very first diet? What eventually happened?

_____

_____

_____

We don't want you to diet. Lose the word from your vocabulary.

Describe your most recent dieting experience.

_____

_____

_____

In what situations are you most prone to graze? (Check all that apply.)

____ when I am lonely

____ when I am bored

____ when I am anxious/stressed

____ when I am afraid

____ when I am idle

___ whenever food is readily available

___ from the time I wake up until the time I hit the hay

___ when I am _____

LEARNING A NEW WAY OF *LIFE*

You'd think we would have it figured out by now. But we don't. Dieting is inherently frustrating because it actually gets us to obsess over food. We end up craving whatever foods the diet forbids us to have. It's not so much "forbidden fruit" as forbidden sweets or starches or fatty fare. We become transfixed by and preoccupied with whatever is off-limits. It's only a matter of time until the siren call of some sinful delicacy wears down our willpower. Can we get a witness?

Because of our past dietary failures and personal hurts, these are the kinds of beliefs we find rattling around in our heads and hearts:

- "You're disgusting. Can't you even get it right for one day?"
- "Why even try? You know you're going to fail. It's just a matter of time."
- "You? Thin? Who are you kidding?"
- "How many times have you tried to lose weight? A thousand? Two thousand?"
- "Why don't you just face facts? You're fat and you'll always be fat."

Write down some messages of the "tapes" that play in your mind.

_____

_____

_____

Consider the following passages of Scripture. These are not nice ideas or warm wishes. They are declarations of eternal, divine truth. God doesn't force us to believe these statements, but if we do—if we base our identity and worth on these biblical precepts—we begin to view God, the world, and ourselves differently. And over time, we begin to act differently (Romans 12:1–2).

"The thief comes only to steal and kill and destroy; I have come that they may have life, and have it to the full." (John 10:10)

See what great love the Father has lavished on us, that we should be called children of God! And that is what we are! (1 John 3:1)

For we are God's masterpiece. He has created us anew in Christ Jesus, so that we can do the good things he planned for us long ago. (Ephesians 2:10 NLT)

. . . Now to him who is able to do immeasurably more than all we ask or imagine, according to his power that is at work within us. (Ephesians 3:20)

For the Spirit God gave us does not make us timid, but gives us power, love and self-discipline. (2 Timothy 1:7)

According to these verses, what is the truth about you?

_____

_____

_____

LIFL Reminders

- You don't need a new diet; you need a new mind-set and lifestyle.
- Remove unhealthy food temptations from your household.
- Drink a lot of water. It's good for you and it can take the edge off your cravings!
- Eat smaller portions and eat slowly.
- Get your body moving.
- Find stress relievers and emptiness fillers other than food: cleaning, exercise, serving others, calling friends, yard work, taking a hot shower, and others.

LOSING IT FOR LIFE

Let's look more closely at why dieting usually ends in disaster and disillusionment.

Check the boxes by the following statements with which you have first-hand experience.

☐ **Dieting means deprivation.**

The cycle of depriving yourself, then giving in, then feeling guilty, which leads to more overeating, is classic. It doesn't work and leads to feelings of failure and shame. And it certainly doesn't address the reasons that you overeat in the first place.

The authors observe: "Diets . . . make food your enemy. And the dietitians' mantra continues to sound: 'There are no forbidden foods.' Anything in moderation will not make you fat!" When we deprive ourselves of certain foods, chances are we'll binge or overeat. Do you agree or disagree with these statements? Why?

_____

_____

_____

☐ **Dieting doesn't fill the empty place.**

Many people overeat because they have emotional needs or want something. But as much as they try, food doesn't fill those empty spaces.

Think of a recent experience (for example, a rejection, a slight, a disappointment, and so forth) in which you reacted by turning to food for comfort. What happened? How were you feeling as you ate? What about afterward?

_____

_____

_____

Be honest. Do you look to God when you are swamped by feelings of emptiness? Why or why not?

_____

_____

_____

> Sometimes overeating is triggered because we feel "empty." We have no active, alive life with God. We don't trust Him to help us handle our difficult feelings and so we eat to fill the void.

☐ **Dieting means missing something.**

We often hunt down foods and eat like a condemned criminal having his or her last meal. How prone are you to fall into this kind of thinking? What foods do you find practically irresistible?

_____

_____

_____

☐ **Dieting gives the control to others instead of you.**

The diet is like Big Brother watching your every move. Add the myriad expert voices telling you to eat only low-fat, high-protein, low carbs, high carbs, only vegetables . . . It's enough to make a person throw in the towel.

If maturity means being responsible for your own choices, then what does it say when we rush out and buy every new dieting book that hits the bookshelves?

_____

_____

_____

☐ **Dieting sets up bingeing.**

To illustrate this point, the authors tell the story of a salesman named Jim (see the story in chapter 3 of the book).

With what in Jim's experience do you relate?

_____

_____

_____

What is the most helpful truth you've discovered in this lesson? Why?

_____

_____

_____

Thinking you are going to miss something sets you up to overeat. What you can't have, you want. This idea goes all the way back to the garden of Eden.

You always have a choice to eat a food, eat less of it, or skip it entirely. A little of something may satisfy your want.

DAY 2
A Proper View of Eating

Since we find so much distortion in our culture concerning food, it's best to look at God's original intention for eating. First, think about your own view of food.

LOOKING AT YOUR *LIFE*

When you were a child, how was food treated or used in your household? For instance, were desserts and treats used a reward? Was the withholding of food used as a punishment? Was food offered as a way of "cheering up" after a bad experience?

_____

_____

What are your most vivid childhood memories of food?

_____

_____

Estimate how much time you spend (on average) weekly in each of the following areas:

_____ planning meals/thinking about what to cook or eat
_____ buying food/grocery shopping
_____ stocking /rearranging food in the pantry/refrigerator
_____ cooking/preparing food
_____ actually eating meals (at home or dining out)
_____ waiting to get your food (either in a restaurant or a fast-food drive-thru lane)
_____ cleaning up after meals

God created us with a physical need to eat and provided food as a way to satisfy that need.

_____ talking about food (good recipes, what you're going to eat, what you did eat, etc.)

_____ snacking

What's your total? Does that seem about right? Excessive? What conclusions can you draw from this exercise?

_____

_____

We don't often hear teaching or sermons on food or eating in a way that honors God. Why is this subject, which is such a major part of everyday life, so seldom talked about or thought about from a biblical perspective?

_____

_____

_____

LEARNING A NEW WAY OF *LIFE*

Food figures prominently in the Bible. The first temptation and sin involved eating; the ending involves a great marriage banquet.

Let's take a quick and broad overview of food as mentioned in the Bible. Eating and drinking were major ingredients of fellowship and hospitality in biblical days. People held feasts, celebrated weddings, invited others for meals, cooked for guests, and used food to nourish, strengthen, and celebrate.

What are your favorite social occasions or holidays that involve big meals? Why?

_____

_____

In the Old Testament, God prescribed seven feasts for the Israelites. These were both solemn assemblies and times of great celebration, intended to commemorate God's deliverance of Israel from Egypt and His constant care in the wilderness. Eating also figured prominently in the sacrificial system that God instructed His people to follow. The promised land was assessed largely on the basis of its fruitfulness (that is, its ability to provide rich supplies of food).

When the Israelites wandered in the wilderness, God provided manna from heaven—a supernatural supply of daily food (Exodus 16). What was God trying to teach His people?

_____

_____

The New Testament recorded that Jesus ate meals with His disciples (including the Last Supper), shared a meal with Lazarus, and was fed by Martha. Preaching in Lystra, the apostle Paul exclaimed: "[God] has shown kindness by giving you rain from heaven and crops in their seasons; he provides you with plenty of food and fills your hearts with joy" (Acts 14:17).

When teaching His followers how to pray, why do you think Jesus included the petition found in Matthew 6:11?

_____

_____

What conclusions can we therefore draw about food and eating?

_____

_____

Food and drink were often a major focal point of miracles—Jesus turned water into wine at a wedding and fed thousands with loaves and fishes on hillsides. In Mark, Jesus compared the coming of His kingdom to a wedding feast. Throughout the Bible, food is discussed symbolically as well as literally and is enjoyed and celebrated.

The resurrected Christ grilled fish on the beach and enjoyed this simple meal with His disciples. He didn't _have_ to do this and yet He did. Why?

_____

_____

In the book of Revelation, the apostle John was given a glimpse into the future at the end of this world. Jesus tells John, "Blessed are those who are invited to the marriage supper of the Lamb" (19:9 NASB). What do you imagine this supper will be like?

_____

_____

"The LORD Almighty will prepare a feast of rich food for all peoples, a banquet of aged wine— the best of meats and the finest of wines" (Isaiah 25:6).

LOSING IT FOR *LIFE*

It is important to have a healthy perspective about food. As physical beings, we need nourishment—vitamins and minerals, fuel to run our human bodies. There is nothing intrinsically wrong or sinful with food. Yet, like all of God's good gifts—rest, wealth, sex, and so forth—food can be abused, misused, or turned into a god. Our goal here is to develop a healthy, biblical perspective on food and eating.

If you had to summarize what God's Word says about food in a few broad principles, how would you do so? Write your summary principles here.

1. _____
2. _____
3. _____
4. _____
5. _____

First Corinthians 10:31 says, "So whether you eat or drink or whatever you do, do it all for the glory of God." How does someone eat for the "glory of God"?

_____

_____

Think about your eating habits for the last couple of days, weeks, or years. In what ways have you glorified God in your attitudes and actions surrounding food? In what specific ways have you not?

_____

_____

DAY 3
What Is Gluttony?

As with most human activities, we can eat and drink to excess. The biblical term for having a ravenous and unrestrained appetite is *gluttony*. A glutton is defined as someone who gorges on food and who is marked by excessive desire. Let's look at what can we learn from Scripture about gluttony, a topic rarely discussed in the American modern church.

LOOKING AT YOUR *LIFE*

When have you heard the word *glutton* used in regular conversation?

_____

_____

When does normal, healthy eating cross over into the realm of gluttony?

_____

_____

The reason we need to understand gluttony is that it can impede our spiritual progress, keeping us from enjoying a victorious spiritual life.

Check any of the following that you personally regard as gluttony:

____ eating three big meals a day

____ making more than one trip to the food bar

____ eating to the point of feel stuffed

____ eating more than a certain amount of calories in a day

____ having frantic late-night binges

____ supersizing meals at fast-food restaurants

____ cleaning one's plate—and also perhaps eating the leftovers off a
spouse's or child's plate

___ having two scoops instead of one

___ going back for seconds

___ inhaling the meal in a very short time

___ eating out of a container or out of the serving dish

___ other: _____

What are your specific criteria for knowing when you've crossed the line into gluttony? (Note: If you don't have any, now might be a good time to take a shot at creating a set of guidelines for knowing when too much of a good thing is too much.)

_____

_____

_____

LEARNING A NEW WAY OF *LIFE*

One of the Bible's direct references to gluttony is found in Proverbs 23, a chapter about the importance of exercising restraint. In Proverbs 23:2–3, Solomon instructs, "Don't gobble your food, don't talk with your mouth full. And don't stuff yourself; bridle your appetite" (MSG). In verse 21 of that same chapter, he states, "Drunks and gluttons will end up on skid row, in a stupor and dressed in rags" (MSG).

How would you summarize the message of these verses?

_____

_____

Jesus talked about how the people tried to discredit His claims to be the promised Messiah by calling Him a glutton. "The Son of Man, on the other hand, feasts and drinks, and you say, 'He's a glutton and a drunkard, and a friend of tax collectors and other sinners!' But wisdom is shown to be right by its results" (Matthew 11:19 NLT).

What does this passage reveal about:

Jesus Christ?

_____

eating and drinking?

_____

In the above instance, gluttony was viewed as a negative behavior trait. Feasting was not a problem, but becoming a lush was. And a lush is not a positive description of anyone. The intent was to criticize Jesus by calling Him a glutton and drunkard—someone who couldn't bridle His appetite or exercise control over His life. Isn't it crazy that the Pharisees applied these labels to Christ? He's God. He's always been in total control of His passions and desires.

Imagine a life free from gluttonous behavior. What would it be like to live moderately? To be free to taste and enjoy a small bit of anything, without going overboard? How—long term—would such a practice change your daily existence?

_____

_____

LOSING IT FOR LIFE

Deuteronomy 21:18–21 weaves together the concepts of gluttony and rebellion. Ponder these verses:

> When a man has a stubborn son, a real rebel who won't do a thing his
> mother and father tell him, and even though they discipline him he still
> won't obey, his father and mother shall forcibly bring him before the leaders
> at the city gate and say to the city fathers, "This son of ours is a stubborn
> rebel; he won't listen to a thing we say. He's a glutton and a drunk" (MSG).

Amazingly, the punishment for this type of rebellion was stoning—to death! (The Bible records no instances of parents having done this.) The consequence was meant to deter rebellion. The point here isn't to suggest an extreme model for dealing with rebellious children. Please don't apply it that way! We believe, however, that Deuteronomy 21 highlights a broad, important principle—rebellion (against authority, whether parental, civil, or eternal) ultimately leads to destruction and negative consequences, consequences that God wanted the children of Israel to avoid for their own good.

Gluttony is one of the so-called Seven Deadly Sins—because it can be harmful to one's relationship with God and others.

Do you eat when you want to rebel? Or when you want to get back at someone—at a spouse, a parent, at God? Are you living a compliant life on the outside but secretly rebelling against something or someone on the inside?

_____

_____

_____

Whether we eat in a passive-aggressive fashion, to lash out or punish someone else, or we eat frantically, out of some irrational fear that we might miss out on "our fair share," gluttony is sin.

Read 1 John 1:9. In your own words, what does it say?

_____

_____

_____

In some cases, angry rebellion is a motive for overeating.

To *confess* means literally to "say the same thing." When we confess our sin, we agree with what God says about it. So, what *does* God say about our sins? First, He says they are an affront to His holy character and standard (Romans 3:23). Second, He says that in Christ our sins are forgiven—all of them (Colossians 2:13). Third, because of the new nature Christ gives us (2 Corinthians 5:17) when we trust Him, sin has no more power over us. We do not have to keep giving in to the same temptations (Romans 6)!

In light of these truths, write out a full confession to God of any acts of gluttony. Claim His promise of complete forgiveness and cleansing.

_____

_____

_____

_____

_____

_____

DAY 4

Our Bodies for the Glory of God

As you read through the biblical references to gluttony, you can understand why more ministers don't preach on this topic! It seems negative and depressing, but it isn't. God created your body. He chose you as His own child. His Spirit lives inside you. Let's explore in this session what it means that our bodies are to be used for the glory of God.

LOOKING AT YOUR *LIFE*

Some troubled youths cut themselves, a practice referred to as *self-mutilation*. What do you think motivates this strange practice against one's body?

_____

_____

The number of people who are choosing to undergo cosmetic surgery is skyrocketing. Why is this one of the biggest growth industries in the Western world?

_____

_____

This may be a difficult or painful exercise. Take some time to think about how you view your body. What do you like about it? Dislike? What body parts or physical features would you change instantly if you could? Why?

_____

_____

"Don't you realize that your body is the temple of the Holy Spirit, who lives in you and was given to you by God? You do not belong to yourself, for God bought you with a high price. So you must honor God with your body" (1 Corinthians 6:19–20 NLT).

129

LEARNING A NEW WAY OF *LIFE*

The shocking claim of the gospel is that God Himself took on human form. The Creator came into His creation in the person of Christ. For thirty-plus years Jesus lived with all the constraints of a human body. How does this fact encourage you?

_____

_____

In a messianic passage referring to the coming Christ, Isaiah 53:2 says, "There was nothing beautiful or majestic about his appearance, nothing to attract us to him" (NLT). How do you respond to this description of Christ?

_____

_____

In Psalm 139, David seems to exult in his body (that is, the precise way God had made him). "You . . . knit me together in my mother's womb. Thank you for making me so wonderfully complex! Your workmanship is marvelous—how well I know it" (vv. 13–14 NLT). Is this how you view yourself? Why or why not?

_____

_____

Our bodies are the dwelling place of the Most High God (1 Corinthians 6:19–20). What does this suggest about how we treat and take care of our bodies? What kinds of things are appropriate? What kinds of things are inappropriate?

_____

_____

When we give our ultimate attention and affection to something— even food— we are guilty of idolatry.

Matthew 6:25 says, "If you decide for God, living a life of God-worship, it follows that you don't fuss about what's on the table at mealtimes or whether the clothes in your closet are in fashion. There is far more to your life than the food you put in your stomach, more to your outer appearance than the clothes you hang on your body" (MSG).

In what ways can our modern preoccupation with food become a kind of idolatry?

_____

_____

LOSING IT FOR *LIFE*

When we become preoccupied with what we will eat, when we look forward to meals more than concentrating on knowing and loving and serving God, we are out of balance. Whenever we get absorbed or obsessed with what we are going to eat, how much we'll be able to have, and how often we can get it, we have ceased following Christ.

Read Matthew 6:33. What does this passage say about:

your priorities?

_____

God's care for those who have right priorities?

_____

A person who decides to be a Christ-follower has the promise that God will meet physical needs as well as emotional and spiritual ones. How can you realistically and practically accept those promises right now—and begin to enjoy them?

_____

_____

Let's say after these last few workbook sessions, you have realized a tendency toward gluttony. Perhaps you habitually overeat. Or you fantasize excessively about food. Or you have let your body, the temple of the living God, get to an unhealthy state. What does all this mean? Does God look upon you with disgust? (Hint: see Romans 8:31–39.)

_____

_____

God wants balance in your life—so go ahead, enjoy eating. Just do not become a glutton. Anything taken to excess can block a vibrant relationship with God. Moderation is key.

    Please understand. You are not condemned by God or by the LIFL community for overeating. God only desires to bring you to improved health, to remove your obsession with food, to prevent negative consequences related to overeating, and to help you enjoy meals and fellowship with others. He wants you to experience the enjoyment of food, the pleasure of taste, and the sensation of a full stomach rather than be bound by guilt, physical discomfort, or negative health consequences related to obesity and bingeing.

The Bible offers the following solutions for idolatry and excess. Spend a few final moments thinking about each of these statements and jotting down any questions, thoughts, or insights you have.

- We get out of spiritual poverty by developing self-control, a fruit of the Spirit (Galatians 5:23).

How developed is this trait in you?

_____

_____

_____

- We are called to practice balance and moderation in all things. "Moderation is better than muscle, self-control better than political power" (Proverbs 16:32 MSG).

In what areas of your life do you see victory and balance?

_____

_____

_____

- A transformed life begins with absolute surrender (Romans 12:1).

What are some signs that a person has truly surrendered his or her life to God?

_____

_____

_____

DAY 5

Distinguishing the Hungers

What is hunger? As part of our ongoing effort to Lose It for Life, we must know the difference between physical, emotional, and spiritual hunger. The three are very different and often confused. Let's explore in more detail.

LOOKING AT YOUR *LIFE*

Speaking of hunger, one person admitted:

> I eat but I'm not really hungry. At least, I don't think I am. I'm not really sure. Sometimes I feel like I could eat everything in the cupboards, like I'm ravenous. So I just do. I never really think about if I'm hungry or not. I think I just really like food, lots of food. And lots of times, I crave things—like cookies. I'll go to the bakery and pretend to be buying a dozen cookies for my kids at school, but really, I plan on eating them all.

In what ways can you relate to this kind of hunger, this kind of craving?

_____

_____

When do you experience it most?

_____

_____

We have other needs and desires, apart from those of our physical bodies. Among those are the needs to be safe, to belong, to be loved, to be esteemed, and to grow.

Write briefly about a time in your life when you felt spiritually ravenous—when you were hungry to know God.

_____

_____

Write briefly about a recent time when you felt starved for emotional connection, when loneliness hit you intensely. What did you do?

_____

_____

LEARNING A NEW WAY OF *LIFE*

Physical hunger is normal, a natural God-given sensation and a cue that our human bodies needs refueling.

What is the hungriest you can ever remember being? Put another way, what is the longest period you've ever gone without food? Describe that time.

_____

_____

Food is used like a drug— distracting, numbing, and helping us avoid the reality of hurt and pain or the emptiness of an unmet need.

What are the indicators of true physical hunger?

_____

_____

How would you define *emotional hunger*? What are the symptoms of this common phenomenon?

_____

_____

In the *LIFL* book, the authors distinguish between physical hunger and emotional hunger.

Physical Hunger	Emotional Hunger
Builds gradually	Hits suddenly, "starving"
Stomach starts to rumble and growl	Anxiety; but there is no real physical symptom of feeling hungry
Feel full and stop eating	Overeat even if feeling full
Different foods will satisfy	Crave very specific food; nothing else satisfies
Physically feel empty in pit of stomach	Mouth and mind are tasting the food
Need to eat but can wait	Eat now to ease whatever is happening
Eat and feel fine	Eat and feel guilt and shame
Four to five hours since last meal; feel light-headed, low energy	Upset and want to eat now
Choose foods purposefully	Automatic or absentminded eating

Where do you see yourself (your own experience and habits) in this chart?

_____

_____

When do you tend to be an emotional eater? In what ways?

_____

_____

During the Sermon on the Mount, Jesus said, "Blessed are you who hunger now, for you will be satisfied" (Luke 6:21). The Greek word for "hunger" is _peinas_, meaning to be hungry, to be famished, to be starved. What does it mean to hunger for God? What does it look like and feel like to be satisfied in God?

_____

_____

The authors suggest that often we are spiritually starving but don't feed our hunger the right way. We become distracted with and chase after other things that can't and won't fill that spiritual void. In what ways and at what stages in your life has this been your experience?

_____

_____

Author Beth Moore says, "Victory is not determined as much by what we've been delivered _from_ as by what we've been delivered _to._"[3] You won't be victorious over food and overeating eating unless you look to God to satisfy you. Nothing else will really do. God wants to deliver you from the need to overeat. He wants you to find your purpose, move in His power, and live a life of overcoming. His way of doing that is to offer Himself to you. He is your deliverer. He offers relationship, intimacy, and abundant life, peace, joy and so much more. The "more" He offers will satisfy. Listen, He wants you, chose you, and is waiting to fill your mouth with good things.

What do these words and claims stir in you?

_____

_____

_____

The following scriptures speak of the great hope we have in Christ:

For everything that was written in the past was written to teach us, so that through the endurance taught in the Scriptures and the encouragement they provide we might have hope. (Romans 15:4)

May the God of hope fill you with all joy and peace as you trust in him, so that you may overflow with hope by the power of the Holy Spirit. (Romans 15:13)

I pray that the eyes of your heart may be enlightened in order that you may know the hope to which he has called you, the riches of his glorious inheritance in his holy people. (Ephesians 1:18)

What would it be like to overflow with hope? How do you think you'd be different if you developed and maintained a rich, intimate daily walk with Jesus?

_____

_____

LOSING IT FOR _LIFE_

Every time we eat, certain "triggers" or "cues" precede our eating. For example, a physical trigger is usually something like a rumbling stomach, a headache, dizziness, weakness, or low energy. Some common emotional triggers are feeling upset, bored, hurt, angry, disappointed, lonely, happy, and so forth.

By learning to distinguish these various cues, we begin to get a handle on our eating. One way to do this is to keep a record. Remember, a big component of the LIFL plan is using a food journal to document what we eat, when we eat it, and why we do so.

As you develop this habit, you are asked to try to describe the motive for your eating. If you notice that many of your daily eating episodes stem from emotional hunger, then we have work to do. The goal of LIFL is to learn to eat in response to physical cues, not emotional ones.

The next time you eat, take a guess at which type of hunger you are experiencing. List the three columns shown below.

- In the first column, check which hunger you think you are having.
- In the second column, record your feelings, physical sensations, emotions, and thoughts right before you wanted to eat.
- In the third column, write how you felt after you ate. Read what you listed and decide if you checked the correct hunger.

A blank copy of this chart is provided in Appendix B. Here's an example.

What we often think is hunger for food or even emotional hunger may actually be a hunger for more of God!

Physical or Emotional Hunger?	Before I ate, I felt: *(Feelings and thoughts)*	After I ate, I felt: *(Feelings and thoughts)*
Emotional	Upset and mad, wanted to eat, stomach tense from anger	Tired, immediately uncomfortable
Physical	Ate four hours ago, light-headed, stomach growling	Satisfied, energized

If you aren't sure what you are feeling or thinking when you eat, focus on the experience of eating and try to become attuned to your physical and emotional state. The goal is to stay in the moment of eating and avoid the common habit of eating without thinking. Here's an additional exercise to try:

- Sixty seconds before you eat, sit quietly (no distractions) and think, *What am I feeling and what am I thinking about right now?* Record this.
- Then look at what you are about to eat. Notice how it tastes. Do you like what you are eating? Do you like the feel of it in your mouth? How does it feel in your stomach?
- After you finish, take another sixty seconds and write down how you feel—energized, tired, unsatisfied, content, etc.

This short exercise will put you in touch with the experience of eating. It will slow you down and help you pay attention to all the sensations involved in eating. Many times after emotional eating, you'll feel tired and sluggish or won't feel satisfied. That's because eating wasn't what you needed to do. In addition, when you choose sugary foods, your blood sugar rises and falls, which makes you feel tired. The goal is to stop eating when you aren't physically hungry, and stop stuffing food in when you are upset or feeling emotional.

The authors offer this encouragement:

God has so much more for you. He doesn't want you dragging through life being defeated by your weight. He wants to give you good things—more of His power, more of His Spirit, more of His love and compassion. The urgency you feel to fill up with food, to overeat, could be the Holy Spirit urging you to satisfy your spiritual hunger through God. Are you afraid you won't get what you need? Not to worry. God has enough to go around for all of us. His resources are limitless. He is the Living Water that never runs dry. He is the Bread of Life who promises eternal life. The fullness He has for you cannot be found in the temporal things of this world. And once you experience His fullness, you'll never hunger in the same way again!

Hunger for more of God. God is the originator and giver of all true satisfaction. Perhaps you've tried to find satisfaction in many other ways. Nothing completely fulfills but more of God. Spiritual hunger is a good because God is waiting for us to open our mouths, like little birds, so that He can fill them.

Do you dare believe these promises? Write out a prayer below that expresses your spiritual hunger. Offer it sincerely to God. Then take a few simple steps of faith.

_____

_____

_____

The important thing is to discover exactly what triggers you to overeat. Write down these cues and study them.

4

The Doctor Is "In"

Early on, we mentioned that one size does not fit all when it comes to losing weight and keeping it off. In this chapter, we want to focus on physical influences that affect weight loss and maintenance. Your physical body is unique and it must be factored in to any program tailored specifically for you. For example, if you have a family history of obesity, you have a greater chance of being obese than someone who does not. This reality doesn't doom you to be overweight, but it is an influence you should recognize.

Whatever your history or genetic picture, be aware that physical influences can speed up or slow down the work. The better informed you are, the more patient you will be with yourself when it comes to achieving your goals. Although you may not be able to control all the factors that led to becoming overweight, you do have control over how you respond to them.

As you consider this chapter, try not to get hung up on the fairness of the genetic hand you may have been dealt. Think of life as a card game—it's not so much the hand you are dealt that influences a win; it's how you play that hand! Your genetic history is part of who you are. Your biology may create more challenges. However, it won't stop you from being successful. By taking care of your body, monitoring your health, and making lifestyle changes, you can and will Lose It for Life.

WEARING THE GENES THAT FIT

Heredity plays a role in what you weigh. If you have a family history of obesity, pay special attention to your food intake and other factors that affect weight gain, because your chances of becoming obese increase by about 30 percent.[1] Being overweight and/or obese runs in families. Researchers are still trying to decide how much of family obesity is due to shared genes or shared family eating and exercise habits. However, twin studies indicate that genetic factors do play a role. Having overweight family members isn't a guarantee that you'll be overweight, but this fact does increase your chances.

BASAL METABOLIC RATE

People also inherit basal metabolic rates. Basal metabolic rate (BMR) is the number of calories you would burn if you stayed in bed all day (not a recommendation we are making). The lower the rate, the more difficult it is to lose weight. BMR is affected by height—lower for short versus tall people—and by weight—the more fatty body tissue you have, the lower the BMR. In contrast, the more lean body tissue you have, the higher the BMR. As you will read in chapter 7 on exercise, building lean body tissue is one of the goals of regular exercise and can help raise BMR.[2]

As you age, you may begin to gain weight even though your eating habits do not change. This is because the body's metabolism slows down with aging. In other words, your body requires fewer calories to do the same work. So eating the same amount of food without changing your activity level can lead to gradual weight gain.

In addition, fever, stress, heat, and cold all raise BMR. Fasting, starving, and malnutrition lower it. Dieting and skipping meals can trick your body into thinking it is starving—thereby slowing down weight loss instead of increasing it! This is the best reason not to "diet." BMR is regulated by the thyroid hormone thyroxin. The more thyroxin produced, the higher the BMR. This helps explain why a low thyroid slows down weight loss in some people. If you suspect this might be your problem, have your thyroid level checked.[3] And if you want to find out once and for all if you have a low metabolic rate, you can have it measured by indirect calorimetry. This service is inexpensive and can easily be done at most hospitals (pulmonary department) or by sports medicine clinics. However, low metabolism is usually not the culprit when it comes to weight gain. We know because we have both tried to use it as an excuse for overeating.

When I (Dr. Linda) was a college cheerleader, I was extremely active. There were daily practices and gymnastic classes in addition to games. After road games, the team and cheerleaders would stop at fast-food places and load up on food. My fellow cheerleaders ordered shakes, double burgers, and fries. Since they were thin and we had all just exercised vigorously, I figured I could load up on food, too, and stay thin. Well, I couldn't and began to gain weight. I was sure my metabolism was slower than everyone else's was (even though I never had a problem with it before and was skinny as a child). In reality I needed to take the red pill as I was eating a whole lot more food than the splurges on away-game nights. My metabolism had little to do with my weight gain and more to do with regular late-night eating in the dorm. But for years, I believed I suffered from a low BMR.

I (Steve) had a low BMR growing up that caused me to greatly resent my older brothers, who could eat more than me and remain fit and trim. It didn't seem fair that my body worked against me. But I discovered something that could be a great source of hope for you. My metabolism works for me now. The difference? Then I had little muscle on my frame. Today, after years of regular workouts with weights, I have much more. What I did can work for you! As we age, we lose muscle tissue each year, which lowers our metabolisms. But with weight training and resistance exercises, that rate of loss can be reduced. You can even build muscle tissue and increase your metabolism, enabling you to lose weight easier or to eat more and still maintain the right weight.

Exercise is a gift from God, and it can be utilized to change your future and have one where you are not defined by your weight. There are many things in this world that cannot be influenced or changed on your own power. But you *can* choose to build muscle and raise your own metabolism, which is reason to hope. You can make your body's metabolism work for you rather than against you.

FAT CELL NUMBER AND SIZE

Another physical factor is fat cell number and size. Fat cells begin to triple from birth to six years of age in both boys and girls. The result is a gradual and similar increase in body fat. But after about eight years of age, girls take off at a faster rate than boys. Fat cell size, not number, increases. Between the ages of six and adolescence, fat cell numbers stay constant in normal-weight children. However, in obese children, the number of fat cells can increase. When adolescence hits, girls almost double the rate of increasing fat of boys. More and larger fat cells are increased about the pelvis, buttocks, thighs, and breasts—a phenomenon related to female hormonal changes.

In women of healthy weights, fat accumulation more or less stops after adolescence with no further increase in the number of fat cells. Similarly, in postadolescent males of a healthy weight, fat cells tend not to multiply. You have probably noticed that men tend to store excess fat in their bellies or abdomens. This is a dangerous place to accumulate fat because it is associated with an increased risk in coronary artery disease, elevated triglycerides, hypertension, and cancer.[4] Fat cells that are packed and swell and become large enough to be seen through the skin are called cellulite. As our skin gets thinner with age and becomes less flexible, cellulite becomes more visible. The only help for this is weight loss and regular activity.[5]

Even if a person has a normal number of fat cells, those cells can increase in size and weight throughout life if that person becomes grossly overweight. The number and size of fat cells reflects the amount of fat stored in the body. If you consume more energy than you expend, it is stored in fat cells. When fat cells reach their maximum size, they may divide and create more. Obesity results when fat cells increase in number, size, or both.

If you have a higher-than-normal number of fat cells in your body, you won't lose fat cells by dieting. Fat cells can shrink, but they don't leave the body. Even if you temporarily manage to empty them, they can easily fill up again as you gain weight. This is why it is easier for someone with an excess of fat cells to gain weight. There is only one way to get rid of fat cells: by liposuctioning them out. And although this may get rid of the fat cells, it's not something we are recommending because it isn't a solution to lifestyle changes that may be needed.

THE STRESS FACTOR

You'd have to be living on another planet not to know that stress affects your body in negative ways. One of those negative ways relates to weight gain. While an immediate response to stress may be a loss of appetite, repeated and chronic stress can cause the opposite effect. Here's why.

When you encounter stress, cortisol, along with other hormones, is released. Following a stressful event, the other hormones return to normal levels, but cortisol can remain elevated for a longer time period. Because this hormone provides energy for the body, it can stimulate appetite and result in weight gain that tends to be concentrated in the midsection or abdominal area.

According to Pamela M. Peeke, MD, MPH (Masters of Public Health), a former senior scientist at the National Institutes of Health in Bethesda, Maryland, and an associate clinical professor of medicine at the University of Maryland School of Medicine in Baltimore, three factors affect central fat in women. They are poor lifestyle, declining levels of the hormone estrogen, and chronic stress.[6] The amount of cortisol experienced with stress seems to vary from person to person. If you are some-one who reacts to stress with increased appetite, you may be experiencing elevated cortisol levels. Whether or not your urge to eat is driven by hormones, you can still interrupt the cycle, break the stress, and stop weight gain. Since stress is something we all experience, we all need to learn effective ways to manage or reduce it. Lifestyle changes recommended in this program can help you with stress.

Begin to evaluate what you are doing that may add stress to your life. Are there habits and practices you could change today that would make you feel better? The answer is probably yes. Think about your response to stress in terms of self-care. How will you take care of yourself in order to battle the negative effects of stress?

1. **Do you have effective ways of relaxing?** We all need downtime. Relaxation isn't something you do once a year on a cruise to the Bahamas (although this can't hurt). Relaxing should be a regular, practiced part of your life. You need balance in all things. Even God rested on the seventh day! Relaxation keeps stress from building up and provides an avenue for releasing tension.

2. **Do you regularly exercise?** The benefits of exercise are enormous, and an entire chapter will be devoted to the topic, as it is an essential ingredient to losing weight for life. Exercise can reduce muscle tension and frustra-tion in addition to providing a host of medical helps. Find something you like—bike riding, dancing, skating, basketball, tennis, skiing, walking, Ping-Pong—anything that gets you off that couch and moving!

3. **How sensibly do you eat?** Do you eat good food that provides nutrition and health benefits? Do you skip meals? Eat burgers in the car while talking on your cell phone? Find yourself at the drive-thru regularly? Chapter 6 will address eating habits.

4. **How well do you manage your time?** So many people spend energy on things that are unproductive or take up too much of their time. If you are not meeting deadlines or procrastinate or obsess over projects, you need help. Some people have to learn to move along more efficiently, while others need to slow down and do things correctly. Because our time is limited, it's important to learn to prioritize and be realistic about goals.

5. **Are you getting enough sleep?** This sounds like a simple question, but so many people have terrible sleep habits. Going to bed at a regular time and getting into a sleep routine is essential. A lack of sleep is associated with changes in hormone levels. When cortisol levels remain high from a lack

of sleep, the body craves carbohydrates and foods high in calories and fat. Metabolism then slows down as the body stores fat.[7] And here's an encouraging thought for those to whom it morally applies—sex usually helps people sleep. Now there's a sleep motivator we can live with!

Revisit Your Motivation

We'll say it again: your motivation for losing weight should not be to please someone else. If you are doing this because your physician or spouse is upset with you, this is a setup for potential failure. Decide if you are ready to lose weight for your own personal reasons. How important is it to you to live a life undefined by your weight and not driven by food and eating? How important is it to you that you lead a healthy life?

If you are motivated to work on all parts of your life—spiritual, physical, emotional, and interpersonal—you will do well. You must take ownership of your goal to lose weight and keep it off. No one else can do it for you, but with God's help, you can be successful. It is also helpful to ask the question, "Why do I want to lose weight now?" Since you have probably dieted in the past and have been overweight for months or even years, why are you ready now? Hopefully you are ready to surrender this problem to God and accept the reality of your situation, including taking responsibility for your part of the problem.

Finally, are you experiencing significant stress right now? If so, this may not be the time to try to lose weight. Instead, you may want to concentrate on making lifestyle changes rather than focusing on weight loss. Significant life stress greatly disrupts a person's ability to lose weight for life. If this resonates with you, please reread the material above, and make any lifestyle changes possible, given your current circumstances—any changes that can be made without overtaxing yourself. When your circumstances have stabilized, consider adding a goal of weight loss.

CONFRONTING THE REALITY OF SIZE AND WEIGHT

Another physical factor to consider is how much weight you have to lose. The more you have to lose, the longer it takes. Don't expect to go from 300 pounds to 180 overnight. Begin by setting your weight loss goal at 10 percent of your current body weight, and consider weight loss of one to two pounds a week successful. This is very doable since you can lose weight just by eating 100 calories fewer a day than you need. Over time, this small reduction will result in a gradual yet steady weight loss.

When you are overweight or obese, the last thing you want to do is confront the reality of your size. To do so means to acknowledge what that state is doing to your physical body. One obese client, an elementary school teacher, experienced great heartache when the reality of her growing size became evident to her. While teaching one day, she suddenly realized that she could no longer fit in the aisles between her students' desks.

When she left school that day, she sat in her car in the parking lot and cried. This experience was a wake-up call. Her overeating was out of control. She knew she was gaining weight but had refused to confront the fact, as many overweight people do. Most look in the mirror from their necks up. They fix their hair, do their makeup, and put on a happy face without looking at the rest of their bodies because it is too painful and depressing. Yet taking a full-length view keeps reality in front of you and can be used as an incentive to make changes.

Rather than look in the mirror and verbally beat yourself up, try this: Stand fully unclothed in front of a full-length mirror. Slowly scan your entire body. Feel the various parts. We know this sounds cruel, but it isn't. The goal is to be in touch with the reality of your size and weight. It's important to your health—another subject that is often avoided by overweight people.

Perhaps you don't want to think about the size of your body or what the extra weight is doing to your overall health, but again, awareness is critical. It is too easy to disconnect your eating from your physical body. Instead, intentionally think about that extra weight and the potential health impact it has, and use this to motivate lifestyle changes, not degrade yourself. To do so is to take a very courageous step, as this journal entry indicates:

Last May I weighed 350 pounds. Today I weigh 237 pounds. Do you have any idea how much easier it is to walk, work, drive, and even sleep with a 113-pound weight loss? Looking back, I am amazed that I was able to function as well as I did. I know laziness is one of the stereotypes for obese individuals, but believe me when I say I have never been a lazy person. I have always been a hard worker, one who ran around the office doing the work of three in hopes of being accepted by the "normal folks."

It was tough weighing 350 pounds. It was hard work carrying the extra pounds everywhere I went. I don't think the world realizes what we go through. The good news for today is that I have given up 113 pounds of baggage (physically and emotionally) and my load is becoming lighter each week. My goal is to have as little baggage as possible. It takes hard work, dedication, and complete faith in Jesus Christ, but He will carry our load if we ask Him.

—Cathy

Cathy had to face the reality of her 350-pound frame. It hurt even to walk. Carrying that weight impacted her ability to do everyday tasks. Furthermore, several doctors told her that she wouldn't live long if she didn't make changes. As a single mom who faced the reality staring back at her, Cathy decided she had to do something about it.

LET'S GET A PHYSICAL

I can't go for a physical. It's too humiliating. Last time I tried (years ago), the doctor never looked me in the eye. I could tell he was disgusted with me. The exam was quick and he barely touched me. Then he handed me a 1,200-calorie diet and told me to lose weight, stating matter-of-factly that my weight would probably kill me. I was ashamed and embarrassed. I've tried his diet but can't do it. I do have heart disease in my family, so he wants me to come back. I don't want to go again. I'd rather not think about it.

—Sue

A comprehensive physical examination conducted by a competent physician is necessary to obtain an accurate picture of your health. You do need that physical. However, we advise that you change doctors if you are uncomfortable with your current physician. Happily, Sue did; a follow-up physical by a new doctor revealed that she had type 2 diabetes. She needed medical supervision and intervention.

We suggest you find a physician who is compassionate and sensitive to overweight people. Unfortunately, we've heard too many stories like Sue's in which physicians simply hand patients 1,200-calorie diets and tell them to lose weight. Reality check: if this worked, people would be able to follow this advice and drop weight. In our experiences, this strategy only compounds feelings of failure in an overweight person.

If your physician is insensitive regarding your weight, change doctors and tell your health-care company why you are doing so. As an overweight person, you already have to contend with ridicule and stigma from the public. You don't need to put up with either from your health-care provider. One of my (Dr. Linda's) physicians has a framed plaque on his wall that I have received permission to copy here. I love what Dr. Su wrote:

Let a doctor be called as a healer, not the health care provider.
Let the patient be treated as the healed, not the health care consumer.
Medicine is not a commercial business but a professional practice based strongly on a doctor-patient relationship of compassion, understanding, and respect.[8]

Find a doctor like Dr. Su who won't treat you like a consumer, but who will show you compassion and be a part of the healing. A physician can monitor your medical conditions, work with you on improving your health, support your efforts to make changes, be aware of the issues involved in your weight-loss maintenance, and encourage a holistic approach.

In addition, keep in mind that some illnesses can lead to obesity or a tendency to gain weight. These include hypothyroidism, Cushing's syndrome, depression, and specific neurological problems that can lead to overeating. Also, certain medications may have side effects that cause weight gain, including steroids and some antidepressants. A doctor can evaluate whether there are underlying medical conditions that may be causing you to gain weight or will make weight loss more difficult. This is information you need to know.

The following section lists the health risks commonly associated with being overweight and obese. This list is not comprehensive. It only touches on main concerns. Of course, there may be other health issues or conditions that require medical supervision and treatment as well. This list is not meant to scare you or make you fearful. Knowing that our tendency is to deny health risks, reading this list is a necessary step as we consider our health. Use this information to motivate and to accept the reality of your health if you make no changes. Keep in mind that even modest weight loss improves your health.

COMMON HEALTH RISKS ASSOCIATED WITH BEING OVERWEIGHT AND OBESE

Type 2 Diabetes

This type of diabetes is also referred to as adult onset or non-insulin-dependent diabetes and is the most common in the United States. It is a disease in which blood sugar levels are above normal and can cause early death, heart disease, kidney disease, stroke, and blindness.

If you are overweight, your risk for type 2 diabetes increases. In fact, about 80 percent of people with this disease are overweight.[9] One thought is that extra weight may put stress on the cells that produce insulin (a hormone that carries sugar from the blood to the cells). The extra stress may make the cells less effective and cause problems. Losing weight and exercising can lower your risk for type 2 diabetes and possibly reduce your current medication if you are already diagnosed.

Heart Disease and Stroke

Heart disease and stroke are caused when your heart, circulation, or blood flow do not operate normally. When this happens, you can have a heart attack, congestive heart failure, sudden cardiac death, angina (chest pain), or abnormal heart rhythm. Heart disease is the leading cause of death in the United States, and death from a stroke places third.[10]

Being overweight puts you more at risk for factors related to heart disease and stroke, including high blood pressure, high levels of triglycerides, high "bad" cholesterol (LDL), and low "good" cholesterol (HDL). Also, obesity is related to inflammation in blood vessels and throughout the body, which is also a risk for heart disease.[11]

By losing between 5 and 15 percent of your body weight, you can lower your risk for both health problems. Think about it! When as little as ten pounds of weight loss can make a difference, it's really not much weight to lose.

Cancer

Cancer touches all of us in some way and is the second leading cause of death in this country. Perhaps you have a friend or family member suffering from one form or another, or you have been diagnosed with cancer yourself. This disease occurs when cells in one part of the body grow out of control or abnormally. Cancer can spread to other parts of the body as well.

When you are overweight, your risk of developing certain types of cancers increases, including colon, esophageal, uterine, postmenopausal breast cancer (women), and kidney. Researchers aren't sure why being overweight is a factor in increased risk, but one possibility is that fat cells make hormones that might affect cell growth.[12] The current thinking is that preventing weight gain, eating healthily, and being physically active may lower your risk for cancer.

Sleep Apnea

Sleep apnea occurs when a person stops breathing for short periods during the night. The result is usually daytime sleepiness, difficulty concentrating, and even heart failure. Usually weight loss improves this condition because it decreases the neck size and inflammation.[13] Research tells us this condition is more prevalent for people who are overweight. One reason is that an overweight person may have fat stored in the neck area that can make the airway for breathing smaller. These fat stores can also result in the neck becoming more inflamed, which can put a person at a greater risk for sleep apnea. As a result, breathing can be difficult, loud (snoring), or even stop altogether.

Osteoarthritis

Osteoarthritis is a joint disorder in which the tissues that protect joint bones and cartilage gradually wear away. Most commonly affected are the joints of the knees, hips, and lower back. The more weight you carry, the more pressure you put on your joints and cartilage. Additional weight may also increase blood levels of body substances that cause inflammation, which may in turn increase the risk for osteoarthritis.

Again, weight loss can remove some of the stress on your knees, hips, and lower back.[14]

Gallbladder Disease

When you are overweight, your risk for gallbladder disease and gallstones increases. This is partly due to the fact that more cholesterol is being produced, which is an associated risk factor. Being overweight can also make your gallbladder enlarged or unable to work efficiently.[15]

If you've ever had a gallstone (a cluster of solid material—mostly cholesterol—that forms in the gallbladder), you know pain! People who lose a lot of weight very quickly (more than three pounds a week) increase their chances of developing gallstones. Often clients who try very low-calorie diets have an increase in gallbladder disease. The message here is to shoot for modest, consistent weight loss of one-half to two pounds a week to prevent an increased risk.

Fatty Liver Disease

Even the name of this illness is unappealing! Fatty liver disease results from the buildup of fat cells in the liver that causes injury and inflammation. It can cause severe liver damage, cirrhosis (scar tissue in the liver that blocks blood flow), and liver failure. It sounds serious, and it is. Most people know about this condition because of the link it has to alcohol. But you can get this disease without drinking any alcohol when you are overweight. Overweight people who are prediabetic (have higher blood sugar) are more at risk. Weight loss helps control blood sugar, which hopefully helps avoid the buildup of fat. Avoiding alcohol helps as well.[16]

ESTABLISH YOUR GOAL

A great place to begin is to establish goals. In terms of healthy weight loss, determine how much weight you want to lose. As you decide on a number or weight range, your goal should meet the following criteria:

1. **Specific.** "I want to be thin" is an example of a nonspecific goal. It is too vague. "I'd like to lose twenty pounds" is specific.
2. **Attainable.** Select a goal that you can actually reach. For example, if you've

been 300 pounds most of your adult life and your lowest adult weight was 190 pounds, then do not select a goal weight of 125 pounds. Most likely, you won't reach that goal. But to set a goal of weighing 190 pounds is reasonable given that you have once achieved that weight as an adult. You can always reset your goal once you've reached 190 pounds if you feel there is more you can lose.

When deciding on a weight-loss goal, it helps to review your weight history. Use your lowest adult weight as a guideline. Another good rule of thumb is to make 10 percent of your current weight your weight-loss goal. When you reach that goal, you can reset your goal for another 10 percent. In our experience, attainable goals build success and confidence. And the meeting of short-term goals brings a sense of accomplishment along the way.

3. **Forgivable**. In other words, don't be rigid. Be flexible in case you aimed too high. Be open to renegotiating your goals as you go. And when you falter, give yourself permission to rethink the goal and begin again. Sometimes a goal is difficult to achieve because all the issues that go into making that goal haven't been considered. For many people, successful weight loss and maintenance requires lasting changes in all areas of life, something we don't always think about when we want to lose weight.

If you are anxious, don't be. Losing as little as 5 percent of your body weight helps. Just remember that slow and steady weight loss is the healthy way to Lose It for Life. No crash diets, starving yourself, or dropping weight too fast. The goal is to make changes that will last. And please, don't ignore the signs and symptoms your physical body may be telling you. Live in the reality that extra weight puts you more at risk for health problems. There is no better reason to lose those extra pounds. Pay attention to your body. It's the only one you have this side of heaven!

METROPOLITAN LIFE INSURANCE CHARTS[17]

These charts are not the end-all when it comes to determining a healthy weight. They are, however, a good tool with which to estimate what weight might be in a healthy range for you. (For more information on these tables, see endnote.)

Height & Weight Table For Women

Height	Small Frame	Medium Frame	Large Frame
4´ 10˝	102–111	109–121	118–131
4´ 11˝	103–113	111–123	120–134
5´ 0˝	104–115	113–126	122–137
5´ 1˝	106–118	115–129	125–140
5´ 2˝	108–121	118–132	128–143
5´ 3˝	111–124	121–135	131–147
5´ 4˝	114–127	124–138	134–151
5´ 5˝	117–130	127–141	137–155
5´ 6˝	120–133	130–144	140–159
5´ 7˝	123–136	133–147	143–163
5´ 8˝	126–139	136–150	146–167
5´ 9˝	129–142	139–153	149–170
5´ 10˝	132–145	142–156	152–173
5´ 11˝	135–148	145–159	155–176
6´ 0˝	138–151	148–162	158–179

Weights at ages 25-59 based on lowest mortality. Weight in pounds according to frame (in indoor clothing weighing 3 lbs.; shoes with 1˝ heels).

Height & Weight Table For Men

Height	Small Frame	Medium Frame	Large Frame
5′ 2″	128–134	131–141	138–150
5′ 3″	130–136	133–143	140–153
5′ 4″	132–138	135–145	142–156
5′ 5″	134–140	137–148	144–160
5′ 6″	136–142	139–151	146–164
5′ 7″	138–145	142–154	149–168
5′ 8″	140–148	145–157	152–172
5′ 9″	142–151	148–160	155–176
5′ 10″	144–154	151–163	158–180
5′ 11″	146–157	154–166	161–184
6′ 0″	149–160	157–170	164–188
6′ 1″	152–164	160–174	168–192
6′ 2″	155–168	164–178	172–197
6′ 3″	158–172	167–182	176–202
6′ 4″	162–176	171–187	181–207

Weights at ages 25-59 based on lowest mortality. Weight in pounds according to frame (in indoor clothing weighing 5 lbs.; shoes with 1″ heels).

Workbook Week 4

THE DOCTOR IS "IN"

DAY 1

The Unique You

Our goal isn't merely losing weight; it is keeping it off and embracing a healthier overall lifestyle. To do that, we need to think through the various physical influences and factors that affect weight loss and general health. That's our goal for these five workbook lessons.

LOOKING AT YOUR *LIFE*

Early on we mentioned that "one size does not fit all." Your physical body is unique and your one-of-a-kind individuality must be factored in. Any successful eating/exercise plan will have to be tailored specifically for you.

Take a few minutes to do a family medical history and weight assessment. What are some of the health issues or diseases that have cropped up in your immediate and extended family?

_____

_____

What close relatives struggle with their weight?

_____

_____

In your opinion, who is the healthiest individual in your immediate or extended family? What are his or her eating habits and exercise routine?

_____

_____

If you have a family history of obesity, you have a greater chance of being obese. This doesn't doom you to be overweight, but it is an influence you should recognize.

Which parent are you most like in your body shape/type?

_____

_____

Let's broaden that parental comparison. Put a check mark by which parent you most resemble in the following categories:

Dad	Mom	Both	Neither	Category
				basic temperament/ personality
				personal preferences
				social skills
				hobbies/leisure pursuits
				political views
				religious/spiritual beliefs
				work ethic
				facial features
				manner of speaking
				sense of humor
				good habits
				bad habits
				way of responding to stress
				handling money
				eating habits

Your genetic history is part of who you are. But it's not so much the hand you are dealt but how you play that hand that counts!

LEARNING A NEW WAY OF *LIFE*

God's creation reveals astonishing diversity. Each person has one-of-a-kind fingerprints, distinct DNA, exclusive personal history, inimitable background, singular life experiences, and so forth.

What conclusions can we draw from this diversity? What does it say about us as human beings? About God?

_____

_____

What does this fact suggest about the way we must each approach eating, exercise, and so forth?

_____

_____

Which of your friends or acquaintances have successfully overcome an obvious family predisposition to being heavy? Call them up. Ask them why they think they managed to avoid the family curse. Write their responses here.

_____

_____

Whatever your history or genetic picture, be aware that physical influences can speed up or slow down the work. The better informed you are, the more patient you will be with yourself when it comes to achieving your goals. Although you may not be able to control all the factors that led to being overweight, you do have control over how you respond to them.

LOSING IT FOR *LIFE*

Heredity plays a role in what you weigh. If you have a family history of obesity, pay special attention to your food intake and other factors that affect weight gain. Your chances of becoming obese increase by about 30 percent.[18] Researchers are still trying to decide how much of family obesity is due to shared genes or shared family eating and exercise habits. Studies of twins, however, indicate that genetic factors do account for something.

What do you know about your metabolism? What questions do you have?

_____

_____

Among other things, we inherit something called a "basal metabolic rate" (BMR). This figure is the calculated number of calories you would burn if you stayed in bed all day (a practice not recommended!). The lower one's BMR, the more difficult it is to lose weight. BMR is affected by height and weight (shorter folks with more fatty body tissue burn less calories). In contrast, the more lean one's body tissue, the higher the BMR. (Note: This is why the LIFL plan encourages regular, vigorous exercise—both aerobic and strength-training.) Building lean body tissue can help raise your metabolism.[19]

For most people, the real culprit isn't a thyroid problem, but an overeating and underexercising problem.

What are your current exercise and fitness habits?

_____

_____

In the following chart, put a check mark by the factors that raise your BMR (metabolism) and the factors that lower your BMR. (When you finish, see the answers below.)

Factor	Raises Metabolism	Lowers Metabolism
Aging		
Fever		
Stress		
Heat		
Cold		
Fasting		
Starving/malnutrition		
Dieting/skipping meals		

(Answers: Aging, fasting, starving and malnutrition, and dieting and skipping meals lower BMR. Fever, stress, heat, and cold all raise BMR.)

Why would dieting and skipping meals *lower* one's metabolism?

_____

_____

Your biology may create more challenges. However, it won't stop you from being successful. By taking care of your body you can and will Lose It for Life.

Statement: "It is better to eat one big meal every evening than to eat throughout the day." Agree or disagree? Why?

_____

_____

BMR is also regulated by the thyroid hormone *thyroxin*. The less thyroxin produced, the lower one's metabolism. This condition is a problem for a small number people and may need to be checked.[20] If you suspect you have an underactive thyroid, you can have it measured by indirect calorimetry. This service is inexpensive and can easily be done at a pulmonary department at most hospitals or by sports medicine clinics.

What do you know about the role of fat cells in weight loss/management?

_____

_____

Take the following Fat Cell True/False Quiz.

T or F?	Statement
1.	The number of fat cells we have and their size is a determining factor in how much we weigh and what we look like.
2.	In postadolescent healthy women fat cell accumulation more or less stops—that is, there is no further increase in the number of fat cells.
3.	When fat cells reach their maximum size, they can divide and create more.
4.	Obesity results when fat cells increase in number, size, or both.

5.	Cellulite is a common circulatory condition that changes the appearance of the deepest layers of epidermis and is treatable with skin creams.
6	The number and size of fat cells reflects the amount of fat stored in the body.
7.	In losing weight and dieting, we actually lose some of our largest, heaviest fat cells.

(Answers: 1. T; 2. T; 3. T; 4. T; 5. F [When fat cells swell and become large enough to be seen through the skin—this is cellulite. As our skin gets thinner with age and less flexible, cellulite becomes more visible. The only help for this is weight loss and regular activity.[21]]; 6. T; 7. F. [Fat cells shrink. They don't leave the body. Even if you temporarily manage to empty them, they can easily fill up and you gain weight again. This is why it is easier for someone with an excess of fat cells to gain weight.])

If you have a higher number of fat cells in your body, you won't lose fat cells by dieting. There is only one way to get rid of fat cells—via liposuction. This is not something LIFL recommends because cosmetic surgery doesn't address lifestyle changes needed.

What's the most surprising thing you've learned here? The most interesting thing?

_____

_____

— DAY 2 —
The Stress Factor

You'd have to be living on another planet not to know that stress affects our bodies in negative ways. Sometimes when we mishandle stress, we end up mis-using food—and we gain weight. Let's explore this in more detail.

LOOKING AT YOUR *LIFE*

While an immediate response to stress may be a loss of appetite, repeated and chronic stress can cause just the opposite.

What is your best definition or description of *stress*?

_____

_____

What is a dictionary definition of *stress*?

_____

_____

What are the most stressful situations in your life currently? (Note: If your life is rather calm and stress-free right now, think back over the last year.) You may wish to answer in terms of the following categories:

	Potential Area of Stress	Specific Stressful Situation
My finances		
My marriage/marital status		

My job/career situation		
My health (or lack of health)		
My children		
My parents		
My social situation		
My church involvement		
Academic demands		
Other		

Which of the following responses are your most common reactions to stress? (Circle any that apply.)

I talk to friends.	I graze.	I binge.	I get angry.	I drink.
I (try to) escape.	I pray.	I complain.	I exercise.	I sleep.
I lose the urge to eat.	I shop.	I pace.	I bite my nails.	I cry.
I eat my favorite food.	I panic.	I get manic.	I throw things.	I snap.
I become controlling.	I lose control.	I worship.	I eat a snack.	I yell.

How effective are your typical responses to stress?

_____

_____

LEARNING A NEW WAY OF *LIFE*

When life gets stressful, our bodies naturally release a hormone called cortisol. During times of ongoing stress, cortisol levels can remain elevated. Since this hormone provides energy for our bodies, it stimulates appetite, making us susceptible to weight gain—especially in the midsection or abdominal area. Pamela

Peeke, a former senior scientist at the National Institutes of Health in Bethesda, Maryland, has concluded that three factors affect central fat in women: a poor lifestyle, declining levels of the hormone estrogen, and chronic stress.[22]

What spiritual truths can we apply to these biological realities?

_____

_____

Read Deuteronomy 20:1–4. What "secret" did Moses give the people of Israel as a way to overcome the stress of facing an overwhelming task?

_____

_____

_____

Spend some time reading and pondering Psalm 18. What did David do when facing a heap of trouble from a host of enemies?

_____

_____

_____

What does 1 Peter 5:7 say to those in trouble? How exactly does a person do this?

_____

_____

> **If you react to stress with a greatly increased appetite, you may be experiencing higher than normal cortisol levels.**

LOSING IT FOR *LIFE*

Because stress is something everyone experiences, we would be wise to learn effective ways to manage or reduce it.

Consider: Some strains and pressures and trials are beyond our control. Facing financial stress because your company suddenly decided to eliminate two thousand jobs is one thing. Facing financial stress because your credit-card spending is wildly out of control is a whole different matter. What could you start doing (or stop doing) today that would make your life less stressful?

_____

_____

We'll end this lesson with five questions designed to help you think about your response to stress in terms of self-care.

What are your most effective ways of relaxing? (Note: Leisure pursuits, hobbies, and so forth keep stress from building up and provide an avenue for releasing tension.)

_____

_____

What current exercise routine do you follow? (Note: Exercise can reduce muscle tension and frustration in addition to providing a host of medical helps.)

_____

_____

What is your diet like? Are you eating sensibly? (Note: Our bodies need good, healthy foods that provide certain vitamins and minerals.)

_____

_____

How well are you managing your time? (Note: Having healthy priorities and realistic goals can be a great stress-reducer.)

_____

_____

How much and how well are you sleeping? (Note: It is important to go to bed at a regular time and get into a sleep routine.)

_____

_____

Relaxing should be a regular, practiced part of your life.

Inadequate sleep results in higher cortisol levels, which causes your run-down body to crave carbohydrates and foods high in calories and fat.

Confronting Reality

After realizing we need to change and deciding that—by the grace of God—we will do so, the next step is taking a realistic, unblinking self-assessment. That's the focus of this lesson.

LOOKING AT YOUR *LIFE*

How tall are you? And how much did you weigh the last time you stepped on the scales?

_____

_____

How much did you weigh when you graduated from high school or turned eighteen?

_____

_____

The more you have to lose, the longer it takes. Don't expect to go from 300 pounds to 180 overnight.

What's the most you've ever weighed? The least (as an adult)?

_____

_____

What size clothes do you wear?

Men	Women
Shirt:	Blouse: _____
Knit: _____	
Dress: _____	
Pants:	Pants: _____
Waist: _____	
Inseam: _____	Dress: _____
Suit: _____	

What do you usually do when you pass a large mirror in the hall, or somewhere else? Why?

_____

_____

LEARNING A NEW WAY OF *LIFE*

You've probably heard the following observations:

- "The unexamined life is not worth living."
- "You cannot possibly get to where you need to be until you first know where you are."
- "Know thyself."
- "If you want to change the world, start by looking in the mirror."

What other sage advice can you recall that urges people to live with healthy self-awareness?

_____

_____

_____

In 2 Corinthians 13:5 the apostle Paul says, "Examine yourselves." In the context of that passage, he is speaking specifically of spiritual assessment. How and why is this a good principle and practice for all of life?

_____

_____

_____

Proverbs 27:12 says, "The prudent see danger and take refuge, but the simple keep going and pay the penalty." What are the implications of this verse for an overweight person with unhealthy eating and exercise habits?

_____

_____

_____

When we are overweight or obese, the last thing we want to do is confront the reality of our size and what it is doing to our body and our health.

Why do you think so many people are reluctant to develop the habits of regularly taking stock of their lives or conducting a personal inventory? Why do we resist so strongly the practices that could end up enhancing or even saving our lives?

_____

_____

_____

LOSING IT FOR _LIFE_

Many overweight people avoid taking a good, hard, honest look at their physical bodies. Most look in the mirror only from their necks up. They fix their hair, do their makeup, and put on a happy face. When we are overweight, looking at the entire body is painful and depressing. Taking a full-length view, however, keeps reality in front of us and can be used as incentive to make changes.

In the _LIFL_ book, the authors ask you to stand fully unclothed in front of a full-length mirror, and "slowly scan your entire body." What kinds of feelings does this challenge evoke within you? Put words to your emotions.

_____

_____

_____

Begin by setting your weight loss goal at 10 percent of your current weight. You can lose weight just by eating 100 calories fewer a day than you need.

Want to take a tremendous step of faith? Follow their counsel. Get the facts. Face reality. Do it. Go ahead. Turn on all the lights so that nothing is hidden, so that the truth is vividly clear for you to see. Afterward, pull out your pictures or photo album and, with God's help, study yourself objectively. Next, go step on the scales and see exactly where you are. Record your thoughts here:

_____

_____

_____

Are we trying to be cruel? No! The goal is to be in touch with the reality of your size and weight. We want you to think about your extra weight and the negative health impact it is having on you. Believe it or not, you can use this to motivate lifestyle changes, not degrade yourself.

Years ago, a popular magazine published a cartoon showing a small group of Chinese individuals standing in the midst of a vast landscape. The caption read, "Well, we have a heck of a wall to build. I suggest we get started."

Funny—in a profound way. What a great reminder that every amazing accomplishment once was nothing but a mere idea, a dream. Yet with a clear plan and lots of hard work and diligence, dreams can and do become reality.

Do this simple exercise. Borrow a child's backpack and fill it up with heavy objects (ten to twenty pounds). Strap it on and do housework or yardwork or walk—for thirty minutes. How do you feel after lugging around this small bit of extra weight?

_____

_____

_____

Now imagine how much more energy you would have and how much better you would feel if you lost those twenty or eighty or two hundred extra pounds of fat you're now carrying!

DAY 4

Let's Get Physical

Do we really need doctors? Why can't we just read the *LIFL* book and work on our weight in private? Is a medical checkup really necessary? That's the focus of this workbook lesson.

LOOKING AT YOUR *LIFE*

A comprehensive physical examination conducted by a competent physician is often necessary to obtain an accurate picture of your health.

In your struggle with weight, who is your most sympathetic and understanding ally? Who is your "drill sergeant" (the person who pushes you and tries to motivate you to success)?

_____

_____

_____

Write about your experiences with the medical profession (doctor visits, hospital stays, and so forth). Do you have positive memories or negative thoughts when you think about your lifetime health-care history? Why?

_____

_____

_____

Describe your personal physician. What is he or she like? What qualities do you like and admire? What qualities/traits do you wish he or she had?

_____

_____

_____

LEARNING A NEW WAY OF *LIFE*

Proverbs 15:22 says, "Plans fail for lack of counsel, but with many advisers they succeed."

Write about a time when you embarked upon an ambitious project (for example, a home improvement project, a craft project, and so forth) without first gathering all the facts or getting the necessary information. What happened? What did you learn?

_____

_____

_____

In what areas of your life are you typically quick to seek counsel or consult experts? In what areas are you reluctant to ask more knowledgeable heads for help? Why?

_____

_____

_____

Consider these nuggets from the book of Proverbs that speak about "war":

Plans are established by seeking advice; so if you wage war, obtain guidance. (20:18)

Surely you need guidance to wage war, and victory is won through many advisers. (24:6)

What do these verses suggest about our own perpetual "war" against fat and obesity? About the need for plans, and guidance, and getting wise advice?

_____

_____

_____

_____

President Coolidge observed, "I not only use all the brains I have, but all I can borrow." What is the value of seeking out expert, professional, medical help when we're not actually sick? Personally, how could you benefit from consulting with a good doctor?

A good physician will monitor your medical conditions, support your efforts to make changes, and encourage a holistic approach.

List the upside of such a decision.

_____

_____

_____

LOSING IT FOR *LIFE*

When is the last time you had a thorough physical? If it's been a long while, list the specific reasons you hesitate to have a regular checkup.

_____

_____

_____

_____

As an overweight person, you already have to contend with ridicule and stigma from the public. You don't need to put up with either from health-care providers.

In the *LIFL* book, Dr. Linda described a plaque hanging on her doctor's wall that says: "Let a doctor be called as a healer, not the health care provider. Let the patient be treated as the healed, not the health care consumer. Medicine is not a commercial business but a professional practice based strongly on a doctor-patient relationship of compassion, understanding, and respect."[23]

How might your experience be different if you were under the care of such a doctor?

_____

_____

_____

What, realistically, can a physician do for his or her patients? What unrealistic expectations do patients sometimes put upon their doctors?

_____

_____

_____

Unfortunately, we hear too many stories in which doctors simply hand their patients 1,200-calorie diets and tell them to lose weight. If this worked, people would be able to follow this advice and drop weight. In our experience, this strategy only compounds feelings of failure. If your physician is insensitive regarding your weight, change doctors and tell your health-care company why you are doing so.

We all but guarantee that someone in your immediate network of acquaintances will know a good doctor or be able to point you to someone who does. If you don't currently have one, make it your goal to find a physician who is compassionate and sensitive to overweight people.

Brainstorm some ways you will begin this process.

_____

_____

_____

DAY 5
The Risks of Obesity

This session will cover some of the most common health risks associated with being overweight. This will not be a comprehensive discussion. We will touch only on main concerns. Our goal is not to scare you or make you fearful but to better inform you. Use this lesson to find the motivation to make healthy changes.

Remember that even modest weight loss improves your health.

LOOKING AT YOUR *LIFE*

In a prior lesson, we asked you for a family medical history. What about your own personal medical condition? What known health issues do you currently face?

_____

_____

What medications do you currently take and for what conditions?

_____

_____

What potential health risks worry you most and why?

_____

_____

LEARNING A NEW WAY OF *LIFE*

We've quoted this passage before and probably will quote it again in this workbook because it speaks directly to the issues we are discussing: "Do you not know that your bodies are temples of the Holy Spirit, who is in you, whom you have received from God? You are not your own; you were bought at a price. Therefore honor God with your bodies" (1 Corinthians 6:19–20).

What are the implications of this truth? What does it say to the person who simply lets himself or herself go?

_____

_____

Proverbs 6:6–11 presents an interesting passage about ants—how they wisely work now so as to have a better future:

> Go to the ant, you sluggard;
> consider its ways and be wise!
> It has no commander,
> no overseer or ruler,
> yet it stores its provisions in summer
> and gathers its food at harvest.
>
> How long will you lie there, you sluggard?
> When will you get up from your sleep?
> A little sleep, a little slumber,
> a little folding of the hands to rest—
> and poverty will come on you like a thief
> and scarcity like an armed man.

The point seems to be that the lazy refusal to lift a finger now can lead to big trouble later. How does this principle apply to the subject of weight loss and health?

_____

_____

Read Luke 12:16–21. While this parable most pointedly addresses a person's failure to care for his or her spiritual life, it more broadly highlights the foolishness of living a shortsighted life. How does this kind of narrow thinking (living only for the moment) often spill over into the way we care for (or fail to care for) our bodies?

_____

_____

"Dear friend, I pray that you may enjoy good health and that all may go well with you, even as your soul is getting along well" (3 John 2).

LOSING IT FOR *LIFE*

Overweight people are foolish to ignore physical warning signs and the findings of modern science. We need to live in the reality that extra weight puts us more at risk for certain health problems. Let's look at the most common health risks of being overweight.

Type 2 Diabetes

(Also referred to as adult onset or non-insulin-dependent diabetes; a disease in which blood sugar levels are above normal.)
Did you know . . . ?

- Type 2 diabetes can cause early death, heart disease, kidney disease, stroke, and blindness.
- 80 percent of people with this disease are overweight.[24]
- Losing weight and exercising can lower your risk for type 2 diabetes.

Heart Disease and Stroke

(Caused when your heart and circulation or blood flow does not operate normally.)
Did you know . . . ?

- Heart disease is the leading cause of death in the United States.[25]
- Strokes are the third leading cause of death in the United States.[26]
- Losing just 5 to 15 percent of your weight can lower your risk for both health problems.

Cancer

(Occurs when cells in one part of the body grow abnormally or out of control.)
Did you know . . . ?

- When you are overweight, your risk of developing certain types of cancers increases.

- Eating healthy foods and being physically active may lower your risk for cancer.

Sleep Apnea

(When a person stops breathing for short periods during the night.)
Did you know . . . ?

- This condition is more prevalent for people who are overweight.
- Fat stored in the neck area can make the airway for breathing smaller.
- Weight loss improves this condition because it decreases the neck size and inflammation.[27]

Osteoarthritis

(A joint disorder in which the tissues that protect joint bones and cartilage wear away.)
Did you know . . . ?

- The more weight you carry, the more pressure you put on your joints and cartilage.
- Excess weight increases joint inflammation, which increases risk for osteoarthritis.

Gallbladder Disease

(Caused when the gallbladder is enlarged or unable to work efficiently.)
Did you know . . . ?

- Overweight people produce more cholesterol, which puts strain on the gallbladder.
- Being overweight means your gallbladder could be enlarged and not work efficiently.[28]
- Losing weight too quickly increases one's chance of developing gallstones.

Are you anxious? Don't be. Losing as little as 5 percent of your body weight helps. Remember to lose weight slowly and safely.

Fatty Liver Disease

(Results from the buildup of fat cells in the liver, causing injury and inflammation.)

Did you know . . . ?

- Fatty liver disease can cause cirrhosis (scar tissue in the liver that blocks blood flow) and liver failure.
- Weight loss helps control blood sugar, which helps avoid the buildup of fat in the liver. Avoiding alcohol helps as well.[29]

What new things did you learn? What fears do you have? What new resolve?

_____

_____

_____

_____

PART TWO

CHANGING HOW YOU THINK, FEEL, AND LIVE

God loves you just the way you are,
but he refuses to leave you that way.

—Max Lucado

5

Nutrition Transformed

"You are what you eat!" Hopefully not, or today I would be soup, which would make me warm, delicious, and filling. The good news? There is a more scientific approach to the subject of food and what it does for us. Our LIFL goal is to transform your ho-hum style or habit of eating what may or may not be good for you into a keen awareness and appreciation of why you eat, what you eat, how you eat, and whether you enjoy what goes into your mouth. The transformation will likely make you feel better and also result in a healthier lifestyle.

The first step is to peruse your food journal from Appendix A. If you have not yet tried this exercise, it isn't too late. If you were to start a journal today and follow through for just three days, you would see patterns begin to emerge that point to the decisions you make about the food you eat. So start today!

Your journal provides specifics about your food choices and how much of those foods you eat. As you read through your journal, you will undoubtedly note food choices that are not healthy and need attention. For example, if you see that you usually have a high-calorie sugar snack (such as a doughnut) around 2:00 p.m. each day, target that snacktime. By substituting a lower-calorie, nutritious snack such as low-fat yogurt, for example, you have made a significant change, because small changes implemented daily make a *big* difference over time.

One of my (Steve's) old eating patterns that needed attention was my frequent morning stops at McDonald's for breakfast. Almost every day I used to start my day with one or more Egg McMuffins (with a lot of jam on the side) and a large soft drink. The surge of sugar, caffeine, cholesterol, grease, and over 1,500 calories ruined any hopes I had of healthy living. Added to that was a fried fruit pie around 10:00 a.m.

I didn't change overnight. But I recognized that I could make a huge impact by changing even one aspect of my eating habits. So I stopped drinking soft drinks and started drinking tea. That slight change alone eliminated hundreds of calories each day. Switching beverages also helped keep my blood sugar more stable, which lowered my cravings. I stopped going to McDonald's altogether and started eating eggs and tomatoes or peanut butter on toast with a glass of nonfat milk. The impact of this change was huge. I felt better and the weight began to come down just from that one change. If you have some poor eating habits, changing only one of them can have dramatic impact. In truth, the worse your eating habits are, the more material you have to work with in making small changes that produce big impact.

You don't have to count calories specifically to Lose It for Life. You will lose weight if you only cut back on calories. For example, if you cut back on just 100 calories a day (such as saying no to a cookie or a third of a candy bar), you would lose approximately ten pounds in a year's time, which can be a big difference! Reducing your portion size and making smarter food choices are two of the easiest and most painless methods to cut calories. Also helpful is to understand the basics about how your body uses food. If you are more comfortable with a complete plan, we provide two possibilities: the Smart Low-Carb Weight-Loss Plan and the Walker's Weight-Loss Plan (see Appendix D).

RISING TO THE CHALLENGE

Four separate verbs make up our overall strategy for healthy eating: reduce, increase, substitute, and eliminate, forming the acronym RISE. And isn't it interesting that the reason we have hope and can overcome difficulties is because of a *risen* Savior? Jesus rose above every challenge and struggle He faced. Even death could not stop Him—He is risen and sits at the right hand of the Father! This fact alone encourages us to an eternal hope and power to live daily in His victory.

Reduce white sugar and flour, white rice, potatoes, any and all white
processed starches and fat, and refined carbohydrates.
Increase vegetables, lean meats, and fruits low in carbs and high in fiber.
Substitute healthy foods for empty calories and poor nutritional foods.
Eliminate junk food and trans fat.

REDUCE

Sugar and Refined Carbohydrates

When there is too much of it, sugar turns to fat. Here's the general idea behind reducing sugar and simple or refined carbohydrates. Our bodies need sugar to function. All carbohydrates contain sugar. However, sugar exists in different forms, some of which are easier to digest than others. The faster sugar is absorbed into the body, the more insulin is produced, creating a rise in blood sugar. *Insulin* is the hormone responsible for circulating sugar into the bloodstream to either be used by organs now or stored for later use. So your body takes the sugar from carbohydrates and converts it to fuel that, when stored, is called "body fat." The more fuel you have stored, the more body fat you have!

Generally speaking, the more food is processed, the faster it is absorbed. When sugars and starches are absorbed quickly into your bloodstream, it is easy to become overweight. Sugar and refined carbohydrates cause rapid changes in blood sugar because they are absorbed quickly. They also stimulate hunger, which may entice you to eat more often.

Our goal is to eat more foods that cause a gradual rise in blood sugar and avoid those that cause blood sugar to spike quickly. One way to become familiar with which foods are healthy regarding sugar is to look at a resource index. In the 1970s, Dr. David Jenkins introduced a new way of categorizing foods—the glycemic index (GI), which measures carbohydrates in foods on a scale from 0 to 100, according to the amount blood sugar rises after eating the food. The lower the score, the longer it takes that food to raise your blood sugar. Therefore, you want to choose foods that are low on the glycemic index. Appendix C lists the glycemic index for a number of foods.

When you significantly reduce or even eliminate high-glycemic foods, you will increase your chances of losing weight. Numerous studies show the significance of the GI in weight control.

Low-glycemic foods:

- satisfy your hunger longer, minimize your food cravings better, and help you lose weight.
- result in a lower rise in blood sugar levels after eating and improve diabetes control.
- can enhance your physical endurance and also help refuel carbohydrate stores after exercise.

Food choices you can make to lower the glycemic index of your eating plan include choosing breakfast cereals with oats, barley, and bran. Eat breads that are "grainy" with whole seeds—no white bread—and include all types of fruit and vegetables (except potatoes) in your daily menu. Load up on salad vegetables (a vinaigrette dressing is fine) because they have a very low glycemic index count.

Many of us eat high-glycemic carbohydrates in the morning for breakfast (doughnuts, bagels, white bread toast, and sugary cereals). These carbohydrates may actually make us feel hungrier by midmorning. This idea is being tested and still debated. However, if you find that you are hungry a few hours after breakfast, switch to proteins or a high-fiber cereal and see if it helps.

Fats (Especially the Bad Kind)

Reducing fat should be a part of your meal plan, but it's important to distinguish between the different types of fat. The unsaturated and non-trans fats are the "good" fats. They include olive, canola, and peanut oil, and omega-3 polyunsaturated fat that is found in fish and fish oil capsules. These fats are actually beneficial in a diet in that they help prevent heart disease and stroke. Read food labels and try to stay within the range of no more than 25 percent of your calories coming from fat. You want to cut back on the trans fats, which will be covered in more detail in the "Eliminate" section.

INCREASE

Fiber

Fiber is the indigestible portion of plant food. It is also an important aid in losing weight because it works to slow the absorption of sugar. It is found mostly in fresh fruits and vegetables, whole grains, and legumes. Fiber slows down digestion, leads to feeling satisfied longer, and decreases appetite. Since we can't digest fiber, the bulk it provides makes you feel full.

Choose high-fiber foods over low-fiber foods. There are any number of high-fiber multigrain breakfast cereals available, not to mention barley, whole wheat bread, and fruits such as pears and raspberries. Eat four servings a week of legumes such as beans, peas, and lentils. Good ways to get these servings include bean or lentil salad, vegetable chili, low-fat refried beans, baked beans, or bean burritos. All it takes to get the recommended dose of fiber daily (20–35 grams) is adding an apple, orange, or one cup of lentils to your meal plan.[1]

Another way to look at this is to eat "big" food. Big food means eating food that has the most volume (nutritional value) with the least amount of calories and carbs. A piece of chocolate cake would be a very "small" food. It has a lot of fat, sugar, calories, and carbs, but very little volume (nutritional value). You can have your cake and eat it too, but it will help if the rest of the day you are eating nutritious, big foods with much larger volumes.

Fill Up and Chill Out

Are you getting enough water? One way to know is to check whether you have any of these symptoms: bad breath, pasty mouth or tongue, intestinal cramping, dark-colored or smelly urine, difficult bowel movements, dry skin, or headaches. If so, add more water to your daily eating plan.

Include nonalcoholic, noncaffeinated, and noncarbonated hydrating liquids such as water, herbal teas, soy or rice drinks (watch the sugar content in these!), and nonfat milk. Alcohol, caffeinated drinks, and carbonated beverages actually dehydrate the body. Drink a 1:1 ratio of water for each of these types of beverages you consume, or simply replace these drinks with water or another hydrating liquid. If you stopped drinking regular soda, for instance, in favor of water, you would reduce sugar and calories by 140–150 calories each time. That small change can add up to about fifteen pounds a year!

We recommend you obtain a favorite water bottle. Fill it with water and keep it with you as a continual reminder to keep on drinking! You may also want to drink an additional glass of water before meals in order to curb your appetite.

If you have difficulty getting in enough water, here is a schedule for drinking water throughout the day that may help:

Begin your day	12 ounces of water
Before lunch	12 ounces of water
After lunch	12 ounces of water
Right before dinner	12 ounces of water
After dinner (but two hours before bedtime)	12 ounces of water

Here's a great tip about drinking cold water. Your body needs to warm up cold liquids in order to maintain an internal body temperature, and this process of warming liquids burns calories. According to Jay T. Kearney, former director of sports science and the technology division at the US Olympic Training Center, drinking eight glasses of ice water a day burns about sixty calories.[2] So chill out and fill up!

Dairy

There is good news when it comes to increasing low-fat and nonfat dairy foods in your diet. Foods like hard cheese, yogurt, and milk (consumed in moderation) appear to speed up your metabolism. According to researcher Michael Zemel, calcium found in dairy foods plays a key role in weight loss. When calcium is in the blood, it signals fat cells to stop storing fat and burn it.[3] Therefore, including four low-fat dairy servings a day is a good idea for weight loss and building strong bones. Again, our recommendation is that you make your dairy choices low-fat. Typically we don't recommend this strategy for other foods because low-fat, processed foods are such because they replace fat with carbohydrates. But when it comes to dairy, low-fat is best.

SUBSTITUTE

Obviously you want to substitute low-fat, healthy foods for high-fat foods of little nutritional value, and low-glycemic foods for higher ones. For example, substitute low-fat, fruit-flavored yogurt for a cinnamon bagel, a cup of sliced cantaloupe for dried apricots (dried fruits are high in sugar), vegetables and low-calorie dip for potato chips and dip, and a bean burrito in a whole wheat tortilla wrap for a beef burrito.

And it's a good idea to try new foods. Our tastes change as we age. There may be food items you didn't like as a child that you may enjoy as an adult. For many people, broccoli is one of those foods. Those vegetables you didn't like as a kid often prove to be good adult choices because they are low in fat and low on the glycemic index.

Food substitution is especially important in maintaining weight loss. The best blueberry muffins in my (Steve's) town became a great midmorning snack when I moved to Laguna Beach. But my weight began creeping up almost immediately with that new little habit. Substituting a blueberry bagel for the muffin eliminated fat and sugar and proved satisfying. Sugar-free ice cream hits the spot when I want something cold and sweet. Mustard on turkey sandwiches replaced mayonnaise until I discovered a reduced-fat mayonnaise that I liked. There are many substitutes on the market for the poor choices that we gradually turn into habits.

ELIMINATE

Trans Fat

As you already know, fats and proteins slow down sugar absorption. Yet not all fats are the same. One type of fat is downright dangerous, so try to eliminate it as much as possible: "trans fat" or trans-fatty acid. Trans-fatty acid is created when hydrogen is bubbled through oil to produce a margarine that doesn't melt at room temperature. Adding trans fat to a food increases its shelf life and often gives food a good flavor.[4] However, trans fat contributes to obesity, a weakened immune system, diabetes, and coronary heart disease because it raises bad cholesterol and blood fats. It also may promote muscle loss and increase your risk for cancer.[5]

Did you know that about 40 percent of the food on grocery store shelves contains partially hydrogenated vegetable oils, which contain trans-fatty acid? (Fortunately there are stores like Wild Oats that won't carry a product if it has hydrogenated fat in it!) In the past, these fats have not had to be listed on many products, but the Food and Drug Administration now requires trans fat to be listed below the saturated fat line of a product.[6] Since trans fat is so unhealthy, there are no safe recommended upper limits of consumption. The best strategy is to eliminate it whenever you can.

Check labels to see if foods contain any trans fats. Also, look at the ingredient list of a product. The higher up in the list that you see the words "hydrogenated" or "partially hydrogenated," the more trans fat the food contains. So pick foods where it is lower in the list or not there at all. Organic food is better than processed food. Make small choices, such as switching to low-fat milk instead of nondairy creamer in your coffee, or using olive oil, sesame oil, or butter-flavored spray instead of margarine. And choose baked chips over those that are fried. Be creative and take small steps when making these changes. Keep in mind that every poor eating habit you change is helping your overall picture of health.

One important note: there is a distant cousin of trans fat called CLA (conjugated linoleic acid) that naturally occurs in dairy and beef. It is not related to partially hydrogenated oils but is similar in structure. New studies show that CLA may actually be helpful in fighting off the very thing its cousin brings about.[7]

MENU RECOMMENDATIONS

Healthy eating can be greatly helped with the addition of a menu of nutritious, tasty food choices. Here are a few suggestions to get started:

Breakfast

Eat an energy-building breakfast that gives you a good start for the day! Make it a priority to eat some protein, as it will help curb your hunger between meals. When using milk, consider using a lower-fat-percentage grade milk or even skim milk. And when making pancakes or waffles, consider using low- or no-fat yogurt or buttermilk.

Also consider adding fruit and whole wheat flour to pancake or muffin mixes. Fruit is a great addition to whole-grain cereals too. Also, eggs are fine to eat for breakfast, when eaten in moderation. Make omelets or scrambled eggs by using Egg Beaters or egg whites. Throw in some diced vegetables for a tasty breakfast.

Lunch

Make the usual turkey on whole-grain bread more exciting by adding cut-up red peppers and a couple of pea pods for nutrients. Eliminate or reduce the mayonnaise altogether and opt instead for mustard or Lemonaise Lite. Try to squeeze in more veggies to your daily menu by eating a spinach salad. Rediscover soup—healthy soup, that is! Though it takes time to eat, the fact that you are slowed down may help keep you from overeating.

Dinner

Eat fish a couple of times a week, especially albacore tuna and salmon. Consider having a vegetarian meal one or two nights a week as well. If you are new to vegetarian cooking, try stir-frying some veggies with tofu in sesame oil; or cook up whole-wheat spaghetti with peas and chopped tomatoes and sprinkle with low-fat or soy parmesan cheese.

When eating meat, try meat strips in place of a full cut of meat. Use sliced beef or chicken to make fajitas by grilling marinated meat with onions, peppers, and tomatoes. Or consider making shish kebabs by cutting up meat or chunks of fish alongside fruit or vegetable chunks. Broil or grill the kebabs and serve with brown rice.

Snacks

A cup of strawberries meets your quota for two servings of fruit and provides all the vitamin C needs for a day. Blueberries are loaded with antioxidants and contain a compound called pterostilbene, which may even lower your cholesterol. And there is a reason that an apple a day keeps the doctor away—it is nature's perfect fruit! You should eat one to two apples every day.

DESIGNING YOUR OWN MEAL PLAN

To lose weight, your goal is to burn more calories a day than you eat. You can design your own plan tailored to your likes and dislikes or choose instead one of the two plans we have provided.

Calorie Count

Whichever plan you choose, the first step is to determine your current calorie intake. Here's an easy way to find out that number. First, decide how active you are. *Sedentary* means you have a job or lifestyle that involves mostly sitting, standing, or light walking; you exercise once a week. *Active* means your job or lifestyle requires more activity than light walking (such as full-time housecleaning or construction work), or you get forty-five to sixty minutes of aerobic exercise three times a week. *Very Active* means you get aerobic exercise for at least forty-five to sixty minutes four or more times a week.

Choose the description that best fits your current lifestyle, and then locate your activity factor from the table below:

You are a:	Your factor is:
Sedentary woman	12
Sedentary man	14

You are a(n):	Your factor is:
Active woman	15
Active man	17
Very active woman	18
Very active man	20

Next, multiply your activity factor by your current weight in pounds. The resulting number is the approximate number of calories you need to maintain your current weight. An example for an active woman who weighs 150 pounds would look like this: *15 x 150 = 2,250 calories.* So if this 150-pound woman wanted to lose weight, she would need to restrict her calorie intake to fewer than 2,250 calories.

If you prefer to not be on a strict plan but want to watch labels instead, we recommend simply reducing your current calorie intake by 500 to 1,000 calories each day. This will lead to safe, effective weight loss of one to two pounds per week. Please note that you should *never* go below 1,500 calories per day unless under the supervision of a doctor.

TWO PERSONAL PLANS

Included in Appendix D are two weight-loss plans: the Smart Low-Carb Weight-Loss Plan and the Walker's Weight-Loss Plan. For both plans, consult the following chart to plan meals; it's important to eat the number of servings listed for each food group. Appendix D includes meal plans and recipes for both plans.

The average diet is full of carbohydrates that take up an estimated 50 to 60 percent of the total number of calories consumed. Based on the calorie level you just calculated, check the table below to find out the approximate number of grams of carbohydrates in your current diet. You might be surprised by the number. This table assumes that 55 percent of the calories in your diet come from carbohydrates, but if your diet is more heavily weighted in carbohydrates, these figures may even be on the low side.

Daily Calories	Carbs (grams)
1,800	248
2,000	275
2,400	330
2,800	385

If you feel you are cutting back carbohydrates too soon, eat 180 grams a day instead of 125. Stay on this schedule for several weeks before switching to 125 grams a day. Most people who consume a low-fat diet will likely lose weight by cutting their carbohydrate intake to 125 grams daily.

HANDLING CRAVINGS

Sugar

Have you ever said, "I'm addicted to sugar"? Well, you may not be too far from the truth. New studies (mostly in animals) show that a habit of overeating sweets may share some characteristics of serious addictions.[8] There is no direct proof yet, but the theory involves the activation of natural opioids in the brain. There is enough similarity that researchers are studying the connection between cravings and brain chemistry.

Dr. Bart Hoebel, a psychologist at Princeton University who conducts animal studies, reports, "People with a genetic predisposition for addiction can become overly dependent on sugar, particularly if they periodically stop eating and then binge." His research indicates that abstinence can bring about withdrawal symptoms similar to drug addiction. An article on Hoebel's research states, "The taste of sugar makes the brain release natural opioids, and the bingeing causes dopamine release."[9] While sugar cravings are yet to be understood, there is possibly some connection to brain chemistry and dependency. According to Dr. Braly, medical director of York Nutritional Laboratories and author of *Food Allergy Relief*, "People with food cravings may actually have neurochemical and hormonal imbalances that trigger these cravings."[10]

While the jury is still out as to whether sugar is truly addictive, one way to circumvent the problem is to simply avoid sugar altogether or find a way to deal with cravings. Distraction is a good answer. If you remove yourself from a situation in which sugary foods are available and wait forty-five minutes to an hour, the craving will probably go away. If you are still thinking about a food item after that much time, have a small amount of it. Other ways to distract yourself are to use physical exercise, relaxation exercises like deep breathing, or involvement in a new activity, such as reading.

For some people, there is little question that sugar is addictive. Perhaps the best alternative, if you cannot stop with a small treat, is to forgo the treat altogether. Sugar is not a food group we have to have. This is a hard journey to travel, and you will have to resolve potential feelings of deprivation, but it may be the only way you can succeed at long-term weight loss.

Chocolate

Give me chocolate or give me death! People crave chocolate more than any other food. Research investigating both the physiological and psychological basis of chocolate cravings remains inconclusive. It is most likely a combination of both. If you are going to eat chocolate, eat small amounts and choose dark chocolate because it has less sugar and fat. Apparently the cocoa in dark chocolate, a plant derivative, has been shown to have antioxidant benefits.[11] However, a little goes a long way because chocolate is calorie dense.

CHANGING YOUR BEHAVIOR

Eat Breakfast

We can't tell you how many people think losing weight is about skipping breakfast. And they couldn't be more wrong if they tried! A wealth of research supports the fact that eating breakfast is key to losing weight and maintaining a healthy lifestyle. Eating breakfast:

- has been linked to having a lower body mass, compared to people who skip the meal.
- reduces a person's risk of obesity and insulin resistance.
- is a proven strategy to maintain long-term weight loss.
- improves grades and behavior among schoolchildren.[12]

Weigh Yourself Regularly

Weigh yourself daily? No way! It sounds counterintuitive, but the members of the National Weight Control Registry, a group of more than 4,500 successful dieters who have lost at least thirty pounds and kept it off for at least one year, say weighing regularly helps keep the weight off.[13] Weekly weigh-ins are characteristic of 75 percent of members, while 44.5 percent weigh daily.

Even though we can usually tell by the fit or looseness of our clothing, the scale is used to self-monitor as a guard against those pounds creeping back without our awareness. Keeping a daily account of your weight will give you the feedback you need to cut back or maintain your weight. Once you notice a three- to five-pound weight gain, it's time to cut back and increase your exercise. Remember, if you overeat at one meal, you can cut back on the next meal.

Every new day is a chance to start afresh. As we are reminded in Lamentations 3:22–24 (MSG), "God's loyal love couldn't have run out, his merciful love couldn't have dried up. They're created new every morning. How great your faithfulness! I'm sticking with God (I say it over and over). He's all I've got left." We need to apply His "new mercies" to our lives daily and walk in victory.

Control Portions

Sizes have really increased in the last few years. Just think about fast-food chains. Nearly everything you buy can be supersized for just a few pennies more. And foods that don't appear in multiples can also be sized too big for one serving. For example, one Noah's bagel constitutes four servings from the bread group. Next time you order pasta in a restaurant, look to see if the portion size is about half a cup (one serving). Most likely you'll be served three or more cups (six servings). And most people clean their plates in restaurants—after all, they've paid for the food!

According to nutrition researcher Lisa Young of New York State University, portions are about twice as large as they were twenty years ago.[14] So downsize your orders, share an entrée when dining out, and pay attention to the amount of food you eat.

Keep in mind, however, that it is a mistake to reduce your portions to the point that you feel deprived or even hungry at the end of a meal. Instead, the solution is to eat more foods that have a lower calorie density and a high volume of nutrition. Change out small-volume foods for big-volume foods. You won't pack on the weight if you load up on veggies and low-calorie soups, but you will feel full!

Replace a Meal

Here's a tip you may want to try from time to time. Replace one of your meals with a portion-controlled food or commercial liquid diet drink. If you aren't sure how much you've been overeating, use a meal substitute for a lunch to bring yourself back under control. A meal replacement tells you exactly how many calories you are getting, so there is no guesswork to do. Just eat or drink up and get back on your regular plan.

Eat More Often

Gently changing *how* you eat produces a positive effect on *what* you eat. Be sure to eat an energy-building breakfast that gets you off to a good start! Eat more meals throughout the day without changing the amount of calories you are taking in. If you eat six mini meals a day, you don't have to pack in the food in order to "make it" until the next meal four hours later. Instead, eat smaller meals every two hours. In fact, research supports the idea that people who eat smaller, frequent meals are thinner and healthier.[15]

Don't Go Hungry to an Event

If you know you are going to an event like an office party, buffet party, or a celebration such as a wedding, don't go hungry. You will overeat, guaranteed. Instead, plan ahead. Drink a full glass of water and eat a piece of fruit before you leave; this small action will curb your appetite and help you resist the goodies you encounter. Place yourself next to a low-calorie snack if you have the munchies. And if you are asked to bring a food or dish, make it a vegetable tray or some other healthy choice that you can nibble on throughout the event.

Routine Is Good

One of the most common problems encountered when trying to lose weight is dealing with all the food choices available. The more variety you have to choose from, the more likely you will be to overeat. Research bears this out.[16] Establishing an eating routine helps. You don't have to be boring and eat the exact same thing each day, but monotony and following a basic schedule of what to eat does help people stick to their plans.

Don't Cook Foods You Have Trouble Resisting

When you are trying to lose weight, don't cook or bake unhealthy foods you will be tempted to eat. Your family will understand and can live without your famous German chocolate cake! Sometimes we feel guilty "depriving" others of the goodies we have decided to forgo. We shouldn't. Lose the guilt and focus on the fact that our decision to lose weight is helping the family make changes for the better as well. No one will suffer from the absence of fudge brownies for dessert. Trust us; it won't come up in therapy twenty years from now.

Variety May Not Be the Spice of Life

In a recent study, Brian Wansink, a professor of marketing and nutritional science at the University of Illinois at Urbana-Champaign, gives support to the idea that more than willpower is involved in resisting food. The color of food, the way it is displayed, and a person's perception of variety can lead to overeating. He says, "People eat more with their eyes, and their eyes trick their stomachs."[17] Based on his study, he offers these tips to prevent unhealthy overeating:

1. Multiple bowls of the same food give you the perception that there is more variety. Therefore, at parties, avoid multiple bowls.
2. At a buffet or reception, don't have more than two different foods on your plate at a time. In fact, decrease the variety of foods on your plate as much as possible.
3. If you arrange fruits and vegetables on your plate in an unorganized fashion, it will stimulate your appetite.

Create a Safe Eating Environment

It's very important to create an eating atmosphere that is free of anxiety. Mealtime should be enjoyable and relaxing. Unfortunately, this wasn't the case in many of your homes growing up. But now, as an adult, you can take charge of meals and make them pleasant. Engage in pleasant conversation, have soft music playing in the background, or light candles. Make mealtime a positive part of the day. If you eat alone, make your place setting attractive. Enjoy the quiet and concentrate on taking your time and relaxing. Chewing food slowly and eating without rushing will help you savor your food. Proverbs 23:2–3 tells us, "Don't gobble your food, don't talk with your mouth full. And don't stuff yourself; bridle your appetite" (MSG).

You should establish regular mealtimes and eat your meals at the kitchen or dining room table. Eating in front of the TV, on the run, in the car, or while reading a book is a setup for "unconscious" eating. Eating becomes unconscious when you hardly remember doing it! It should not be considered an activity to multitask with. Break the habit of eating in places other than at the table.

Also, make sure you sit down while you eat. This will help break the habit of eating while you cook, clean up, or serve others. A little taste here and there can really add on the pounds. By using the same place settings (pick small plates), you will establish a routine for your meals. It may be psychological that small plates help us eat less, but it works to trick you into thinking you are getting plenty of food.

Another way to create a safe environment is to rid your house of tempting high-fat foods or binge foods. For example, if you have a hard time resisting Oreo cookies, don't buy them. If you are trying not to snack on chips, keep them out of your pantry. You won't be tempted by what is missing, and you will have to eat what is available. So have healthy low-calorie snacks available to munch on for those hungry moments. Go through your pantry and toss out the chips, sodas, and cookies; load up on fruit, nuts, and veggies.

We also advise putting leftovers out of sight right after the meal is over. Don't leave them on the counter. Seal them in foil so you don't look at the food every time you open the refrigerator or freezer door, because when you can't see it, it's less tempting! And remember to distinguish between physical hunger and hunger related to emotions such as boredom or stress. Turn off TV commercials or switch channels when an advertisement gives you a craving. Pass by the magazine food advertisements. There is enough evidence to suggest that looking at pictures of food cues your desire to eat it,[18] so don't look at those pictures!

In addition, you should eat in full view of friends and family. Secret eating gets people in trouble. Sometimes we think that sneaking food or eating in secret doesn't count. But that isn't true, and hiding from the reality only hurts you.

DINING OUT

Let's face it. Few of us eat all our meals at home. In our fast-paced lives, dining out is a reality, but it doesn't have to be a nightmare if you are trying to lose weight. Here are ten tips for dining out compiled by Nanci Hellmich of *USA Today* after she talked with four nutritionists:[19]

1. Order less of something. Ask for half a portion or a junior portion of what's served.
2. Choose a sauce that is red versus white or pink. Red sauces are usually tomato-based and have less fat and fewer calories.

3. Skip the bread basket. Either ask the server not to bring it, to bring it late in the meal, or to only serve one slice of bread.
4. Order soup (broth-based) prior to eating an entrée. It will fill you up.
5. Avoid large portions on the menu and descriptions that sound like trouble, such as "fried," "battered," or "buttery."
6. Order steamed or sautéed vegetables as a side dish.
7. Take half the meal and wrap it up before you even begin to eat it. You won't be tempted to eat past your feelings of fullness if the remainder of the meal isn't on the plate.
8. Split a dessert or only take one bite. If you really want something for yourself, order a cappuccino with low-fat milk and add some sugar (or Splenda). This treat is only about 100 calories!
9. Avoid anything supersized. Order a kid-sized portion if you can.
10. Instead of an entrée, order an appetizer. The portion size is usually smaller and plenty filling.

DINING IN THE SKY

Eating meals on an airplane can create a challenge. If you know a meal will be served on a particular flight, you can request a special meal (low-fat, vegetarian, or seafood) if you call ahead and place an order. Also, many hotels will box up food for you to take on a plane. Or you could walk to a local food market and package a meal or snack to take along. Make sure to drink plenty of water, since airplane travel dehydrates travelers. Avoid coffee and alcohol for this reason.

Eating should be a pleasure. And although losing weight means adjusting eating habits and patterns, it does not have to result in out-of-control feelings of deprivation or frustration. The important thing is to choose an eating plan and foods that will improve your energy and health. Follow the RISE formula to do this—it really works! And remember, small changes that you can stick with are much more powerful than big ones you won't continue. So make changes you can live with to establish healthy eating habits that will last for life.

Workbook Week 5

NUTRITION TRANSFORMED

DAY 1
RISE Above Your Old Habits (Part 1)

When it comes to eating, popular slogans such as "You are what you eat!" don't help very much. We prefer a more scientific, more practical approach to eating. These lessons will help you decide on an eating plan that's right for you. Our goal is to make healthy lifestyle changes regarding food and eating.

If you have poor eating habits, changing only one of them can have a dramatic impact.

LOOKING AT YOUR *LIFE*

"Q: How do you eat an elephant? A: One bite at a time." Obviously no one at LIFL wants anyone to eat an elephant or eat like an elephant! The point of that familiar maxim is that we accomplish big things by doing little things over and over.

What projects have you completed by chipping away and faithfully plodding ahead?

_____

_____

How are you doing with regard to keeping your food journal? What's the experience been like? In what ways has this habit begun to change your mind-set about food and eating?

_____

_____

Skim your journal and note the kinds of foods you eat in a typical day (pick a day from the last couple of weeks). Do certain foods seem to keep finding their way into your mouth at certain times of the day? What type of foods and at what times? What's going on here?

_____

_____

The authors make the point that even small changes in amount (one cookie a day instead of three) and small substitutions in the types of food we eat (an apple instead of a Twinkie) can add up over time to big changes. Have you been able to make small changes like this? Record your thoughts here.

_____

_____

What have you decided about making meal plans? Of the two plans suggested in the _Lose It for Life_ book (the Smart Low-Carb Weight-Loss Plan and the Walker's Weight-Loss Plan), which one is a better fit for you? Why?

_____

_____

LEARNING A NEW WAY OF _LIFE_

LIFL is more comprehensive than a mere diet; it involves lifestyle changes. As we explore areas in our lives that need to change, a one-word strategy will help: RISE. This acronym reminds us of four actions that need to become our regular habits: _Reduce, Increase, Substitute,_ and _Eliminate._ The RISE formula embodies our overall strategy for success, and we will apply it to each area of needed change.

If you doubt your ability to succeed in this, spend a few minutes pondering these Bible passages that speak of God's power. Jot down your thoughts and observations after each passage.

> I pray that the eyes of your heart may be enlightened in order that you may know . . . his incomparably great power for us who believe. That power is the same as the mighty strength he exerted when he raised Christ from the dead and seated him at his right hand in the heavenly realms. (Ephesians 1:18–20)

As we focus on the acronym RISE, it's helpful to remember that we serve a risen Savior. Not even death could stop Jesus—a fact that should fill us with great hope.

_____

_____

I pray that out of his glorious riches he may strengthen you with power through his Spirit in your inner being. (Ephesians 3:16)

_____

_____

His divine power has given us everything we need for a godly life through our knowledge of him who called us by his own glory and goodness. (2 Peter 1:3)

_____

_____

What do these verses tell you about God? About His love and care for you? If God is "able"—if He is "for us"—then what should we expect as we endeavor to change by His power?

_____

_____

When have you seen or experienced the power of God?

_____

_____

LOSING IT FOR _LIFE_

Let's begin applying the RISE strategy to our food choices and eating habits by taking a closer look at foods we need to reduce and foods we ought to increase.

Foods to Reduce

There are exceptions, but generally it is wise to cut back on white foods—white sugar, white flour, white rice, potatoes, etc. How much a part of your diet are these foods?

_____

_____

Take this true/false test about sugar.

True or False?	
1.	Too much sugar turns to fat!
2.	Our bodies need sugar to function.
3.	Most carbohydrates contain sugar.
4.	Sugar exists in different forms, some easier to digest than others.
5.	Your body takes the sugar from carbohydrates and converts it to fuel that is either burned or stored. When it is stored, it's called body fat. The more fuel stored, the more body fat you have.
6.	You can eat as much low-fat stuff as you want without gaining weight.
7.	A candy bar or bag of chips can actually stimulate your hunger by raising your blood sugar levels too quickly.
8.	The so-called glycemic index measures the movement of glaciers in northern Canada.
9.	When you significantly reduce or even eliminate high glycemic foods, you will increase your chances to lose weight.
10.	Some research suggests that sugar may be addictive.

"People with a genetic predisposition for addiction can become overly dependent on sugar, particularly if they periodically stop eating and then binge" (Dr. Bart Hoebel).[20]

(Answers: 1. True; 2. True; 3. False [All carbohydrates contain sugar]; 4. True; 5. True; 6. False [Many low-fat foods are high in carbs, which—if not burned—end up stored as fat]; 7. True; 8. False [The glycemic index measures carbohydrates in food on a scale from 0 to 100 according to the amount your blood sugar rises after eating it]; 9. True; 10. True [New studies, mostly with animal subjects, show that overeating sweets may share some characteristics with serious addictions.][21])

In Appendix C you'll find a glycemic index for a number of foods. Look it over. Which high-glycemic foods are a regular part of your diet?

_____

_____

_____

_____

Write about your own relationship with sugar. How about chocolate? Are you a chocoholic? What are some practical, proven ways a person can resist these kinds of high-glycemic foods?

_____

_____

Foods to Increase

Fiber is a hugely important part of a healthy-eating life plan. Fiber is the indigestible portion of plant food, found mostly in fresh fruits, vegetables, whole grains, and legumes. Fiber can help us lose weight by slowing down the absorption of sugar and our digestive process, thus decreasing our appetite. Since we can't digest fiber, its bulk gives us a full feeling, which can help us eat less.

What are your favorite foods that are rich in fiber?

_____

_____

Your body automatically warms up cold liquids in order to maintain its internal temperature. Drinking eight glasses of ice water a day burns about sixty calories.

Your body automatically warms up cold liquids in order to maintain its internal temperature. Drinking eight glasses of ice water a day burns about sixty calories.[22]

The authors suggest this plan: drink 12 ounces of water when you first wake up, 12 ounces before lunch, 12 ounces after lunch, 12 ounces right before dinner, and 12 ounces after dinner.

Does this water plan seem doable for you? Why or why not?

_____

_____

There is good news when it comes to including dairy in your diet. Hard cheeses, yogurt, and milk appear to speed up our metabolisms. Calcium in the blood signals fat cells to stop storing fat and burn it.[23] Including four dairy servings a day is a good idea for weight loss and for building strong bones.

How much dairy product do you eat? What kinds and how often?

_____

_____

Specifically, what foods are you going to reduce? Which ones do you intend to increase?

_____

_____

DAY 2

RISE Above Your Old Habits (Part 2)

Let's continue the RISE process. We've looked at foods we need to reduce and others we need to increase. In this session, we'll explore the foods we need to substitute and eliminate altogether.

Increase your consumption of vegetables, lean meats, and fruits low in carbohydrates and high in fiber. Select at least one fruit or vegetable each day.

LOOKING AT YOUR *LIFE*

What are your guiltiest pleasures when it comes to eating?

_____

_____

_____

What foods or dishes hold a special place in your heart and mind? Why do you think those items are so enticing to you?

_____

_____

_____

What healthy foods and snacks do you enjoy—that taste good to you?

_____

_____

_____

LEARNING A NEW WAY OF *LIFE*

Check out the following Bible verses that speak about food and eating.

Then God said, "I give you every seed-bearing plant on the face of the whole earth and every tree that has fruit with seed in it. They will be yours for food." (Genesis 1:29)

Everything that lives and moves about will be food for you. Just as I gave you the green plants, I now give you everything. (Genesis 9:3)

He makes grass grow for the cattle, and plants for people to cultivate—bringing forth food from the earth. (Psalm 104:14)

So whether you eat or drink or whatever you do, do it all for the glory of God. (1 Corinthians 10:31)

What general conclusions can you draw from these passages about God? About what we can and should eat? About *how* we should eat?

_____

_____

_____

It's important to remember that LIFL is not a diet. It's a way of life. It's remembering that God is good and that His gifts are good. The key is moderation, not gorging ourselves, and not using food to fill needs it was never intended to fill.

Many, if not most diets absolutely *forbid* certain kinds of food. The LIFL program maintains that no foods are off-limits. What are the positive benefits of this philosophical difference? What are the potential dangers?

_____

_____

_____

"God . . . richly provides us with everything for our enjoyment" (1 Timothy 6:17).

How are you changing as a result of reading, thinking, and applying the LIFL plan?

_____

_____

LOSING IT FOR *LIFE*

LIFL urges us to *reduce* our intake of certain foods and to *increase* our consumption of others. The plan also suggests certain things to substitute or eliminate altogether.

Foods to Substitute

Obviously it is wise to substitute high-fat foods that contain little nutritional value with low-fat healthy foods.

Using your food journal as a guide, list some substitutions you could and should make that would lead to a healthier you.

_____

_____

_____

It is also wise to substitute high-glycemic foods with low ones. Some examples: eating fruit-flavored yogurt instead of a glazed doughnut, vegetables and dip instead of potato chips and dip, a bean burrito instead of a beef burrito, and so forth.

Again, look at the record of your recent eating habits. Using Appendix C, suggest at least five food substitutions you could begin making regularly, that—over time—would result in a big difference.

_____

_____

_____

The authors urge us to try new foods, noting that some food items we didn't like as children we would enjoy now. List personal examples of this.

Foods I Disliked When I Was Younger   When I Learned to Like Them

_____   _____
_____   _____
_____   _____
_____   _____

Now list some other not-so-favorite foods (low in fat and low on the glycemic index) that you will agree to go back and try again.

_____
_____
_____

Foods to Eliminate

We've seen that fats and proteins slow down sugar absorption. Yet we've also noted that not all fats are the same. One type of fat is downright danger-ous, so we want to eliminate it as much as possible. The fat to avoid at all costs is _trans-fatty acid_, also called "trans fat."

Take a short true/false quiz and see how much you remember from the _LIFL_ book about trans fat.

	True or False?
1.	Trans-fatty acid is created when our diets include too much beef and too many carbonated drinks.
2.	Adding trans fat to a food increases its shelf life and often gives it a good flavor.
3.	Too much trans fat can lead to obesity, a weakened immune system, diabetes, coronary heart disease, muscle loss, increased cancer risk, and global warming.
4.	About 40 percent of the food on grocery store shelves contains partially hydrogenated vegetable oils, which contain trans-fatty acid.
5.	The way to tell how much trans fat a food item has is to look at the nutrition label. If you see the words "hydrogenated" or "partially hydrogenated" anywhere near the top of the ingredients list, the food is high in trans fat.

6.	Typically, organic foods have more trans fat than foods processed in modern factories.

(Answers: 1. False ["Trans fat" is a man-made substance produced when hydrogen is bubbled through oil to produce a margarine that doesn't melt at room temperature]; 2. True[24]; 3. False [Everything but the global warming part]; 4. True; 5. True 6. False [The truth is just the opposite; natural foods are healthier than processed ones.])

Where do you see a lot of trans fats in your diet? What particular foods?

_____

_____

_____

There is a distant cousin of trans fat called CLA (conjugated linoleic acid) that naturally occurs in dairy and beef. New studies show that CLA may actually be helpful in fighting off the very thing its cousin brings about.[25]

Take a field trip to your pantry. List the items you find there that are high in trans-fatty acid.

_____

_____

_____

Some practical tips for eliminating the scourge of trans fat: switch to milk instead of nondairy creamer in your coffee, use olive oil or sesame oil or butter-flavored spray instead of margarines, and choose baked chips over fried.

What's the most powerful or helpful thing you've learned in this lesson? Why?

_____

_____

_____

DAY 3

What's on the Menu?

We all *have* to eat. We all *want* to eat. We have myriad choices, but not all choices are wise ones. Our goal in this lesson is to take a look at menus—to begin to formulate a personalized eating plan that is both nutritious and delicious; a plan that will help us drop extra weight and keep it off for life.

LOOKING AT YOUR *LIFE*

Just for fun, think back to school lunches. What do you remember? Did you eat in the cafeteria or bring your lunch? Write a few memories in the space below.

_____

_____

Try to list ten foods that taste good and are good for you. Which ones are part of your regular diet?

_____

_____

_____

Choose fruits and vegetables with vivid colors. You can't go wrong by choosing these nutrient powerhouses.

We can fall into certain eating patterns in which we tend to eat the same dishes time and time again. Consider your own eating habits. In a typical month, what are the meals you eat, what are the snacks you seek out, and what restaurants do you dine in? In other words, what foods comprise the bulk of your personal menu?

Top Ten Meals (Home-Cooked)   **How Many Times Eaten per Month**

_____

_____

_____

_____

_____

Top Ten Snacks   **How Many Times Eaten per Month**

_____

_____

_____

_____

_____

Top Ten Meals (Restaurant)   **How Many Times Eaten per Month**

_____

_____

_____

_____

_____

"So do not worry, saying, 'What shall we eat?' or 'What shall we drink?' or 'What shall we wear?' . . . your heavenly Father knows [what] you need" (Matthew 6:31–32).

Based on what you've learned thus far, what problems do you see with your existing eating habits?

_____

_____

LEARNING A NEW WAY OF *LIFE*

Paul has an interesting paragraph in his letter to the Philippian Christians. He wrote:

Join together in following my example, brothers and sisters, and just as you have us as a model, keep your eyes on those who live as we do. For, as I have often told you before and now tell you again even with tears, many live as enemies of the cross of Christ. Their destiny is destruction, their god is their stomach, and their glory is in their shame. Their mind is set on earthly things. But our citizenship is in heaven. And we eagerly await a Savior from there, the Lord Jesus Christ, who, by the power that enables him to bring everything under his control, will transform our lowly bodies so that they will be like his glorious body. (Philippians 3:17–21)

Notice the phrase "their god is their stomach." In other words, these worldly people are slaves to their own sensual appetites and physical desires. Whatever urges they sense within, they immediately follow and seek to satisfy. Paul contrasts this kind of immediate gratification mind-set and lifestyle with believers who have an eternal perspective.

In what ways can the desire for food become all-consuming—like a "god"?

_____

_____

_____

What's involved in making the switch between "living to eat" and "eating to live"?

_____

_____

_____

Read and ponder Matthew 6:25–34. How do these words of Christ provide new perspective on life (including the role of food)?

_____

_____

LOSING IT FOR *LIFE*

The *LIFL* book contains all kinds of practical ideas for menu development. Which ones strike your fancy? Jot down the tips and suggestions that you'd like to try.

_____

_____

_____

_____

Reduce your current calorie intake by 500 to 1,000 calories a day. This will lead to safe, effective weight loss of one to two pounds per week.

Chapter 5 of *Lose It for Life* helps you calculate your current calorie intake and activity level. Based on the chart in the book, are you sedentary, active, or very active? How many calories do you estimate that you burn daily?

_____

_____

Using the formulas and following the directions in the book, what calorie level intake do you need in order to lose a pound or two a week?

_____

_____

Look at the five-day meal plan in Appendix D. This menu is based on 125 grams of carbs a day. What do you like about this plan?

_____

_____

The Walker's Weight-Loss Plan is featured in Appendix D. Take a few minutes to study the weeklong menu provided there. What's your assessment? How could this work for you?

_____

_____

DAY 4

Common Sense for Uncommon Weight Control

Some people get so immersed in calories and carbs, and in the science of fats and fitness, that they lose sight of simple, basic truths. The goal of this lesson is to remember some commonsense practices that can lead to uncommon success in losing it for life.

LOOKING AT YOUR *LIFE*

A few years ago, a best-selling book offered everyday wisdom gleaned from the lives of regular folks. For example, "I've learned it's possible to do something in a moment that you'll regret for a lifetime." Or "I've learned that when all is said and done, more things are said than done."

Following that same format, what are some lessons you've learned about food and eating in your lifetime? (Ex: "I've learned that I should *never* go grocery shopping when I'm hungry!")

"Get wisdom. Though it cost all you have, get understanding" (Proverbs 4:7).

_____

_____

_____

What's been the most helpful advice or suggestion you've received so far in your participation in the Lose It for Life system? Why?

_____

_____

_____

215

In what specific ways do your LIFL comrades encourage you to keep persevering?

_____

_____

_____

What about your family and friends? What's been their attitude as you have embarked on this new weight-loss/weight management life plan?

_____

_____

_____

Have you been to the LIFL website? If not, take some time right now, log on to the World Wide Web, and surf your way over to www.LoseItForLife.com. You'll find many interesting features and articles.

LEARNING A NEW WAY OF *LIFE*

Just for fun, take this food quiz and test your knowledge of eating habits in Bible times. Match the following questions with the correct answers.

1.	What strange snack did Samson eat?	a. Camels, hares, snakes, ostrich, locusts (Leviticus 11)
2.	What was John the Baptist's weird diet?	b. Cooked goat (Genesis 27:14–18)
3.	What unusual food had the appearance of coriander seed?	c. Fish, cucumbers, melons, leeks, onions and garlic (Numbers 11:5)
4.	What did the Hebrews eat in Egypt?	d. Locusts and honey (Matthew 3:4)
5.	What was on King Solomon's daily menu?	e. Bread, beef, lamb, goat, deer, gazelle, roebuck and choice fowl (1 Kings 4:22–23)

6.	What food did Jacob use to get his brother's birthright?	f. Roasted lamb, unleavened bread, bitter herbs (Exodus 12:1–10)
7.	What meal did Jacob cook to steal his father's blessing?	g. Bread and lentil ("red") stew (Genesis 25:27–34)
8.	What foods did the Mosaic Law forbid the Jews to eat?	h. Honey, out of a lion's carcass (Judges 14:5–9)
9.	What foods were part of the Passover Meal?	i. Almonds (Genesis 43:11)
10.	What food "gift" did the sons of Jacob present to Joseph when they arrived in Egypt to buy grain?	j. Manna (Exodus 16:31)

(Answers: 1. h; 2. d; 3. j; 4. c; 5. e; 6. g; 7. b; 8. a; 9. f; 10. i)

Read Jesus' comments in John 4:32–34. What do you think He meant? In what way is doing God's will "food"?

_____

_____

_____

What are the implications of this for your life?

_____

_____

_____

LOSING IT FOR *LIFE*

What reasons are given in the *LIFL* book for eating breakfast? What's your own experience? How has skipping breakfast helped or hurt you?

_____

_____

_____

We can't tell you how many people think losing weight is about skipping breakfast. They couldn't be more wrong!

Why is weighing yourself regularly a good practice to develop?

_____

_____

_____

Keeping a daily account of your weight will give you the feedback you need to cut back or maintain your weight.

What might happen if you downsize your portions? For example, have two cookies instead of three, eat an 8 oz. steak instead of a 12 oz. steak, or leave some food on your plate when dining out. If you did this consistently for six months, what might happen? How would it make a difference?

_____

_____

_____

If you increased your intake of foods that are lower in calories and higher in density, such as veggies and low-cal soups, what can result?

_____

_____

_____

The authors suggest eating more often. "If you eat six mini meals a day, you don't have to pack in the food in order to 'make it' until the next meal four hours later. Instead, eat smaller meals every two hours. In fact, research supports the idea that people who eat smaller, frequent meals are thinner and healthier."[26]

What are your thoughts about mini meals? Have you tried this? With what results?

_____

_____

_____

When you are trying to lose weight, don't cook or bake or buy rich, fatty foods you will be tempted to eat.

The authors also recommend a regular eating routine, because the more variety you have to choose from, the greater the likelihood of overeating. In what ways have you experienced this fact personally?

_____

_____

_____

Why is it a bad idea to go to a big event hungry?

_____

_____

_____

Handling Dangerous (Food) Situations

We've been looking at the practical things about eating and reminding ourselves of some common food traps and some common sense solutions. Let's continue in that vein, focusing in this short lesson on how to create an overall safer eating environment.

It's very important to create an eating atmosphere that is free of anxiety. Mealtime should be enjoyable and relaxing.

LOOKING AT YOUR *LIFE*

Most of us know ourselves well enough to know our tendencies. In what situations are you most inclined to overeat? Why?

_____

_____

_____

When was the last time you ate so much you felt physically ill?

_____

_____

_____

When was the last time you said no to a tantalizing food temptation? How did you manage to do it? How did you feel afterward?

_____

_____

_____

Describe mealtimes around your house. What's the mood like—before, during, and after? What goes on in your own heart? Why?

_____

_____

_____

_____

LEARNING A NEW WAY OF _LIFE_

If while driving down the highway, you suddenly encountered a series of warning signs (for example, "Bridge out ahead" or "Left lane closed"), you would slow down, right? You'd become more aware, more careful.

Proverbs 22:3 says, "The prudent see danger and take refuge, but the simple keep going and pay the penalty." This verse suggests a very wise principle: Be on the lookout; be smart. Don't make foolish, avoidable decisions that lead to unnecessary grief.

Let's apply that to eating. What are the warning signs for you that you might be entering a "dangerous food zone"?

_____

_____

_____

Proverbs 23:2–3 (MSG) states, "Don't gobble your food, don't talk with your mouth full. And don't stuff yourself; bridle your appetite." Your reaction?

_____

_____

_____

Ponder this amazing verse for a few minutes: "No temptation has overtaken you except what is common to mankind. And God is faithful; he will not let you be tempted beyond what you can bear. But when you are tempted, he will also provide a way out so that you can endure it" (1 Corinthians 10:13).

You can create an eating atmosphere that is soothing and peaceful . . . and conducive to losing weight and keeping it off.

What does this passage promise?

_____

_____

_____

What are some ways out for us when we find ourselves in the midst of tempting sumptuous food situations?

_____

_____

_____

What are the implications of this verse for us as we strive to settle into a healthier lifestyle of eating right and exercising consistently?

_____

_____

_____

LOSING IT FOR *LIFE*

What are some reasons that soft music, candles, and positive conversation can help us develop a new attitude about eating?

Read through the following list of eating habits. Why do you think each of these can be "dangerous" habits sometimes?

Eating too hurriedly

_____

Eating at irregular times

_____

Eating in front of the TV

_____

Eating in the car

_____

Eating while reading

_____

Eating while standing

_____

Eating while you cook

_____

Eating at other places than the dining table or breakfast bar

_____

Which of these habits are you guilty of?

_____

_____

_____

Write a comment or two about each of the following—specifically why they are _wise_ habits.

Chewing food slowly

_____

Putting down your fork between bites

_____

Drinking water with your meal

_____

Eating off a smaller plate

_____

Ridding your house of tempting high-fat foods

_____

Wrapping leftovers in foil rather than plastic wrap

_____

Choose an eating plan and foods that will improve your energy and health. Even just a few changes, over time, will produce a healthier, thinner you.

Putting leftovers away, out of sight

_____

Changing the channel or turning the page when you see a food ad on TV or in a magazine

_____

Eating in front of others

_____

Which three positive habits can you (_will_ you) implement today?

_____

_____

Go back and review the authors' suggestions for dining out, found in chapter 5 of the book. Of the ten tips they give, which two or three will you put into effect the next time you go out to eat?

_____

_____

_____

6

Move It *and* Lose It

You've heard the saying, "Move it or lose it!" We'd like to alter it a bit to, "Move it *and* lose it." That's right. The more you move it, the more you'll lose it—or at least keep from going in the opposite direction! Even though exercise will not turn you into Twiggy (for those of you too young to remember, she was a very skinny model from the 1960s), it is responsible for keeping many people from gaining weight. Members of the National Weight Control Registry report that exercise plays a role in keeping their weight off as well. Most reported exercising about an hour a day.[1]

Okay, so an hour a day sounds like torture to some of you. Not to worry! We are convinced that there is at least one activity you can really enjoy. There isn't a requirement to exercise for sixty minutes straight either. So take a deep breath and relax. Exercise can work for you.

To begin, let's revisit our RISE formula and apply it to exercise.

Reduce your negativity and lackadaisical attitude toward exercise.
Increase your physical activity, water consumption, commitment to exercise, and accountability.
Substitute the right attitude—a cheerful one—if need be, and also the right workout clothing for the wrong apparel.
Eliminate all excuses for not exercising! Exercise isn't optional in Lose It for Life.

Steve's Secret

Exercise is the area of Lose It for Life that was the most transforming for me. Before I finally lost the weight for good, I couldn't jog around the block, and I saw no reason to try. I was so out of shape that even walking up a flight of stairs created intense embarrassment for me. I smoked and was fat and just saw no reason to exercise. I admit it: I hated the very idea of exercising. I saw it as something no one in their right mind would engage in regularly because they wanted to. But all that has changed. I am living proof of the transformation that can occur when a person decides to start exercising and sticks with it.

I went jogging this morning before church and had a great run by the water. Once I was finished, I felt so good knowing I had done something for myself and my health. I now view exercise as a gift from God. It not only helps me control my weight and improve my health, but it also improves the quality of my life.

There is one point that I want to stress. If you struggle with exercising, there is a way to make it better that has proven successful over and over again: find an exercise partner. I have seen people struggle with their weight for decades and then find success because they were held accountable and kept moving. It doesn't cost anything to have a friend who will exercise with you! But it will keep you from turning over and going back to sleep rather than getting up and moving.

If you don't have any friends, or you live in a swamp, or you're in a relationship that won't allow you to have friends, you should know that your excuses are nothing new! So when you are ready, overcome the excuses, get a partner, and realize that you just may have found the key to the long-term weight loss you have been looking for.

Do you absolutely hate the very idea of exercise? Let's take a little quiz and see if you have the right mind-set to get moving. (Use the answer key below to see how ready you are to jump in and begin moving, based on the number of times you answered yes.)

Ready to Exercise?

	Y	N
1. Does the very idea of exercise bore you?	Y	N
2. Are you a pro at finding excuses not to engage in physical activities?	Y	N
3. If a friend invited you to go on a bike ride, would you suggest meeting for lunch instead?	Y	N
4. Do you get tired watching someone else work out?	Y	N
5. Do you choose the elevator over stairs every chance you get?	Y	N
6. Have you given up exercising because you weren't satisfied with previous results?	Y	N
7. Are you waiting to lose weight until you start exercising?	Y	N
8. Do you hate the idea of breaking a sweat?	Y	N
9. Do you resolve to take up exercising year after year but never seem to get around to it?	Y	N
10. When you are running errands, do you often drive rather than walk?	Y	N

0–2: **You're ready to reap the energy-boosting benefits of exercise.** You're actually pro-exercise, but there may be a few things keeping you from fully adopting an active lifestyle. Revisit a sport you enjoyed in your youth. Or choose something new that you've always wanted to learn or do.

3–5: **Your fitness hurdles are mainly attitude induced.** If you have been unhappy with past exercise efforts, you may have expected results too soon. While exercise often feels good in a matter of days, it usually takes a month to see real cardiovascular and strength benefits. For instant encouragement, keep a graph that shows the length and frequency of your workouts.

6–10: **You're on the wrong side of the starting gate**. Your excuses for skipping workouts only cheat yourself. When you're tempted to skip, think about this study from the Veterans' Affairs Palo Alto Health Care System at Stanford University: a person's peak exercise capacity, as measured on a treadmill test, is a more powerful predictor of longevity than health risk factors such as heart disease, high blood pressure, or smoking.[2]

HOW MUCH IS ENOUGH?

Your attitude toward exercising matters—in fact, it's as important as the food you put in your mouth. Since finding time to exercise is usually a factor for most people who struggle to get moving, consider this. According to the results of a series of studies undertaken at the University of Pittsburgh, women who were told to exercise in ten-minute bouts four times a day exercised more and lost more weight than women told to exercise for forty minutes once a day. Most of the women in the study chose walking for their exercise. Those who exercised in short bouts lost about twenty pounds after twenty-six weeks, while those who exercised in longer stretches lost only about thirteen pounds.[3] This fact should be of great encouragement if you struggle to find significant blocks of time in the day to exercise. You also may benefit from this strategy if you are someone who physically hurts when exercising. If you aren't sure what can be done in just ten minutes, turn to Appendix E for our Ten-Minute Workout.

While the above study encourages you to exercise for short periods throughout the day, more recent recommendations from the Institute of Medicine (IOM) provide a different recommendation. In September 2002, the IOM recommended that adults engage in sixty minutes of moderate intense physical exercise, such as brisk walking, every day.[4] The time length differs from the U.S. Surgeon General's 1996 recommendation of thirty minutes of daily exercise. The IOM has increased the daily time because of the increased calorie consumption and weight of most Americans. Twenty to thirty minutes of high-intensity daily exercise would meet their guidelines as well. So while this is a bit of a confusing picture, your best bet is to exercise somewhere between thirty and sixty minutes a day.

A quick note regarding your health—since exercise is so important to your overall success, make sure you are physically ready to begin. According to the President's Council on Physical Fitness and Health, if you are under age thirty-five and in good health, you don't have to see a doctor before beginning an exercise program. However, if you are over thirty-five and have been inactive for several years, you should consult with a doctor.[5] If for any reason you aren't sure how to proceed or have questions about your health, ask your doctor if there are any special concerns that need to be faced before you begin.

BENEFITS OF EXERCISE

There are so many benefits when it comes to exercise. Here are six of the best reasons:

- Exercise helps reduce hidden belly fat, lowering the risk of heart disease, diabetes, stroke, and some types of cancer.[6]
- Exercise prevents muscle from wasting and helps to lose fat.[7]
- Exercise helps the brain deal with stress more effectively.[8]
- Moderate cardiovascular exercise such as thirty minutes of brisk walking a few times a week can improve your memory.[9]
- Exercise helps manage hunger. Research shows that exercising increases control over hunger and food intake. In fact, the physically fit person is often not hungry until several hours after exercise.[10]
- Exercise improves your immune system.[11]

We can't stress this point enough: *when it comes to making exercise a habit, attitude is more than half the battle.* Whatever reasons you have used for avoiding exercise in the past—it's unpleasant, too painful, inconvenient, frustrating, or too time-consuming— the reality is that exercise is necessary if you are serious about being healthy. Regardless of your past experiences, regular physical activity is essential for weight control and developing a healthy lifestyle.

Physical activity increases the number of calories your body uses and promotes the loss of body fat instead of muscle and other nonfat tissue. In addition to promoting weight control, physical activity improves your strength and flexibility, lowers your risk of heart disease, helps control blood pressure and diabetes, can promote a sense of well-being, and can decrease stress.[12]

Finally, it is documented truth that the more sedentary you are, the more likely you are to be overweight. So any activity, however small, is a change in the right direction. Remember to appreciate what you can do, even if you think it's a small amount. Moving any part of your body, even for a short time, can add up to a big difference. And being physically active doesn't have to occur only when you are in sweats and working out at the gym. If money is an issue, cost doesn't have to get in the way. There are many free ways to exercise, either by yourself or with friends. You can find a local school track where you can walk or run, or walk around a mall before the stores open. Parks are a great place to walk or jog, and quite often you can find a time of the day when they are empty if you prefer a little more privacy while you exercise.

Consider smaller day-to-day changes to improve your health over dramatic goals and types of exercise that will not last. Try taking short walking breaks at work a few times a day or marching in place during TV commercials. (Okay, we admit that could be embarrassing, so be careful you don't do it where they might cart you off under the care of mental health workers in white suits!) Taking the stairs instead of the elevator and walking the dog are also good choices. With the convenience of cell phones, walking while catching up with old friends you can't be physically near is now possible, even if you are just pacing around the house!

Parking your vehicle far away from the mall entrance so you can walk the extra distance is another relatively painless choice. If you take the bus or subway to work, get off one stop early and walk! One of the less touted but still very healthy forms of exercise is working around the house—whether you mow the lawn (no riding mowers, please), rake leaves, garden, or spring-clean, you will be moving!

MATCHING EXERCISE WITH WHO YOU ARE

Though you won't be expected to do more than you are capable of doing, exercise is essential to the overall Lose It for Life program. Choose activities that mesh well with who you are and what you like to do, and you'll be more likely to stick to them. And if an activity provides mental relaxation and enjoyment, you'll receive double the benefits! The following quiz will help you identify what activities are a good match for you, based on your personality, workout goals, and schedule. By combining the results of the three parts of this quiz, you'll have figured out your total fitness personality.[13]

What Is My Personality?

Part One: My Personality and Hobbies

(Circle the letter that most represents you.)

1. As a kid, the activities I liked best were:
   a. gymnastics, cheerleading, jump rope, or dance classes.
   b. playing outside—such as building forts or lemonade stands, climbing trees, or exploring the woods.
   c. competitive sports.
   d. playing with dolls, reading, coloring, or art projects.
   e. parties, playing with my friends.

2. My favorite hobbies today are:
   a. anything new and challenging.
   b. outside activities—gardening, walking the dog, watching the stars.
   c. tennis, card or board games, team and/or spectator sports.
   d. reading, movies, needle crafts, painting, or anything that provides an escape.
   e. group activities with friends—participating in a walking club, joining a book group, or just talking.

3. I get motivated to exercise if:
   a. I get a new exercise video or piece of equipment, or I try a new fitness class.
   b. I get a new piece of outside equipment, I discover a new walking or jogging path, or the weather is nice.
   c. I'm presented with some competition.
   d. I find an exercise that I get into to the point that I forget my surroundings.
   e. I exercise in a group.

4. I prefer to exercise:
   a. indoors.
   b. outdoors.
   c. wherever there's a competition.
   d. wherever I am not the center of attention.
   e. in a gym or fitness center, not at home.

Interpreting Your Score (Part One)

If you circled mostly the letter "a" or there is not an emerging pattern within your choices, you are probably a Learner. You're always trying something new and welcome physical and mental challenges. You are most likely an "associative exerciser," meaning you focus on the way your body moves and feels when you exercise. Choose activities that help you explore new moves: aerobics classes, any form of dance, Pilates, seated aerobics, in-line skating, skipping rope, fencing, or any other activity that attracts your interest.

If you circled mostly the letter "b," you would be classified as an Outdoors Person. Fresh air is your energizer. So why not include nature in your exercise routine? Try hiking, biking, nature walking, gardening, swimming laps, or cross-country skiing.

If you circled mostly the letter "c," you are classified as a Competitor. You naturally like one-on-one, competitive types of activities. Try fencing, cardio kickboxing, and spinning classes. If you excelled in or enjoyed a sport when you were younger, take it up again.

If you circled mostly the letter "d," you are classified as Timid. You're a "disassociative exerciser," meaning you fantasize or think of events in your life when you exercise rather than contemplating the exercise itself. You're more like a wallflower than a participant.

You'll like mind/body activities like Pilates and stretching. Also try nature walking or hiking. You'll also probably love exercise classes. Sign up for classes such as aerobics, cardio kickboxing, seated aerobics, spinning, step aerobics, or water aerobics.

If you circled mostly the letter "e," you are classified as a Social Butterfly. As a people-person, you tend to prefer the gym to exercising in your living room. Try aerobics classes, kickboxing, seated aerobics, spinning classes, stretching, step aerobics, and water aerobics. For weight lifting, find a buddy or two and do circuit training.

Part Two: My Workout Style and Goals

(Circle the letter that most represents you.)

1. My primary exercise goal is:
   a. to lose weight or tone up.
   b. to relax and relieve stress.
   c. to have fun.
   d. depends on how I feel.

2. I prefer:
   a. a lot of structure in my workout.
   b. some structure, but not too much.
   c. no structure.
   d. depends on my mood.

3. I prefer to exercise:
   a. alone.
   b. with one other person.
   c. in a group.
   d. depends on my mood.

Interpreting Your Score (Part Two)

If you circled mostly the letter "a" or a mixture of letters, you're classified as a Gung-Ho Exerciser. You don't mess around when you work out. You're there to lose weight and tone up—period. You'll benefit most from doing a specific activity, like cycling, aerobics, or using an elliptical machine, treadmill, or stair climber, at a moderate intensity. For optimal weight loss benefits, you should burn 2,000 calories a week. One way to achieve this would be to perform thirty minutes of aerobic-based exercise daily, combined with three sessions of weight training per week.

If you circled mostly the letter "b," you would be classified as a Leisurely Exerciser. Your main exercise objectives are to relax and de-stress. To relax, try stretching. Studies have shown a direct relationship between physical activity and stress reduction. Hop on the treadmill or head outside and walk for five minutes, run slowly for thirty seconds, and then run fast for thirty seconds, repeating this sequence for about thirty minutes. Circuit weight training is another great interval workout. You do all your reps; then you rest; then you do a few more, and then you rest.

If you circled mostly the letter "c," you are classified as a Fun-Loving Exerciser. Fifty straight minutes on the treadmill is not your bag—there's no room in your fun-filled life. You'll be most likely to stick to activities that are already an integral part of your schedule. Grab your in-line skates and circle the neighborhood. Put on your favorite music CD and dance around the living room. And you can make your weight routine more amusing by doing circuit weight training.

If you circled mostly the letter "d," you are classified as a Flexible Exerciser. Exercise turns you on, but routine doesn't. You'd rather fly by the seat of your gym shorts, which is fine. To add variety, use the elliptical machine one day, the treadmill the next, and the cross-country skiing machine the next.

Part Three: My Lifestyle and Schedule

(Circle the letter that most represents you.)

1. I have the most energy:
   a. in the morning.
   b. in the middle of the day.
   c. in the evening or at night.
   d. my energy level fluctuates.

2. I have the most time:
   a. in the morning.
   b. in the middle of the day.
   c. in the evening.
   d. depends on the day.

3. I'm most likely to:
   a. go to bed early and get up early.
   b. go to bed and get up at the same time every day, but not particularly early or late.
   c. go to bed late and get up late.
   d. depends on the day.

Interpreting Your Score (Part Three)

If you circled mostly the letter "a" or a mixture of letters, you're classified as a Morning Dove. You like to get chores out of the way as soon as you get up because that's when you have the most energy. Whether you go to the gym before you start your day or head outside for a dawn walk, you'll have an extra edge over those who hit the snooze button a few more times.

If you circled mostly the letter "b," you would be classified as a Midday Duck. You'd rather plop down on an exercise bike than in front of a sandwich when noon rolls around. Whether you're at home or work, exercise is a great way to break up your day.

If you circled mostly the letter "c," you are classified as a Night Owl. You haven't seen a sunrise since that all-night party in 1974. If you have more energy at night, use that time to exercise. Just don't do it too close to bedtime, or you'll have trouble sleeping.

If you circled mostly the letter "d," you are classified as a Flexible Bird. The best time of day for you to exercise varies with your schedule. So just go with it and don't try to set yourself up with an intense schedule. But do push yourself to exercise as often as possible!

SAFETY TIPS

Drink Plenty of Water

Whenever you exercise, make hydrating your body a priority. Water is beneficial to every cell and organ in your body. It cushions your joints, improves your bowel functions, and keeps your body cool. Drink it before, during, and after exercise.

Pay Attention to Your Body During Exercise

If you become out of breath while exercising, slow down. You should be able to talk while you exercise and not be gasping for air. Do not ignore pain or discomfort when you exercise, as you could do harm to your body. If you notice any of the following signs,[14] stop exercising immediately and contact your health-care provider:

- Shortness of breath
- Pain or pressure in the midchest area, left side of your neck, left shoulder, or left arm
- Dizziness or nausea
- Breaking out in a cold sweat
- Muscle cramps or pain in your joints, feet, ankles, or legs

Wear Appropriate Clothing

When you exercise, it helps to wear clothes that are lightweight and loose-fitting so you can move easily. Wear supportive athletic shoes for weight-bearing activities. And when your shoes need to be replaced, don't put it off. If you are a woman, a good support bra is an essential piece of workout equipment. For all clothing, choose fabrics that absorb sweat and remove it from the skin. Never wear rubber or plastic suits, as these could hold the sweat on your skin and make your body overheat.

When exercising outdoors, wear a knit hat to keep you warm in cold weather. A baseball cap is a good choice when the weather is hot in order to shade your face and keep you cool. And don't forget the sunscreen when you venture outside!

It Gets Easier with Time

If you still feel a bit overwhelmed by adding exercise to your daily routine, this journal entry from Cathy may motivate you. She hated to exercise. It hurt! And the embarrassment was almost too much to bear, but she really wanted to Lose It for Life.

> I am down to 272. That is 78 pounds gone forever! I am doing a lot better on my softball team. I am the catcher. About a month ago, I could barely squat down to catch the pitch. And once I was down, I hated to have to stand back up. I actually got dizzy and saw stars because I was so out of shape. I would basically stay down unless I absolutely had to get up to get the ball.
>
> Things have definitely changed for the better! I played a doubleheader last Thursday night and another doubleheader on Friday. I can now squat down for every pitch, and I quickly stand back up to throw the ball back to the pitcher. I love it! I feel like a regular person, athletic and all! I received comments and hugs from the other players—they said I was the best catcher our team has ever had, and they said they're proud of me for sticking with it.

THE FIRST STEP

Consistent exercise will take commitment. Don't be afraid of that word, however. You can do this with God's help and the help of others. Success is at the end of many tasks, like healthy eating, getting enough sleep, and spending time with the Lord each day. Boundaries and accountability are necessary.

We take care of ourselves by setting boundaries with our time and energy so that there is time for the priorities, such as healthy eating and exercising. Decide that your fitness, nutrition, spiritual, and personal time are nonnegotiable. This means exercising should not be the first thing you take out of your schedule if life's "stuff" gets in the way. Make every effort to stay with your routine. There is grace for those times when we allow life to crowd out our personal commitments, but we must make it a priority to get back on track and make time for exercise.

If you do not carve out time for your physical, spiritual, and personal needs, you will burn out, bum out, and bail out by acting out. Overeating, overworking, drinking, anger, depression, worry, and anxiety are all symptoms of burnout. Create good habits and routines for exercise, nutrition, and spiritual and personal time so you won't burn out.

Check Your Heart Rate

Pace yourself. Remember to slow down if you're too out of breath to carry on a conversation. Before you begin, you should know how to take your heart rate. It's a great measure of intensity during aerobic exercise.

Your resting heart rate can be taken after sitting quietly for five minutes. Count your pulse for 10 seconds and multiply that number by six to get your heart's per-minute rate. For example, if your resting heart rate for 10 seconds is 13 beats, your heart's per-minute rate is 78 (13 x 6 = 78). When you exercise, check your pulse rate five seconds after interrupting your activity. Your target heart rate is calculated by taking the maximum heart rate and multiplying it by 70 percent. Your maximum heart rate is figured by taking 220 minus your age.[15] For example, if you are 40 years old, your maximum heart rate is 180 (220 − 40 = 180). Then multiply 180 by 70% to arrive at your target heart rate of 126 beats per minute (180 x 70% = 126). In order to really benefit from exercising, you should raise your heart rate and sustain it at your target heart rate for 12 to 15 minutes. So, if you're 40 years old, you should exercise in a manner that will keep your heart rate at 126 beats per minute for 12 to 15 minutes. The goal is to maintain 55 to 85 percent of your maximum heart rate for 20 to 60 minutes.

The more intense the workout, the shorter it needs to be (but not less than 20 minutes).

If you find yourself unable to exercise consistently, you need more accountability! Find someone who has the discipline you're lacking and ask him or her to help you. Draw help from this person and make the most of his or her presence and encouragement to provide the structure you need until you are able to provide it for yourself. As you begin a new exercise program, start slowly. Your body needs time to get used to your new activity. Fitness doesn't happen overnight. Be patient and give the process time to work.

We suggest setting short- and long-term goals for your exercise routine. If you have difficulty exercising, a good short-term goal may be to walk for five minutes at least two days per week for two weeks. A long-term goal may be to walk forty minutes most days of the week after nine months. Writing down your progress in a journal is an excellent way to track goals and stay on track. Though you may not feel like you are making progress within a given week, when you look back at where you started, you may be pleasantly surprised!

As was stressed earlier, support is a key factor in staying motivated. An exercise buddy can cheer you on and hold you accountable. For women in particular, it's a good way to feel safe while exercising outdoors.

ESTABLISH A ROUTINE

The goal is to find whatever is necessary—tools, books, therapists, or personal trainers—to help you establish a routine you can do for the rest of your life. If you approach a routine with this mind-set, finding a pace that is workable will be easier and you will be more likely to stick with it. Don't give up if you miss a few days. Just pick up where you left off and jump right back into the routine.

Five Keys to Success in Your Exercise Program

1. **Make exercise convenient**. Try to fit it into your lunch hour or even while you're watching TV. Just get started and remind yourself of what you hope to gain.
2. **Make it fun**. There is nothing worse than being bored or hating what you are doing. Find something you enjoy. If you like to play tennis, do that. If walking is your thing, walk every chance you get. Rollerblade with your children, hike with a friend, or get out your bike and start riding around your neighborhood.
3. **Enjoy variety**. Mix it up. You don't have to walk every day! You can take a bike ride one day, walk the next, and Rollerblade in the park the third day.
4. **Add music to the routine**. Listening to music may make exercising more enjoyable, and it often adds extra motivation to a workout. Choose your favorite tunes and see if the addition doesn't liven up your workout.
5. **Exercise with a partner or friend**. As was mentioned above, a partner can provide accountability and encouragement. When you commit to someone else, you have added motivation to make the time and fulfill your commitment, but you also add fun! If you prefer a solo workout, that's fine too. Just decide what works best for you and get moving.

Warm-ups and Cool-downs[16]

It's important to warm up and cool down for at least five minutes as part of your routine. Warming up slowly increases your heart rate, getting more blood to your muscles to ready them for your workout. A cool-down allows your heart to slow down gradually. Your warm-up and cool-down don't have to be complicated. They merely involve going a little more slowly than usual. For example, if you're walking, start at a leisurely pace for five to six minutes and then pick up the pace by pumping your arms.

A cool-down should be built into your routine to slow down little by little. If you've been walking fast, walk slower to cool down. Stretching for a few minutes at the end of a workout is also a good idea. Research suggests that cooling down may protect your heart, relax your muscles, and keep you from getting hurt.

Incorporate Three Types of Exercise

To keep from getting into a rut, purposefully integrate different components of exercise. Variety is the secret to a solid fitness program. We recommend incorporating three components into your program:

1. **Alternate aerobic exercises**. Aerobic exercise burns body fat. Work your muscles differently by integrating more than one aerobic exercise into your routine. All of these aerobic activities can be alternated on any given day: walking, biking, jogging, tennis, or swimming.

    For aerobic exercise, use this routine:

    1. Warm up for about five minutes.
    2. Slowly increase your pace until you reach your target heart zone.
    3. Sustain this zone for twelve to fifteen minutes.
    4. Keep moving in some way or other for ten more minutes.
    5. Cool down for about five minutes.
    6. Slowly decrease your pace and bring your body back to a resting level.
    7. Then stretch the muscles you used for at least three minutes.

2. **Strength training**. Strength training builds strong muscles and bones. To do this, you can exercise at home or a gym or fitness center. Hand weights or even two soup cans are fine for a beginner. Weight training strengthens and tones muscles, and it slows bone loss and builds bone density. Other benefits include improved flexibility and mobility, more controlled blood pressure, and a decrease in lower back, arthritic, and joint pain. We recommend strength training two to three days per week. Target each of the following areas of your body with strength-training exercise: arms, chest, shoulders, abs, back, buttocks, thighs, and calves.

If you are a beginner, use dumbbells rather than barbells. Begin with one hand at a time in order to get a more balanced workout. If you are strength training for fitness, do ten to twelve repetitions (reps) of each exercise for each major muscle group. If you desire to bulk up, do more sets (a set is a series of reps that are done in succession), or use heavier weights and decrease your reps. To provide variety, vary your program for strength training by using free weights one day, resistance bands another day, and machines at the gym a third day.

Always make sure you know the correct posture for the strength-training exercise and that your movements are slow and controlled. It is important to use a weight you can lift at least ten times, but no more than twelve times without tiring. If you can't do an exercise eight times in a row, your weights are too heavy. If it is easy to do the exercise twelve times in a row, your weights are too light.

3. Stretching. Stretching is easy to do yet has many benefits. It can improve your flexibility, blood flow, range of motion, and strength, as well as prevent your muscles from getting tight after doing other exercises. Stretching also relieves tension and stress. It's a great exercise in that you don't have to set aside a special time or place for it. Whether you're at home or at work, you can stand up, push your arms toward the ceiling, and stretch. Stretch slowly and only enough to feel tightness, not pain. If it starts to hurt, stop stretching before the stretch reflex is activated, which causes your muscles to contract instead of extending.

But you shouldn't stretch cold muscles, so do a few warm-ups first. Within your exercise routine, try to include stretching for ten minutes, at least three to five days a week. Repeat each stretch three to five times. Before you begin each exercise, exhale; then relax into the stretch. Hold the stretch for up to thirty seconds—less if you are new to stretching or start to feel uncomfortable. The next section lists stretches to target the various muscles of the body:

Basic Stretches

Neck. In either a standing or sitting position, ease your right ear toward your right shoulder. Gently lower your left shoulder. Slowly move your head closer to your right shoulder with your right hand. Release and then do the other side. When you are finished, shrug your shoulders, hold, and release.

Face forward. Turn your head slowly to the right and stop at the point of resistance. Hold. Gradually bring your head back to the middle. Repeat this head movement toward the left. After you have finished, lower your chin to your chest. Keep your shoulders back. Hold and release.

Shoulders. In either a standing or sitting position, extend your right arm straight across your chest. With your left hand, pull your right elbow into your chest. Hold and release. Then switch arms and repeat.

Next, raise one arm straight up over your head. Stretch it as far as you can without bending your body. Turn the palm of your hand upward and push toward the ceiling several times. Release and repeat with your other arm. For a greater stretching movement, bend to the left at your waist as you reach with your right arm. Hold, release, and switch sides and repeat.

Triceps. In either a standing or sitting position, reach your right arm up behind your head as if to scratch the upper center of your back. (Your arm makes an inverted V by your ear.) Reach over your head with your left hand and slowly lower your right elbow. Hold and release. Switch your arms and repeat.

Biceps. With the palm of your hand up, extend your right arm out in front of you. Using your left hand, take the fingers of your right hand and pull them toward the floor. You'll want to keep your right arm straight in front of you, parallel to the floor. Switch arms and repeat.

Forearms. In a standing or sitting position, extend your right arm out in front of you, placing your palm down. With your other hand, take the fingers of your right hand and pull them slowly toward your shoulder. Hold and release. Switch arms and repeat.

Chest. Standing tall, clasp your hands behind your back. Squeeze your shoulder blades toward each other and lift your chest up and out. If you can, raise your hands and arms. It's important to keep your lower back from arching. Hold, release, and repeat.

Standing in a doorway, rest your right forearm against the doorframe. Bend your right arm in a 90-degree angle at the elbow. Slowly lean forward until you feel a comfortable stretch in your chest muscles. Hold and release. Repeat on the other side.

Back. Lie on your back with your legs extended. Clasping your right knee with your hands, slowly pull it toward your chest as far as you can without feeling discomfort. Hold. Slowly release. Switch legs and repeat. When you are finished, hug both knees to your chest. Hold and release.

Get on your hands and knees with your face and eyes looking forward. Exhale slowly while you allow your head to sag slowly toward the floor. At the same time, arch your back toward the ceiling. Hold in your stomach muscles. Hold and then release, bringing your back to the original position.

To stretch your upper back, extend your arms in front of you at shoulder height while in a standing or sitting position. Clasp your fingers together. Lower your head and turn the palms of your hands out. Round your shoulders and back, extending your arms out even farther. Hold and release.

To stretch the muscles that run alongside your back, stand up and place your feet shoulder-width apart. Link your fingers together and turn your palms upward, reaching toward the ceiling. Slowly bend to one side. Hold, and then return to the middle. Repeat on the other side.

Calves. In a standing position, extend your arms in front of you. Put your hands shoulder-width apart on a wall. Move back a couple of feet. Keeping your legs straight and your feet and heels on the floor, lean into the wall. Hold and release.

Stand on a step. Hold onto a railing or the back of a chair and allow your heels to hang off the edge of the step, lower than the position of your toes. Rise up on your toes slowly and hold for several seconds. Then slowly lower your weight onto your heels.

Ankles. Sitting on a chair, extend your legs in front of you with your feet one or two inches off the ground. Flex your ankles and feet toward you and hold. Then slowly point your toes and feet downward away from you and hold. Release.

INCREASING THE ROUTINE

To continue making headway in your exercise program, eventually you will need to increase the frequency, intensity, and length of workout time. Exercising a little harder each week enables you to improve without spending more time working out. If you want to lose weight and boost your cardio-endurance, increase both the frequency and the duration of your workouts.

For the greatest overall health benefits, experts recommend twenty to thirty minutes of vigorous physical activity, such as aerobic dancing, brisk walking, or swimming three or more times a week, and some type of muscle strengthening activity, such as weight resistance or stretching at least twice a week. However, if you are unable to do this level of activity, you can improve your health by performing thirty minutes or more of moderate-intensity physical activity over the course of a day at least five times each week.[17] Such activity would include walking up stairs, walking all or part of the way to work, using a push mower to cut grass, or playing an active game with children.

Any type of physical activity you choose to do, be they vigorous activities such as running or aerobic dancing, or moderate-intensity activities such as walking or household work, will increase the number of calories your body uses. The key to successful weight control and improved overall health is to make physical activity a part of your daily life.

Research has shown that little bursts of activity throughout the day can increase your calorie burn up to a startling 500 calories or more per day.[18] These little bursts are simple and easy. Try to get up once every hour for a one- or two-minute burst of activity.

- Do standing squats as you blow-dry or curl your hair.
- Pace or march in place while you talk on the phone.
- Take the stairs whenever possible.
- Squeeze your buttock muscles and zip up your abs as you stand in line at the grocery store or while manning the fax machine.

Seven Cardio Workouts That Burn Fat Fast

If you'd like to step up your workout and burn more calories, try these seven ideas for a cardio workout:

1. Bicycling

Calorie burn per fifteen minutes:
Road biking, 136; trail or mountain biking, 145

Did you like to ride a bicycle as a kid? If so, you may want to try road or trail cycling. Cycling is a great no-impact to low-impact activity to help burn calories. Do it long enough and intensely enough in order to keep your heart rate in the fat-burning zone. For rougher terrain, you may want to try a mountain bike. These bikes have wider tires and are heavy. You can also buy a larger seat for your bike to avoid becoming sore. Make sure the bike you buy has a weight rating at least as high as your own weight.

Bicycling enables you to get outdoors and explore your neighborhood and area parks. It's also a great way to get around when you're on vacation. Many cities feature bicycle trails that protect cyclists from traffic. And mountain or trail riding is a great activity to get in touch with nature, but do stay on trails for your safety.

Whether you take to the road or the trail is your decision. Riding on roads will give you a more predictable, steady workout with fewer bumps and unexpected turns, but you will have to deal with traffic. Trail riding offers the potential for a greater workout for your upper body as you maneuver through uneven terrain and bumps.

Be cautious your first time out: be sure you know where you are located so that you can make it back. Use good form to avoid stiffness. When cycling, regularly arch and round your back as you ride. When gripping the handlebar, keep your elbows unlocked. Keeping a loose grip will also keep you from having tingling hands.

2. Cardio kickboxing

Calorie burn per fifteen minutes: 170

Do you want a fun way to relieve fat-generating stress while getting a great workout that burns those calories and tones your major muscles at the same time? Cardio kickboxing provides a positive format to help you release tension and aggression. Because kickboxing is not about kicking higher or punching harder than everyone else, it can easily be modified to suit your needs. The old adage of "no pain, no gain" simply does not apply to this form of exercise. You will finish sessions feeling better both mentally and physically.

Give your body a chance to get used to the movements, even if you're a seasoned exerciser. "Keep your kicks low and don't punch with a lot of intensity," says one instructor certified by the American Council on Exercise. "Listen to your body. If you are tired, take a break. If you get thirsty, drink some water. If you feel discomfort, stop. It's important to pace yourself, but do challenge yourself during the workout."

If you leave class early, remember to cool down and stretch on your own. Kickboxing classes provide a warm-up with a stretch as well as twenty to forty minutes of cardio work that includes kicking and punching drills. Some classes will also have running and skipping, which can be modified by marching in place. Music is a driving force in many cardio kickboxing workouts. Some instructors may be open to you suggesting songs or certain styles of music. The variety within this form of exercise, as well as personal enjoyment, will help you stay with your program.

3. Dancing

Calorie burn per fifteen minutes: jitterbug and tap, 80; country and western, disco, Irish step, line, swing, and flamenco, 75; cha-cha, 50

Do you love to dance the night away? You'll be pleasantly surprised to learn that you burn fifty or more calories for every fifteen minutes you do the cha-cha or the bump. Some forms of dancing burn more calories than others. Slower dances like waltzes can burn up to fifty calories while jazz dancing can burn more than eighty calories for the same fifteen-minute span.

If you're worried about not being able to keep up with the rest of your dance class, feel free to stand back and watch. One dance instructor comments, "Standing behind someone who seems to know what they're doing is a great trick. In a dance class, you're very dependent on the people who are a little more advanced than you."

Before you begin to dance, breathe deeply and shrug off the worries of the day. Mastering the moves will enable you to begin to improvise, create your own movements, and be more expressive. With dance, there are no limits! Choose from any number of ethnic styles or traditional forms to find a form that's right for you.

4. Hiking

Calorie burn per fifteen minutes: 120

You can soothe your soul and burn those calories at the same time by hitting the trail. There's nothing like being surrounded by trees and chirping birds to help you forget that you're burning calories as you walk. If you are a beginner, try a well-traveled, level trail. Have the right footwear, hat, and sunscreen handy. And don't forget to stretch when you finish.

Turn your hike into a special occasion by bringing along a picnic lunch. Relax and enjoy the scenery. There are endless trails that allow you to hike up mountains, along rivers, and even through city parks. Give yourself permission to go at a slower pace if necessary. You are exercising, and whether you walk a little slower for a period of time is irrelevant—what's important is the fact that you are outside and moving around!

5. In-line skating

Calorie burn per fifteen minutes: 84–119, depending on intensity

Zoom off the calories! Tone your troubled spots! You can cover a lot of ground fast with in-line skating. However, just learning how to use the skates is good exercise. It takes a lot of energy to do it correctly when you are a beginner. Take a little extra time and be sure you know how to use the heel brakes on the skates. If you are just starting out, find an empty parking lot with a smooth, level surface. Your neighborhood roads can be quite bumpy, which may cause your shins to hurt. Master the basics and then try a squatting position, or use long, graceful strides, which will make in-line skating feel more like ice-skating than roller-skating. Try going uphill for an even greater burn and overall workout.

6. Swimming laps

Calorie burn per fifteen minutes: 136

Swimming laps is the best choice for a total-body workout and stress reducer. Unlike other activities, water workouts exercise both the upper and lower body. And because of the buoyancy of the water, water exercise doesn't stress your joints the way other activities do. You can bend and move your body in water in ways you can't on land. Swimming is an ideal exercise if you're overweight or recovering from an injury.

To find a pool near you, check out your local YMCA or community center. Also, if you don't want to fight for lane space during your first few sessions, ask when the pool is least crowded. Don't be discouraged if you can do only one or two laps at first. Swim as long as you comfortably can, rest for a few minutes, and then start swimming again. In time, you'll be able to swim farther and longer. Because doing the same stroke lap after lap can get boring, try the breaststroke, freestyle, backstroke, and even the sidestroke for variety and an enjoyable swimming workout.

If you haven't yet learned to swim, you should know that it isn't necessary to know how to swim in order to work out in water. You can do shallow-water exercises without swimming. Just make sure the water level is between your waist and your chest. If the water is too shallow, it will be hard to move your arms underwater. If the water is too deep, it will be hard to keep your feet touching the pool bottom.

7. Step aerobics

Calorie burn per fifteen minutes: 102, depending on your weight

Strengthen and tone your leg and bun muscles while burning calories with step aerobics. You step on and off a platform about two or three feet long that rests on the floor or atop one or more risers. Once you learn the basic moves—getting on and off the platform, over, and across it, you are ready for routines led by an instructor. If you're a beginner, start with a platform height of four to six inches. If your knees are bent more than 90 degrees, your step is too high.

Focus on the arm movements after you have the steps down. Keep your neck and back straight, shoulders back, pelvis tucked, abdominal muscles pulled in, and chest lifted. Lean from your ankles when stepping onto the platform. The music and the group interaction provide extra stimulus for sticking with this form of exercise.

Try Walking

If the above seven options sound a bit too strenuous, there is always walking. Walking is a great form of exercise and something most people can do. Do light stretching before and after you walk, and warm up with five minutes of slow walking. Increase your speed for the next five or more minutes. Then cool down by walking slowly for the last five minutes. Make sure you stand up straight, lift your rib cage, and look straight ahead (but keep your shoulders relaxed). This will let your spine curve in a natural, healthy position. Swing your arms and move at a steady pace. This will also help keep your fingers from swelling.

Walking should be enjoyable. Try walking with a friend or pet, and walk in places you enjoy, like a park or shopping mall. Your walking partner(s) should be able to walk with you on the same schedule and at the same speed. If possible, walk at least three times per week, and add two to three minutes per week to the fast walk. If you walk less than three times per week, increase the fast walk segment more slowly. Over time, make it a goal to walk faster, farther, and for longer periods of time. The more you walk, the better you will feel, and the more calories you will burn.

When you walk, always think about safety. Walk in the daytime or at night in well-lit areas. We recommend walking with another person or in a group, especially at night. You can even notify your local police station of your group's walking time and route, if you desire. Become aware of your surroundings and leave headphones off. And leave your jewelry at home![19]

A Common Problem for Walkers—Heel Pain

It's an annoying reality that all walkers face one day. The older you get, the more likely you are to experience the stabbing heel pain known as plantar fasciitis. That's because, as you grow older, the ligaments in your foot stretch and lose some of their supportive quality. Your foot can then overpronate (lean inward) more easily, stretching tissues on the sole of your foot beyond their

---

normal length. Over time, this tissue (called plantar fascia) becomes inflamed and sometimes even tears, causing pain.[20]

Taking anti-inflammatory medication or simply waiting for the pain to subside on its own won't solve the problem and could, in fact, lead to a more serious injury that may take months to heal. Here are four steps you can take now to stop the throbbing.

1. **Replace your walking shoes before they wear out.** Buy shoes at least every 300 miles (or four or five months) if you walk around fifteen miles per week.
2. **Be sure to stretch.** Tight calf muscles create additional pressure on the tissues under the foot. Get in the habit of stretching regularly before and after your walks. Start by standing about eighteen inches from a wall with your palms on the wall. Extend your right leg back about two feet, and bend your left knee. Keep your right leg straight, pressing your right heel into the ground. Your toes should be pointing forward. Hold for fifteen seconds, and then switch legs. If you experience heel soreness, stretch ten times with each leg, twice a day.
3. **Curb your walks.** If supportive shoes or inserts ease your discomfort (ask for help at your local sports store), then it's fine to continue walking. Just avoid hills or roads that are sloped toward the shoulder. But if your pain is severe, you may have to take time off. Check with your doctor to see if cycling, swimming, or another activity might be a good substitute for your walks.
4. **See a podiatrist or orthopedic specialist.** If you don't notice any improvement within one or two weeks, you should see a doctor.

For some of you, exercise will be your biggest challenge. When you are overweight, exercise is difficult because it physically hurts the body to move all that weight around. Part of the work will be finding movement that isn't painful—like water aerobics, or exercises that don't put pressure on the joints.

We know it's embarrassing to go to a public pool to do aquatic exercise. Putting on a bathing suit in public is not for the fainthearted. Several years ago however, something terrific happened in my community that gave me (Dr. Linda) renewed hope regarding this issue. As I pulled together a multidisciplinary team of health-care providers to work with my obese clients, I listened to the pain, embarrassment, and shame they faced when they tried to exercise. The exercise physiologist on our team responded with a wonderful plan.

We negotiated with a local YMCA for a private room to lead exercise classes. These classes would not be open to the public—only to my clients, but at a much reduced fee. The instructor led the classes in a way that minimized their physical pain yet slowly but steadily got the group moving. In the privacy of that room, organized exercise was finally a fun option. We also set up private hours for use of the swimming pool. In the water, movement was so much easier on their bodies.

I can't tell you how grateful these clients were for the opportunity to exercise without feeling humiliated. They cried, we cried, and the weight began to drop off. Because a few people cared enough to be empathetic and support people with a particular need, these hurting people found healing.

Every one of those clients wanted to make changes, but embarrassment had kept them from trying. Please don't allow negative past experiences to stop you from doing what is in your heart to do. You can be victorious in this journey. God knows your physical and emotional pain and isn't judging you, and there are people who can and will support you in this endeavor.

As you begin to exercise, you may encounter people who don't understand and who may judge you. Yet God sees and knows what you are going through. As Paul admonishes us in Philippians 3:13–14, "Forgetting those things which are behind and reaching forward to those things which are ahead, [we] press toward the goal" (NKJV). Don't focus on what you can't do or how others may perceive you. Instead, reflect on each small step you make and recognize those steps for what they are—individual acts of courage.

Exercise isn't an option if you want to reap the benefits of a healthy life. Whatever your pleasure, there is an activity that is right for you, but it's up to you to find that exercise and to get moving. Whether it's walking, aerobics, weight lifting, stretching, or even taking the stairs instead of the elevator, each small change will make a difference in your health, weight maintenance, and mental health. So get motivated and get moving so you can Lose It for Life!

Workbook Week 6

MOVE IT *AND* LOSE IT

DAY 1
Exercise 101—Do We Have To?

You've heard the saying, "Move it or lose it!" We'd like to alter that a bit to say, "Move it *and* lose it." The more you move your body, the more calories you'll burn and the more fat you'll lose. Exercise may never turn you into an Olympian, but it is a huge part of shedding excess weight and keeping it off. That's our focus in these five sessions.

If exercise sounds like torture to you, don't worry! We are convinced you can find physical activities that you really enjoy.

LOOKING AT YOUR *LIFE*

Begin by examining your attitude toward exercise. Check all the statements that are true of you.

_____ I absolutely *detest* the thought of exercise.

_____ It's tough for me to find the time to exercise.

_____ I frankly don't like to sweat.

_____ I have had some negative exercise experiences in my life.

_____ I'd rather chill out on the couch than engage in physical activities.

_____ Give me the elevator over the stairs any day!

_____ I always fail in my commitments to exercise.

_____ Most of my friends and family are sedentary.

_____ I need to lose weight first—then I'll exercise.

_____ Even a brief walk or small bit of exertion wears me out.

How many check marks do you have? _____

Now evaluate yourself against this scale:

    0–2—**Awesome! You are knocking on the door of great success!**

    3–5—**With just a few minor attitude adjustments, you'll be burning some serious calories!**

    6–10—**Time to think long and hard about some serious questions:** Do you really want to continue living an unhealthy existence of being overweight and tired all the time and living a life that revolves around food? Aren't you hungry for a richer, fuller, happier lifestyle? Wouldn't you rather be "weightless," that is, free from the trap of fat, feeling fit, and finding joy in the Lord rather than in food?

LEARNING A NEW WAY OF *LIFE*

Philippians 4:8 says, "Finally, brothers and sisters, whatever is true, whatever is noble, whatever is right, whatever is pure, whatever is lovely, whatever is admirable—if anything is excellent or praiseworthy—think about such things."

If exercise is good and right for us, how might the verse above apply to our approach to it?

_____

_____

How does your thinking regarding exercise need to change?

_____

_____

We've already applied the RISE formula (Reduce, Increase, Substitute, and Eliminate) to eating. Now let's apply it to exercise. Give some specific examples in each of the following:

When it comes to exercise, I need to reduce . . .

_____

_____

When it comes to exercise, I need to increase . . .

_____

_____

When it comes to exercise, I need to substitute . . .

_____

_____

When it comes to exercise, I need to eliminate . . .

_____

_____

LOSING IT FOR *LIFE*

According to the book, is it better to have several short bursts of exercise daily or longer, once-a-day physical exertions? What's the optimal amount of exercise daily?

_____

_____

Your attitude toward exercising matters. Consider it as important as the food you put in your mouth. Exercise isn't optional in Lose It for Life.

What are the implications of this research as you look at your personal schedule?

_____

_____

List some of the benefits of exercise cited in the *Lose It for Life* book. Which of these facts surprise you the most? Which of these benefits would you most like to see in your life?

_____

_____

We find time—or *make* time—for the things we value and consider important. How can you adjust your schedule so that you can begin exercising on a regular basis?

_____

_____

What would you say to friends who made the following arguments about exercising?

- "Thanks, but I'm going to lose weight by simply dieting."

_____

_____

- "I walked consistently for two weeks and didn't see any results!"

_____

_____

- "Running around the block? Getting on an exercise bike? Exercise is boring!"

_____

_____

- "I don't have time to exercise!"

_____

- "Nobody will exercise with me, and I just can't do it by myself!"

_____

_____

- "Aerobics? Are you kidding? I get winded if I walk to the mailbox!"

_____

_____

- "Money's tight right now—I can't afford a health-club membership."

_____

_____

If you are over thirty-five and have been inactive for several years, you should consult with a doctor first.[21]

Simple (and Sensible) Strategies

Maybe you haven't exercised in years. Maybe a simple stroll around the block wears you out. Maybe you can't afford a health-club membership. Not to worry. Don't let any of that discourage you! You can do this. By God's grace and with common sense and a little effort, you can begin the process of shaping up. That's the focus of this lesson.

LOOKING AT YOUR *LIFE*

Think back to when you were a child. What were you favorite activities? What active games did you play? Which ones were you good at?

_____

_____

What organized sports did you play?

_____

_____

What kind of chores and jobs were you assigned around the house?

_____

_____

If nothing were stopping you (money, being overweight, and so forth), what sport or recreational pursuit would you like to participate in? Why?

_____

_____

Circle the following descriptions that apply to you. "I'm more motivated to exercise . . ."

First thing in the morning	Midday	Afternoon	After work/Evening
By myself With others	Against others (that is, in competitive situations)		
Inside Outside	At a health club		
If the activity is purposeful If the activity is mindless If I buy some new video or exercise equipment			
If the activity is new	If the activity is something I'm good at		

Why is it important to understand yourself, your likes, dislikes, and passions when trying to create an exercise regimen?

_____

_____

LEARNING A NEW WAY OF _LIFE_

Any worthwhile endeavor takes time, and we have to start where we are. Whether you are 25 or 250 pounds overweight, so be it. Your weight is what it is—but not for long. We're going to get you moving. And you're going to learn to like it, because in time you're going to start feeling better and looking better.

The laws of physics tell us, "A body at rest tends to remain at rest; a body in motion tends to remain in motion." Why is that worth mentioning here? What's the point?

_____

_____

"The longest journey begins with the first step" (Chinese proverb).

In the book of Proverbs, a "sluggard" is a person with no discipline or motivation, in short, a foolish failure. He or she is lazy in every way—mentally, spiritually, morally, financially, and so forth. A sluggard takes the path of least resistance. Some descriptive examples:

- "How long will you lie there, you sluggard? When will you get up from your sleep?" (Proverbs 6:9).
- "Lazy hands make for poverty, but diligent hands bring wealth" (Proverbs 10:4).
- "As a door turns on its hinges, so a sluggard turns on his bed. A sluggard buries his hand in the dish; he is too lazy to bring it back to his mouth" (Proverbs 26:14–15).
- "A sluggard's appetite is never filled, but the desires of the diligent are fully satisfied" (Proverbs 13:4).
- "The way of the sluggard is blocked with thorns, but the path of the upright is a highway" (Proverbs 15:19).

What is the overall picture painted here? Do you *like* being around this kind of person? Do you *want* to be a sluggish, aimless individual, existing and not accomplishing anything?

_____

_____

Laziness is often a primary reason we fail to exercise. What other reasons might we have for not engaging in physical activity?

_____

_____

Choose physical activities that mesh well with who you are and what you like to do. You'll be more likely to stick to them.

LOSING IT FOR *LIFE*

Exercise is much broader than what you do in a health club or something that requires special equipment. In all sorts of ingenious, simple ways, we can move our bodies and burn calories daily. The *LIFL* book listed some creative examples of this: getting up to change the TV channel instead of using a remote, getting off the bus or subway one stop early and walking the rest of the way, walking around while you talk on the cordless phone, and so forth.

Think for a few moments about your everyday life. Brainstorm ten ways to avoid becoming an inactive couch potato, to begin moving and speed up the old metabolism.

_____

_____

_____

_____

_____

What sorts of activities would be ideal for a person who likes new things, new physical and/or mental challenges?

_____

_____

What kind of workout regimen would you recommend for a person who gets bored easily or hates too much routine and structure? Why?

_____

_____

What are the pros and cons of exercising early in the morning? At lunch? In the evening?

_____

_____

_____

What are your conclusions at the end of this lesson?

_____

_____

If you're an outdoorsy type person, include nature in your exercise routine. Try hiking, biking, nature walking, gardening, lap swimming, or cross-country skiing.

DAY 3
Safety Reminders

Here's what you *don't* need—deciding to get active only to injure yourself (a pulled muscle, a strained back, and so forth). This puts you in worse shape than before you started to Lose It for Life! The object of this lesson is to look at some basic safeguards for exercise success.

LOOKING AT YOUR *LIFE*

Don't focus on what you can't do. Don't worry about how others may perceive you. Instead, ask God for courage and then do something.

What's your all-time worst exercise or sports injury? What is your "Achilles' heel" (a vulnerable or weak spot) when it comes to physical training?

_____

_____

We've all heard the phrase "no pain, no gain" used in reference to exercise. To what extent is this advice true? When does this sentiment go too far?

_____

_____

Do you grunt or groan involuntarily when you bend over or squat or exert yourself? What does this mean, if anything?

_____

_____

Rank from 1 to 10 these fitness fiascos by their severity *to you* (1 = "no big deal"; 10 = "earth-shattering").

___ Spraining an ankle

___ Pulling a hamstring

___ Breaking in new pair running/walking shoes

___ Tripping and falling off a treadmill in front of a bunch of strangers at a health club

___ Getting shin splints

___ Getting athlete's foot

___ Developing blisters on your feet

___ Being chased on your bike by a vicious dog

___ Getting drilled in the "caboose" with a hard-hit racquetball

___ Dropping some weights on your foot

Whenever you exercise, drink plenty of water before, during, and after exercising to keep your body hydrated.

LEARNING A NEW WAY OF *LIFE*

Jeremiah 29:11 says, "'For I know the plans I have for you,' declares the LORD, 'plans to prosper you and not to harm you, plans to give you hope and a future.'" This verse technically applies to the Old Testament people of God. The prophet Jeremiah spoke it to the Jewish nation just before they experienced judgment at the hands of Babylon. God wanted His people to know that He wasn't finished with them. After a time of exile would come restoration and a glorious future.

What comfort can people of God today draw from this verse? What does it suggest about the character of God, His control of our lives, and His heart for His children?

_____

_____

_____

Exercise helps manage hunger. Research shows that increased exercise increases control over hunger and food intake.[22]

Given glimpses of the Almighty like this one, how do you know that God wants to see you succeed in your LIFL venture? Why?

_____

_____

_____

Read Philippians 4:6–7 and 1 Peter 5:7. What are these passages about? What relevance do they have as you contemplate (perhaps anxiously) embarking on a more rigorous exercise routine?

_____

_____

_____

If God has knowledge of seemingly trivial facts such as how many hairs we have on our heads (Luke 12:6–7), then what can we conclude about His keeping track of our efforts to burn calories and get in better shape?

_____

_____

_____

LOSING IT FOR _LIFE_

The _LIFL_ book mentions the importance of paying attention to our bodies when we exercise. Five physical warning signs (signals to stop exercising) are given in chapter 6. List them here.

_____

_____

_____

Which of those red flags, if any, have you experienced lately?

_____

_____

_____

_____

Why is lightweight, loose-fitting clothing important to wear when you exercise?

_____

_____

Which of the following do you have and routinely use?

      ___ Personal support (an athletic bra for women, athletic supporter for men)
      ___ Well-fitting shoes designed for the kind of activity in which you are engaging
      ___ A hat for warmth in winter, and sunlight/heat protection in summer
      ___ Sunscreen for outdoor activities
      ___ Sweat suits that absorb perspiration, removing it from your skin

The authors make the case that exercise really *does* get easier over time. Has this been your experience? Give some examples.

_____

_____

_____

DAY 4

Getting Started

How tragic that for many people exercise is a hated or dreaded part of life. Moving your body (that is, burning calories, building muscle, losing weight, and so forth) can and should become a joyous and life-enhancing activity. That's our goal. In this session we'll find motivation to get going.

LOOKING AT YOUR *LIFE*

Think about your schedule. When are your most convenient or most ideal exercise slots? Why is convenience an important factor in physical fitness success?

_____

_____

What activities do you most enjoy? What sports do you truly dislike and why? Why is having fun an important part of your exercise success?

_____

_____

Are you the kind of person who likes variety—in your diet, or your clothes, or on vacation? How might a varied exercise regimen help you reach your goals?

_____

_____

An exercise partner can provide accountability and encouragement.

Think about your circle of friends and acquaintances. Which friend(s) do you seek out when you . . .

want to laugh?

_____

want to be challenged in your thinking—want a good intellectual exchange?

_____

want to be encouraged and inspired?

_____

need some support?

_____

are looking for wisdom or counsel?

_____

How could you combine some of these friendships with your exercise needs and goals?

_____

_____

LEARNING A NEW WAY OF *LIFE*

Don't forget Paul's words in 1 Timothy 4:8: "Physical training is good, but training for godliness is much better, promising benefits in this life and in the life to come" (NLT).

What conclusions can we/should we draw from this verse?

_____

_____

What are the limits of physical exercise? In other words, what can it do for us and *not* do for us?

_____

_____

_____

You may decide you prefer to work out alone because it's the one place in your schedule you can have peace and quiet.

What spiritual exercises are part of your daily routine? Why are these disciplines important?

_____

_____

_____

LOSING IT FOR _LIFE_

As you can see, the decision to exercise will take _commitment_. Don't be afraid of that word. You can do this with God's help and the help of others.

Three kinds of exercise are important for all-around fitness. These are listed in chapter 6. Do you remember what they are and why each is important? Give some examples of each.

_____

_____

_____

Some people who haven't exercised for many years are put off by the thought of strength training. Maybe it conjures up images of smelly gyms and muscle-bound bodybuilders. What are some strength-training exercises you can do that don't require a set of weights?

_____

_____

_____

If you do not carve out time for your physical, spiritual, and personal needs, you will burn out, bum out, and bail out by acting out.

What muscles in your body are especially weak?

_____

_____

_____

Why is stretching important?

_____

_____

_____

The *LIFL* book suggests that we put our fitness goals and routine on paper and set some strict boundaries to guard that time. Why is this an important step? Have you done this? If not, stop and do so now.

_____

_____

_____

Why is it important to start slowly with any new exercise routine?

_____

_____

_____

What good purpose can an exercise journal serve?

_____

_____

_____

DAY 5
Options Galore!

Aren't you glad to have so many food options? Imagine a life in which we ate gruel—and only gruel—every single day. Thank the Lord for so much variety! In the same way, there are lots of possibilities for exercise. We conclude this week of lessons with a final look at your fitness options and a few reminders.

Any kind of activity is good, but experts recommend twenty to thirty minutes of vigorous aerobic activity three or more times a week.

LOOKING AT YOUR *LIFE*

Describe your experiences of the following activities when you were a kid. When did you do these activities? How did you feel when you did them?

Riding a bike

_____

_____

Skating

_____

_____

Dancing

_____

_____

Hiking

_____

_____

Do you agree that "variety is the spice of life"? Or are you the kind of person who becomes overwhelmed when presented with a broad array of options? Why?

_____

_____

What's a sport or leisure pursuit you've always wanted to try? Why does it intrigue you?

_____

_____

Swimming or water aerobics is an excellent way to burn calories and strengthen the heart. The buoyancy of the water helps reduce stress on the joints. Is swimming something you like? If not, what is difficult about it for you?

_____

_____

LEARNING A NEW WAY OF *LIFE*

We humans tend to be superficial, focusing mostly on externals. God looks deeper (1 Samuel 16:7). He's more concerned with the condition of our souls.

As you add exercise to your busy schedule, how can you also make sure you maintain a close relationship with God? Any ideas for doing both at once (that is, exercising physically and spiritually)?

_____

_____

The key to successful weight control and improved overall health is making physical activity a part of your daily life.

If you're a mom or a dad, if you're a church member, if you have a circle of friends, if you have bills to pay, and so forth, you always have a zillion things you could be doing other than exercise. With an endless number of needs around you, you may even feel it's selfish to think of carving out thirty to forty-five minutes a day for yourself (specifically for your own physical and spiritual health and well-being).

What do the following passages say about taking time alone?

Matthew 4:13:

_____

_____

Mark 1:35:

_____

_____

Mark 6:31:

_____

_____

Luke 5:16:

_____

_____

We must take care of ourselves by setting boundaries with our time and energy so we have time for important personal priorities, like eating right and exercising. It is important to decide in advance that your fitness, nutrition, spiritual, and personal time is nonnegotiable. You are no good to anyone else if your own body and soul are falling apart.

LOSING IT FOR _LIFE_

Why do the authors suggest that beginners slowly and gradually increase the frequency, intensity, and length of their workouts?

_____

_____

_____

The authors recommend engaging in short bursts of exercise each day. Check the boxes of the ones you think are doable for you.

☐ Marching or running in place   ☐ Crossovers

☐ Kicks   ☐ Punches

☐ Jump rope   ☐ Jump squats

☐ Waist twists   ☐ Jack-in-the-box

If those exercises seem a bit too strenuous, which of the following ones seem more suited to you?

☐ Doing standing squats as you blow-dry or curl your hair

☐ Pacing or marching in place while you talk on the phone

☐ Taking the stairs, instead of the elevator, whenever possible

☐ Squeezing your buttock muscles as you stand at the stove or fold laundry

☐ Doing leg-raises while you watch TV

☐ Zipping in your abs while you iron

☐ Putting on lively music and dancing while you mop

☐ Using a push mower instead of a riding mower

What other simple, creative ways can you find to get your heart pumping while you are going about mundane tasks?

_____

_____

_____

What are some of the advantages and benefits of cycling?

_____

_____

What are some of the advantages and benefits of walking?

_____

_____

_____

What's the difference between walking and hiking? Which do you prefer and why?

_____

_____

_____

Why are the right shoes such an important part of a walking exercise regimen?

_____

_____

_____

When should a person consult his or her physician before starting a new fitness program?

_____

_____

_____

It's time to get moving! Perhaps exercise will be your biggest challenge. If you are overweight, it hurts both physically and emotionally to move your body. But you can start slow. Take baby steps. Be patient. Remember you're not in a race; you're embarking on a new lifestyle. Give yourself plenty of grace (God does!).

And remember this great truth: "Let us not become weary in doing good, for at the proper time we will reap a harvest if we do not give up" (Galatians 6:9). Technically the verse is speaking about doing good to others, but the deeper principle still holds. Doing right, over time, ultimately results in good results.

7

Coming Out (of the Eating Closet)

November 21, 2003—What a week! Hands down, this has been one of the toughest weeks I've faced since embarking on this healthy lifestyle journey. Needless to say, my emotions have been all over the place. In the past, I have always stuffed away the sad or emotional times by eating large amounts of comfort food until I was emotionally numb, i.e., safe. I have now stopped medicating with food, and it's incredible to actually "feel" my emotions—good and bad. Of course, some days I want to run to the refrigerator and comfort myself with food. But, amazing as it sounds, this is when I'm learning to press into God even harder and ask Him to walk me through the emotions at hand. I can't share all I've gone through this week, but I can say it's a miracle I have not gone back to my old ways. It's confirmation to me that the Lord has begun a good work in my life. I am now down 92 pounds. I have 8 pounds to go until I reach the halfway mark. Praise God.

December 17, 2003—Imagine living your life numb. Never really experiencing true happiness, joy, sadness, etc. In this state, life just sort of passes you by while you exist. Sadly enough, this is how I have lived most of my life. I've learned that this was how I protected myself from past hurts, humiliations, letdowns, and unforgiveness in my life. The good news is that with the Lord's constant guiding in this journey, I have made a U-turn. Let me tell you, it is an incredible thing to feel, to really live life experiencing the good and the not-so-good times. It is so much better than simply existing in a numb state, day after day after day.

I have also realized that not only did I not want to feel, but I was uncomfortable when my kids felt too. I have always said things like "stop crying," or "you're okay, it's not that bad," when my kids were hurting. I thought I was protecting them, but I now realize that I should have allowed them to feel their emotions. It's healthy to have good days and bad days. It's healthy to let them cry it out when they hurt, to scream out when excited, and to voice their fears when afraid. From now on, I am asking the Lord to help my kids and me learn to face our emotions and walk through them head on, so we can continue to grow and become the people God created us to be.

—Cathy

Cathy has come out of the eating closet! For the first time in a long time, she is beginning to feel emotions she used to numb out with food. And sometimes she feels overwhelmed, like a dam is breaking and she'll be swept away by the force of her emotions. But we love Cathy's new response—to press into God even harder and know He will walk her through the emotions she feels. God is faithful and can be trusted. He may not always remove Cathy from difficulty, but He promises His comfort, peace, and presence no matter what.

What is so encouraging about this brave sister in the Lord is that she is not asking God to remove her feelings or the feelings of her children. Cathy is beyond "the quick fix, instant solution" God concept that typifies the spiritual move many people make. Instead, she is asking God to help her and her kids face the feelings and allow the experience to produce growth. This truly is how we can continue to grow and become the people God created us to be. There is no lifestyle, no matter how healthy, that will free you from negative emotions or horrible pain. But you can find a way to face those moments, resolve them, and grow from the experience, if you allow God to help you.

THE GIFT OF EMOTIONAL PAIN

One of our favorite physicians is Dr. Paul Brand, a man who dedicated his life to helping people with leprosy. What struck him while working with these patients was their inability to feel pain—literally, the patients would become injured and not know it! Because pain is an important warning signal that something is wrong, Dr. Brand spent his life trying to find a way to give his patients the "gift of pain."

Physical pain is necessary to our functioning. It is part of God's design for our bodies because it signals there is a problem to which we should attend. Emotional pain is similar. It signals there is a problem God wants to heal. Cathy is learning this for the first time in her life. Rather than protect herself from emotional pain by using food as her numbing agent, she is taking courageous steps to walk through past hurts and problems. When we see emotional pain as the symptom that leads us to depend on God and turn to Him for healing, we begin to understand its purpose.

Granted, you may be thinking, *If emotional pain is a gift, please don't give it to me!* But think about the times in your life when you have grown the most. Were they during the mountaintop experiences or in the lows of the valleys? Most of us grow during valley experiences, those difficult times in our lives when we can turn one of two ways—toward a more intimate relationship with God or away from Him. And when we choose to go to God, we grow and mature.

Cathy is leaving a legacy for her children. She is breaking a family pattern and teaching her children to feel emotional pain and deal with it. What a gift to give the next generation! As this family learns to feel the good and the bad, they will realize they can tolerate much more than they ever thought possible. No longer will they have to hide from emotional feelings, because they have found freedom!

ARE YOU AN EMOTIONAL EATER?

Cathy admits she is an emotional eater. She anesthetizes herself with food so she doesn't have to feel negative emotions. Like so many overeaters, this woman was unaware that emotions were at the root of her hunger. Perhaps you are like Cathy and haven't made the connection between overeating and emotions. If not, now is the time to take a deeper look at your relationship with food. The twenty questions below will help you decide if you are an emotional eater.

1. Do I think about food often or all the time?
2. Do I eat to relieve tension, worry, or upset feelings?
3. Do I eat when I am bored?
4. Do I continue to eat after I feel full, sometimes to the point of feeling sick?
5. Do I use eating to relieve anxiety?
6. Do I eat without thinking?
7. Do I feel I have to clean my plate?
8. Do I eat in secret or hide food?
9. Do I eat quickly, shoveling in the food?

10. Do I feel guilty after I eat?
11. Do I eat small portions in front of people, but go back for more food when people aren't around?
12. Do I binge (eat large amounts of food in a short time)?
13. Can I eat one serving, or do I eat the entire amount (a bag of cookies or the entire half-gallon of ice cream)?
14. Do I feel out of control and impulsive when eating?
15. Do I eat when I am not physically hungry?
16. Do I lie to myself about how much I really eat?
17. Do I have trouble tolerating negative feelings?
18. Do I have impulse problems in other areas of my life (for example, shopping, gambling, sex, alcohol, pornography, or drugs)?
19. Have I been on numerous diets over the years?
20. Do I experience constant weight fluctuations?

If you answered yes to all of these, well, you are probably so depressed you are eating right now, or you are crying so hard you cannot read on. If you answered yes to several of these questions, chances are you are an emotional eater. This means that feelings often trigger your desire to eat. This is not an easy topic, but it is imperative to get to the root of why you are eating. In fact, it is the key to unlocking your weight problem—*when* you stop eating depends on *why* you are eating.

Emotional eating can be learned early as a child. Food can be used to comfort, or it can become a trusted friend. Children often use food in response to physical or sexual abuse, or growing up in the home of an alcoholic or mentally ill parent, or in response to any number of difficult circumstances. When boundaries are violated, as in cases of abuse, or nurturing is unstable or unpredictable, as in cases of neglect and addiction, or loss is experienced in significant ways, as in situations involving divorce or death, children often turn to food for comfort. Eating calms the anxiety, numbs out trauma and abuse, and soothes the troubled soul.

Other people become emotional eaters as a result of trauma or stress experienced later in life. The trigger might be an unhealthy relationship, death, illness, or a job loss. In my own case, I (Dr. Linda) used food to cope with my brother's death. He was killed when the airplane he was on exploded over New Delhi, India. (We now believe the plane was the target of a terrorist bomb.) It happened the summer before I left for college. Between the trauma of his death and beginning my freshman year of college out of state, the losses were great. I unconsciously used food to soothe myself from all the stress and emotional pain I carried, and I gained thirty pounds before realizing that eating was my new coping mechanism.

I remember feeling unprotected when my brother was killed. We were a Christian family! Where was God when that plane went down? The enemy, during a time of incredible hurt and loss, implants doubt about who God is and how He loves and cares for us. Like Eve, I listened to that gnawing, twisted voice. I made a vow never to be dependent on a man, and I wouldn't allow that kind of hurt to happen again. I would take control of my life. God could come along for the ride, but He had to take the backseat, because in my mind, He was no longer trustworthy.

Even though I grieved my brother's death, those unspoken vows caused marital problems in the early years of my marriage. What I didn't realize was how captive I was to fear. Freedom came when I renounced those old vows and then challenged the lie of my unbelief. In prayer, I asked Jesus to speak His truth to me.

As I waited before the Lord in prayer, I heard Him tell me that my life was in His hands. There is not a day I live that He hasn't numbered; in fact, my life had been in His control all along. I had to trust Him, despite my lack of understanding. I didn't have to understand my brother's death, but I did have to trust that "all things work together for good to those who love God" (Romans 8:28 NKJV). My faith was on trial, and my unbelief and doubt were choking the spiritual intimacy I desperately needed.

WHAT IS THE ANSWER?

Our lives, our eating, and our emotions all have spiritual ramifications. You can rely on God. God won't protect you from horrible situations or difficult emotions, but He does sustain and protect His children from hopelessness. God knows what you need, always. And through the pain and struggle of this journey, He will deliver you, if you are willing.

One of the biggest barriers to moving forward in the things God has for us is getting stuck in our emotional pain and allowing it to move us away from God. When we experience trials or suffering, we might not loudly reject God, but we may very well begin to doubt who He is and whether He truly loves and cares for us. We all have experienced hurts and disappointments in our lives. For some of us, we've had deep traumas or abuse. For others, we've experienced lost dreams, disappointments, heartaches, and relationship problems. Certainly, there is no shortage of emotional pain. And unfortunately, all that suffering can lead us down the road to anxiety, depression, and eating problems.

The reality is that putting your trust in anything or anyone but God will block your intimacy with Him. Our earthly supports, whether people or merchandise, gradually disappoint or fade away. We live in uncertain times. God wants you to look to Him first for security. He came to bring peace and comfort to those who mourn.

> He has the power to heal the brokenhearted,
> to proclaim liberty to the captive,
> to open the prison doors to those who are bound,
> to give beauty to ashes,
> and the garment of praise for the spirit of heaviness,
> that we might be called trees of righteousness,
> the planting of the Lord, that *He might be glorified.*
> (adapted from Isaiah 61:1–3; emphasis added)

Let your emotional pain lead you to Him. Become His tree planted with deep roots, trusting Him, knowing Him, so that He can transform your pain for His glory. God wants us to come to Him no matter what—so don't allow your losses and pain to turn you away from Him. The answers are found in Him. "For in Him we live and move and have our being" (Acts 17:28 NKJV).

Your loss might be the work of the enemy and something God allowed to happen. But just look at the story of Job. Job was righteous in God's eyes. He was faithful and yet lost everything because God allowed it. Job's story illustrates how we can obey God and be right in the center of His will and yet still experience great loss. And when this happens, it is very hard to understand, and harder still to accept.

Turning to food is but one choice for covering up emotional pain. But once emotional eating becomes habitual, you have to break the connection between emotions and food to get back on track. Those emotions need to be revisited, felt intensely, grieved, and released. If you struggle with emotional pain and are using food to cover up the hurt, pour out your heart to the Lord as Hannah did in 1 Samuel 1. And remember that Christ has taken your grief and carried your sorrow (Isaiah 53). He identifies with what you are going through. He intimately knows every tear you cry, and He can handle your intense feelings.

In addition to pouring out your heart to God, find someone who will listen and can be trusted with your pain. This may be a good friend, a counselor, a family member, or your spouse. The Bible instructs us to "bear one another's burdens" (Galatians 6:2 NKJV) and to intercede in prayer on behalf of others. Allow trusted people in your life to be a part of your healing journey. Often they have words of encouragement or scriptures that will uplift you and offer hope when you are feeling down.

RISE ABOVE EMOTIONAL EATING

As you already know, physical hunger is rarely the trigger for overeating. Overeating can be stimulated by seeing food, thinking certain thoughts, learning behavior patterns, and feeling certain emotions. We must learn to:

1. identify the emotions associated with the urge to overeat.
2. feel those emotions and manage them, instead of allowing them to manage us.
3. work through emotional pain, grieve it, and allow God to transform it.

We can assure you that people who learn to respond to emotional difficulties without using food to numb or escape feelings have a better and longer weight-loss maintenance record than those who only deal with eating and exercise. Both research and clinical experience support this reality. This is a difficult road to take, because a learned way of coping needs to be unlearned. You may feel flooded with emotions that you haven't felt in a long time, thanks to eating covering them up, but the rewards are well worth the effort.

To RISE above the challenge, here's what to expect:

Reduce stress where and when you can; also eating in response to negative feelings and stress.

Increase confession, your ability to tolerate negative feelings, confrontation of tough issues, and assertiveness.

Substitute new ways to deal with emotions for eating, such as grieving for overeating.

Eliminate fear, feelings of rejection and shame, and hopelessness.

IDENTIFY THE FEELINGS

When you have the urge to eat, try to identify what you feel. This sounds easy enough, but if you have been taught to ignore feelings, particularly negative emotions like anger, envy, or pride, it may be more difficult. Negative emotions are part of our human condition and must be dealt with in a healthy and biblical way. Emotions aren't wrong or bad, but what you do with an emotion counts.

I (Steve) heard a comedian do a comedy routine around the fact that there are about two thousand emotions and men are only able to feel between three or four, or only know what three or four are! I hope it is not that bad for us men. It is so important that we learn to identify what feelings we are experiencing.

After my divorce I began to feel deep emotional pain like I had never experienced before. I hurt at the core of who I was. I did not try to eat or drink it away. The pain was too intense and destroyed my desire for anything. I cried and sometimes wailed in my despair. Initially, I told myself all I was feeling was a generic pain that all experience. It wasn't until just a few months ago that I really got in touch with what that pain really was: pure fear to the degree I would even label it terror. I was afraid of what would happen to my daughter. I was afraid of what would happen to my ministry. I was afraid of everything that could go wrong as a result of the divorce. My faith was at an all-time low while my fear raged on. And because I did not identify the fear as the source of my pain, I didn't deal with it in the counseling I was involved with. As a result, that fear stayed with me for far too long. It was only when I acknowledged it and addressed my lack of faith that the fear subsided and my pain had a purpose.

I hope you come to identify the feelings you have and then start to deal with them openly and honestly so they will no longer control any part of your life. The end result will be that you are no longer an emotional eater compelled to eat in a futile effort to medicate the emptiness within your soul.

Anger

Anger is the most reported emotion tied to overeating. People eat when they are angry! Anger feels uncomfortable and is often confused with a need to eat. It's interesting to note that women, more so than men, have trouble acknowledging anger. This may have to do with parent training (nice girls don't get mad), corporate game-playing rules (just look pretty and don't say anything), or other societal messages women receive.

Though it is sometimes viewed as bad, anger is a biblical reality. Cain was so angry, he murdered his brother (Genesis 4:5–8); Simeon and Levi took revenge for their sister's rape (Genesis 49:5–7); Herod was angry toward the wise men for deceiving him (Matthew 2:16); the people of Nazareth were angry with Jesus (Luke 4:28); and Paul felt anger toward Ananias (Acts 23:1–3). The list goes on and on. Keep in mind that when Jesus took the form of man, He experienced every emotion, including anger.

The biblical directive given in Ephesians 4:26 (NASB) is, "Be angry, and yet do not sin." This scripture affirms anger as part of our human nature but also tells us not to sin in response to that emotion. Yet anger will not go away on its own. To be rid of it requires recognizing anger, acknowledging you have it, and then dealing with it according to these biblical guidelines:

James 1:19—Be quick to listen, slow to speak and slow to become angry.

Proverbs 29:11—Fools give full vent to their rage, but the wise bring calm in the end.

Proverbs 15:1—A gentle answer turns away wrath, but a harsh word stirs up anger.

Matthew 6:14—For if you forgive other people when they sin against you, your heavenly Father will also forgive you.

Psalm 4:4—Be angry, and do not sin. Meditate within your heart on your bed, and be still. (NKJV)

1 Peter 5:7—Cast all your anxiety on him because he cares for you.

Proverbs 22:24—Don't hang out with angry people; don't keep company with hotheads. (MSG)

Fatigue

Many of us overeat when we are tired. Food is often used to energize us. If you are a workaholic, you've probably used food to keep your energy level up. Or maybe you use food to ease tension from being overly tired. If you've had a horrendous day at the office, have overdone it by drinking too much coffee and snacking on chocolate for quick recharging, you may crave carbohydrates at night to calm you down. Overeating happens more often when we are tired and our defenses are down. We take a careless attitude and dive into snacking.

If you are tired, rest is what you need. Food may give you a temporary surge, but you will end up feeling more sluggish and still tired in the long run. Rest, exercise, and eat well. Eating when you are tired only compounds your problems. Rest is biblical—even God rested after creating the world.

Psalm 37:7—Rest in the LORD and wait patiently for Him. (NKJV)

Matthew 11:28–30—Are you tired? Worn out? Burned out on religion? Come to me. Get away with me and you'll recover your life. I'll show you how to take a real rest. Walk with me and work with me—watch how I do it. Learn the unforced rhythms of grace. I won't lay anything heavy or ill-fitting on you. Keep company with me and you'll learn to live freely and lightly. (MSG)

Hebrews 4:1—For as long, then, as that promise of resting in him pulls us on to God's goal for us, we need to be careful that we're not disqualified. (MSG)

Hebrews 4:9—The promise of "arrival" and "rest" is still there for God's people. (MSG)

Depression

When you feel down, it's easy to try to eat those feelings away. People who eat when they feel depressed usually go for dairy products like ice cream or cheese—and of course, chocolate! These foods tend to provide a boost by giving the brain a neurochemical lift. But eating doesn't take away depression; it only masks it.

Your most powerful weapon against depression is praise. We are told in Isaiah 61:3 to put on a garment of praise for a spirit of despair. Don't wait to feel like you want to praise. Do it no matter what you feel like. Praise God for who He is. Praise is the antidote to feeling down. Let His praise be in your mouth continuously (Psalm 34:1), and the Lord will lift your spirit.

If you struggle with clinical depression, there is nothing wrong with going on an antidepressant to help stabilize your mood and correct brain chemistry. Taking medication does not demonstrate a lack of faith. Antidepressants are simply agents used to get you living well again by restoring proper brain functioning. All healing comes through God, but He does use miracles and medicine to accomplish His purposes. You may need to see a doctor and/or a therapist to help with depression.

Loneliness

When you are lonely, you may overeat instead of engaging in activities that could end your loneliness. Food can become a trusted friend that is always with you and always available. Therefore, you must find other ways to deal with loneliness. Join an organization, volunteer your time, enroll in a class, become active with a charity, attend a church function, or make the first move and call someone you'd like to befriend.

The Duchess of York, Sarah Ferguson, lost her mother to a divorce when she was twelve years old. Her mother left her and her father to marry another man and move to Argentina. Since that time, Sarah describes herself as an emotional eater. "I overate to compensate for my feelings. I didn't want to express to my mother that I was angry or sad that she'd left me."[1] She admits that she was blind to the emotional triggers that set off her eating as an adult. Loneliness can be that trigger.

Inadequacy

When you don't feel good about yourself, you can eat to cover up feelings of inadequacy. Most people wrestle with self-doubt from time to time, but if you have a constant feeling of being inadequate, you may be tying your eating to that feeling. We are all inadequate because we are human. You must learn to accept your weaknesses and flaws and not dwell on them. And when you feel inadequate or weak, it helps to know that God is strong and can work through you anyway.

Make a list of your strengths and weaknesses. Try to focus on those things you do well. Then ask God to help you with your weaknesses. By His Spirit, He is able to accomplish much, even with your limitations (Zechariah 4:6). Turning to food will not help you accomplish anything. In fact, it leads to more feelings of inadequacy because of weight gain.

This is an area that has plagued me (Steve) since I was a child. My first problem was an obsession with others and comparing myself to them, trying to figure out where I was on the food chain. I wanted so much and to do so much while always feeling I had too little. It wasn't until I finally realized that the curse of not being as talented or having as much as others was actually a gift.

The gift was knowing that God had done things through me in spite of my inadequacies rather than because of my strengths. It was a gift to see that although I did not measure up, God used me to become part of His kingdom-building project. If you start to look at your emotions and find that inadequacy is at the top of the list, give up on trying to feel better about yourself and start focusing on feeling better about God. Look at what God has done through you. Look at what God has allowed to happen in your life even though you did not have it all together or have all that others had.

Insecurity

If you eat because you feel insecure, no amount of food will change that feeling. The only place you are truly secure is in your relationship with God. A multitude of scriptures speak to who we are in Christ—we are loved, forgiven, saved by grace through faith, joint heirs with Christ, blessed with all spiritual blessings, sons and daughters of God, complete in Him, and so much more. It may help you to do a study on scriptures related to our security in Christ. Here are a few to get you started:

Psalm 34:4—I sought the LORD, and he answered me; he delivered me from all my fears.

Deuteronomy 31:8—The LORD himself goes before you and will be with you; he will never leave you nor forsake you. Do not be afraid; do not be discouraged.

Romans 8:28—And we know that in all things God works for the good of those who love him, who have been called according to his purpose.

2 Corinthians 1:21–22—Now it is God who makes both us and you stand firm in Christ. He anointed us, set his seal of ownership on us, and put his Spirit in our hearts as a deposit, guaranteeing what is to come.

Guilt

Guilt is only healthy when it relates to sin. We should feel guilty when we go against God's Word and sin. But once we confess that sin, it is gone and forgotten. To hang on to guilt serves no good purpose and can be cause for overeating. Jesus does not accuse (John 5:45) or condemn you (Romans 8:1). When you own your mistakes and take responsibility, you must let go of condemnation and unhealthy guilt—to not do so is to ignore the power of the blood covenant over past sins. You may intellectually know that Jesus died on the cross to take your sins yet be unable to get past your mistakes. So you walk around carrying tremendous guilt and shame, yet Christ died so you could give Him these sins and burdens. Hand them over and walk with your head held high.

In 2 Corinthians 7:9–10 we see what God is really after when we do something wrong:

Now I [Paul] am happy, not because you were made sorry, but because your sorrow led you to repentance. For you became sorrowful as God intended. . . . Godly sorrow brings repentance that leads to salvation and leaves no regret, but worldly sorrow brings death.

Godly sorrow moves us to change. It motivates us toward God and relationship with Him. So feel the guilt, confess it, and then turn it into a spiritual experience of godly sorrow that increases your character.

Shame

Shame takes you nowhere but the refrigerator. Shame comes when you've done something improper or wrong and you internalize "badness" because of it. Shame says, "I *am* a mistake," not "I *made* a mistake." Shame often develops from a message that you are bad, weak, or unloved. Parents, teachers, friends, boyfriends, spouses, and coworkers can humiliate, belittle, and criticize rather than deal with inappropriate behavior a better way. If you struggle with shame from overeating, you aren't alone. Read this journal entry:

> A few years ago I went with a group of friends to a theme park. We waited in line for almost an hour to ride their largest roller coaster, and our excitement level was huge by the time we actually took our seats on the ride. I'll never forget what happened next.
>
> Each car held four people. For some reason the car I was in was having a problem with the safety bar locking. The ride operator came by to assist us. He pushed the bar down, attempting to safely lock us in. As he did this, I felt extreme pain as the bar pinched an area of my outer thigh against the metal seat. He didn't realize it was my large legs causing the problem, so he continued to jiggle and pushed down on the bar a few more times with all his strength. The pain was excruciating, and I could feel the blood running down my leg, but I was frozen with shame and unable to speak.
>
> The young ride operator finally realized what the problem was and, in front of everyone, said, "I'm sorry, you're too big for this ride." I was crushed. I climbed out of the ride embarrassed and ashamed, trying not to limp, and acted like it was no big deal. Some people were laughing and snickering and others looked mortified. I started laughing and pretended not to care about what had just happened. I told my friends to go without me and, once the roller coaster was out of sight, I slipped away and cried alone. As you can imagine, I have not felt very comfortable going on carnival rides since.
>
> —Cathy

Experiencing this kind of insensitivity can leave scars. We want you to be free of the hurt right now and not have to wait to be thinner! If you've read this entry and are feeling shame right now, here's what we want you to do. Embrace that shame and allow yourself to feel it. Understand, it's going to feel awful, but don't push it away or try to avoid it. Then ask the Lord to show you the source of that pain—a cruel word, a disappointing look, a moment of rejection. Let your mind go wherever the Holy Spirit takes you.

With that memory in mind, try to think *why* you feel shame. What thought comes to your mind? Is it *I am a bad person* or *I don't deserve to be treated nicely*? Be honest with what you are thinking. The thought is most likely a lie. Once you've identified the lie, ask Jesus to speak His truth to you. Wait and allow Him to speak truth. What do you see or hear Him say? His truth will set you free from that shame. Then, forgive the person who did or said something that created that feeling of shame.

Shame is a deep internal response of feeling unworthy in another person's eyes. It can be experienced through unkind words and actions. But understand something important. Jesus does not shame you. He sees you as worthy and valuable! He does not judge you by your weight. When He sees the shame you experience, He urges you to bring it to the cross. He died for it.

The life lived with God is a great adventure, much like the roller-coaster ride. It is filled with ups and downs to be experienced. When you experience the downside, find your worth in Him and hand over the shame. He's with you on this journey and won't ask you to step out of the car. Instead, He'll ride alongside, whether you fit in the car or not. And He's whispering in your ear, *Enjoy the ride. Shame is not on you! I took it to the cross!*

Many women with lifelong weight problems were molested at a young age. They felt the shame of that molestation for years and fed the pain with food. They medicated the horror with carbohydrates and anything that would give them some sense of comfort. Essentially they took the shame of another and put it onto themselves. Though innocent, they lived out a sentence of shame that the guilty should have experienced. If this is your story, please release your shame to God. Give it up, let it go, and experience the love and acceptance that God has for you now and has always had for you.

Jealousy

People eat out of jealousy when they compare themselves to others and look only at the appearance of others. To assume because others are thin that they are happy and living a good life is to be deceived. Jesus tells us to "stop judging by mere *appearances*, but instead judge correctly" (John 7:24; emphasis added). He is not impressed with people who *seem* to be important. And Paul, in Galatians 2:6, follows Christ by saying, "As for those who were held in high esteem—whatever they were makes no difference to me; God does not show favoritism—they added nothing to my message." So stop comparing yourself to others. Jealousy is a very unproductive emotion.

Happiness

When things are going well, some people turn to food in order to fill up on those happy emotions. Happiness is something to be gobbled up before it disappears. Others feel they don't deserve to be happy and eat to sabotage happy feelings. We frequently see this when people are beginning to be successful with weight loss.

It's wonderful to be happy, but those feelings come and go and can't be relied upon as a gauge for eating. So when you are happy, celebrate in other ways, like calling a friend, getting a massage, buying fresh flowers, or enjoying the stars on a clear night. And recognize that while happiness comes and goes, you always have joy in the Lord; joy is your strength.

Psalm 19:8—The precepts of the Lord are right, giving joy to the heart. The commands of the Lord are radiant, giving light to the eyes.

James 5:13—Is anyone among you in trouble? Let them pray. Is anyone happy? Let them sing songs of praise.

Acts 14:17—He has shown kindness by giving you rain from heaven and crops in their seasons; he provides you with plenty of food and fills your hearts with joy.

Psalm 28:7—The Lord is my strength and my shield; my heart trusts in him, and he helps me. My heart leaps for joy, and with my song I praise him.

Anxiety, Worry, and Fear

Food is used to relax. In today's world, there are endless situations over which to worry. Psalm 139:23–24 says, "Search me, God, and know my heart; test me and know my anxious thoughts. See if there is any offensive way in me, and lead me in the way everlasting." God knows if we are anxious! He wants us to stop feeling responsible and worried for those things we can't control. Jesus tells us not to worry even about our basic needs in life (Matthew 6:25–34).

Worry paralyzes our faith and draws our attention away from the faithfulness of God. Paul tells us to be anxious about nothing (Philippians 4:6) and then explains how we can accomplish this—by thanking God and sharing our concerns with Him through prayer. That is to be followed by meditating on God's goodness. The result is His supernatural peace resting on us.

Numerous times in the Bible we are told to hold fast against fear.

1 John 4:18—There is no room in love for fear. Well-formed love banishes fear. Since fear is crippling, a fearful life—fear of death, fear of judgment—is one not yet fully formed in love. (MSG)

Isaiah 35:4—Tell fearful souls, "Courage! Take heart! GOD is here, right here, on his way to put things right and redress all wrongs. He's on his way! He'll save you!" (MSG)

Disappointment/Hurt

There are so many opportunities to be disappointed with others that we could spend our whole lives eating in response to this one emotion. People make mistakes, betray us, are self-centered, and don't always look out for our best interests. Thus, our faith and confidence must be in the Lord. Even then, we may feel let down or hurt, even by God, and overeat as a result.

If this is the case, there is a problem of trust. He orders your steps and will allow difficulty in your life for a purpose. However, God's promise is to be with you through tough times. Focus on what you can learn from disappointment, but trust God to work it for your own good in His due time and in His way.

Isaiah 26:3–4—You will keep in perfect peace those whose minds are steadfast, because they trust in you. Trust in the LORD forever, for the LORD, the LORD himself, is the Rock eternal.

Emptiness

So many people go through life feeling empty and without purpose. Eating becomes a way to try and fill that empty place inside, but nothing will fill that void like an authentic relationship with God. He desires to draw close and be with you. He wants to fill you with good things and has a plan and purpose for you specifically. Engage with God in a new way. Be filled with His Word and when you feel empty, hunger and thirst for righteousness. His promise is that we will be filled if we "hunger and thirst for righteousness" (Matthew 5:6). We must fill the emptiness that only God can fill so that our lives are not controlled by our appetites for other things, because nothing but God can come close to fulfilling us. Emptiness leads us to fill our lives with everything but the one thing we truly need—God.

Procrastination

Eating is a great way to delay unpleasant tasks or to waste time. Perhaps you eat to avoid doing things you'd rather not do. But think about it! Has food ever made an unpleasant task go away? No! The task will still be there when you finish eating. It's best to tackle a task head on, delegate it to someone else, or decide not to do the task at all.

Boredom

When there is nothing to do, eating is an activity that can fill time. Thinking about what you will eat next is a way of filling time that might otherwise be spent thinking of other unpleasant things. Food then becomes an obsession. If you are unsure how you would spend your time if you weren't eating, cooking, or planning meals, you may need to address this reason. Perhaps you will need to develop hobbies or find other ways to relax. For some people, this means trying new things and getting comfortable with relaxation.

Rejection

Food doesn't make rejection go away. Read this journal entry and see if it rings true for you.

The things I am learning about myself are incredible—specifically, why I have acted and/or reacted to people and situations the way I have. I realize that I have lived most of my life with a thick, protective bubble around myself. You know, the kind of person who has many casual friends, but hardly any close ones. The kind of person who seems really tough on the outside, but if you dig a little deeper, you find they aren't the person you first thought. I've also learned that even at 350 pounds, I was a marathon runner. Not the type of runner who wins races, but the type of runner who runs from people, churches, love, constructive criticism, and, if I'm really honest, reality.

In taking a closer look, I see that at a very young age I learned I couldn't trust people to love, protect, nurture, or even meet my most basic needs. When I tried to get these needs met by asking, I was repeatedly rejected. Even a small child will eventually stop asking for help if it means experiencing less pain for the moment. This pattern of rejection became a lifestyle. And, eventually, I found a substitute for these basic needs in my life. The substitute was food.

Praise God, the walls around me are beginning to fall. The thick protective bubble is thinning, and my run has slowed to a walk. I believe the Lord is going to heal me in these areas, and the root fear of rejection will no longer have a hold in my life.

—Cathy

Rejection is hard to handle whether you weigh 120 pounds or 300 pounds. It is especially difficult to swallow when it comes from those who are supposed to love us. One way to deal with rejection is to do what Cathy did—to try not to feel it and cover it up by eating. When people let you down, food can become your friend. It is always available, tastes good, and satisfies for the moment. But no matter how many times you shove a slice of pizza down your throat, the pain won't go away. The hurt still lingers beneath the layers of fat.

To be healed, you must face rejection. Feel it with all your soul. Pour out your heart to the Lord. Once you've allowed yourself to really feel the pain of rejection, pray and ask God to take it. Then ask Christ to speak His truth to you. You see, the enemy uses emotional pain to implant lies—that no one will want or love you; that people will only hurt you; that if only you were thinner . . . all lies!

The truth is that there is Someone who will never reject you and is completely trustworthy. Your acceptance has nothing to do with your actions or your weight. Jesus unconditionally loves you because you are His. Know that Jesus Christ identifies with your pain. According to Isaiah 53, Christ was despised, rejected, and a man of sorrow. Because of His great love for you, He suffered the pain of rejection. On the cross, it was crucified once and for all. Once you allow His truth to soak your spirit, you can give up the pain of rejection and accept God's unfailing love.

If you've suffered a number of rejections, try to understand that those people were probably not rejecting you personally as much as the concept of you or what you represented. If you suffered parental rejection, for example, your parents probably rejected the concept of having a child with needs, rather than rejecting you as an individual. Rejection still hurts, but it may be easier to forgive someone once you realize that person had problems of his or her own that were taken out on you. Whatever the case, you will need to forgive those who rejected you.

Loss of Control

Isn't it interesting that when we feel out of control, we eat out of control? We actually create the very thing we fear. We fear we'll lose control, so we try to control the people around us or our circumstances. Of course, we can't do that and end up feeling out of control and then stuff food inside. Here's the reality: if you think you have control, you need that red pill again. Control is elusive and no amount of eating will change that. You are not in control, so you might as well surrender to the One who is.

EXPRESS YOUR FEELINGS

Once you have identified your feelings, you must learn to express them directly rather than medicating them with food. Feelings can be expressed by talking them out to a friend, writing them in a journal like Cathy did, and/or by crying and giving direct vent to feelings. For example, you might say out loud, "I am so sad right now because I feel ignored." Give verbal expression to your feelings instead of swallowing them or stuffing them away. Allow yourself to feel whatever the feeling is until the intensity subsides. Then determine if there is a need behind the feeling, such as a need to be loved, accepted, approved of, or respected. Many times the urge to eat represents an unmet need. Get to the heart of the feeling and decide if you are being realistic. If you must grieve a loss or work on ways to get your needs met, don't eat to feel better. Deal with the feelings.

CONFESSION—GOOD FOR THE SOUL

Once you become more comfortable identifying feelings and allowing yourself to feel them, you need to be honest about what is going on inside of you. There is sickness in secrecy. The sinning psalmist said, "When I kept silent, my bones wasted away . . ." (32:3). When we are willing to be open, healing becomes possible. By breaking our silence and speaking the truth about ourselves aloud to another person, we move out of the darkness and bring secrets into the light. Confessing our sins and talking about the wrongs done to us is another key to spiritual healing and health.

It is clearly important to God that men and women verbally express the struggles hidden in their hearts. Verbalization gives substance to inarticulate thoughts, and words affirm the realities of which we have become aware. Even on the key issue of Christian salvation, belief is to be affirmed with spoken words. Paul wrote, "If you declare with your mouth, 'Jesus is Lord,' and believe in your heart that God raised him from the dead, you will be saved. For it is with your heart that you believe and are justified, and it is with your mouth that you profess your faith and are saved" (Romans 10:9–10).

Unexpressed thoughts do not allow others to give input or challenge us to see the truth. When we confess our thoughts, we put others in the position of advising us, praying for us, and sharing our struggles. We must be careful, however; confession requires confidentiality. It is an invitation to intimacy and involves trust in both God and another person—a trust that is absolutely necessary for us to be able to truly reveal our secrets.

Openness is an outward act of trust that enables us to cleanse our souls from the inside out. If you want to break free from emotional eating, you must confess the need that is not being met and be honest about what you truly feel. Pretending not to have anger or not to be jealous will not help you heal, but honesty brings about authentic change. Confession means we:

- submit ourselves to God's ways of handling secrets
- are willing to overcome our fear of rejection by revealing our failures to another person and admitting we need help from fellow believers
- reject our habit of self-protective secretiveness
- admit to at least one other person that we have fallen short of God's best, be it through character defects or judgment errors
- stop trying to mask our true feelings and put our vague sense of guilt into written or spoken words, without making excuses

By openly confessing our flaws and struggles, there is hope for healing. Admit what you really feel and where you struggle emotionally. Come out of the eating closet and identify your hurts and losses. Do what James 5:16 commands: "Confess your sins to each other and pray for each other so that you can live together whole and healed" (MSG).

Have more than one person to talk to about your struggles so you don't overburden a person. Also, you won't feel guilty asking for help multiple times if you can spread around the need. Find someone who is a good listener, humble, trustworthy, evidences a quiet godliness, and is stable and positive. You want to avoid people with personal agendas, controlling personalities, or those who are needy, unstable, or sexually attractive to you. If you are married, it's better to find a same-sex confidant so that sexual tension will not be an issue. Lastly, remember to treat this person as a friend, not a therapist.

KEEP A PRAYER JOURNAL

We also recommend keeping a prayer journal, a tool to help document prayer requests and answers to prayer. They also are an excellent way to track your emotional swings. Whatever you feel, take it to God in prayer. Don't edit your feelings; just record them honestly. If you aren't sure how to begin, try this meaningful exercise:

1. Spend time in the Word or a devotional reading.
2. Write down a key verse or main idea from the reading.
3. Write out your prayer requests in response to what you have read.
4. Spend time in prayer.
5. Wait for a personal word from the Lord. (This step takes time to develop.) Wait before the Lord in silence and allow Him to speak to you. Then write down what you believe you hear in your spirit. Don't be surprised if you think you don't hear anything at first. Most people report that it takes time to learn how to be quiet before the Lord and listen for His voice. With time, you will develop your spiritual hearing.

SUBSTITUTE A NEW BEHAVIOR FOR EATING

Pain is not optional, but misery is. You can't always control pain, but you can do something about misery. If you are looking for a quick fix to emotional pain, you're reading the wrong book! Healing is often progressive because it requires changes in your character and actions. The way you cope with emotional pain must change if you decide to no longer eat your way through it.

Keeping a record of what you do when you become emotionally upset is a good way to watch your progress—perhaps in a journal. The journey to finding new alternatives to eating might look like this:

Event: Received an upsetting phone call from my ex
Emotion: Very hurt
Reaction: Went to the refrigerator and opened the door to eat

Now, think of a new way to cope with that feeling. What behavior could you substitute for eating?

New Behavior: Call a friend and let her pray with me

Here's another example:

Event: Heard someone gossip about me at church
Emotion: Anger

Reaction: Stopped for fries at a fast-food restaurant
New Behavior: Gently confront the person who did the gossiping

To help yourself choose alternatives to eating, make a list of twenty behaviors you can substitute for eating the next time an intense emotion triggers that desire. Your list should include things you can do while driving, being at home, at work, or on the go. Post the list on your refrigerator and make a copy to take with you. Every time you are tempted to eat because you feel an unpleasant emotion, pull out your list and choose a new thing to do. Feel free to borrow ideas from this list:

- Take a short walk and cool down.
- Listen to calming music.
- Take three deep breaths.
- Distract yourself with something in the room or car.
- Take a bubble bath.
- Call a friend.
- Count to twenty.
- Take a short nap.
- Pray and ask God to help you.
- Turn up the radio and get lost in the music.
- Stand up and do some stretches.
- Go to the bathroom, even if it's only to splash water on your face.
- Play with your dog.
- Play with your child.
- Watch a funny movie.
- Go somewhere quiet and practice deep muscle relaxation.
- Clean something.
- Run up and down the stairs to release tension.
- Work on a crossword puzzle.
- Play a video game.

March 29, 2004—Incredible! I just made it through an entire week in which food has not been an issue. I'm serious! I haven't wasted one minute wondering what I'm going to have for dinner the next day. I haven't been secretly imagining what unhealthy food snacks I'd devour if no one was around to see me. Food just hasn't been the primary thing on my mind. I even went to New York this weekend just for fun. I had a blast doing the whole tourist thing, and it wasn't about the food. I never thought this could be possible. I feel like the food handcuffs have somehow been released, and I'm now a free woman. Praise God for weeks like this.

—Cathy

Maybe you've been hurt by a cruel divorce, an abusive father, a betraying friend, or an insulting boss. Whatever the cause of your hurt, it's time to stop using food as an emotional crutch and let the pain surface. When you do, you might experience intense feelings of anger or fear, but there will not be healing until you face those feelings.

Just let the feelings come, and ask God to help you understand exactly why you feel as you do. Don't try to edit your thoughts. Whatever comes in to your mind, grab that thought. Most likely it is a lie that was implanted at the time of the emotional pain when you first experienced those feelings. Try to identify the lie, and once you find it, ask Jesus to speak His truth to you. Wait and listen for His voice, whether it comes in the form of a whisper of His Spirit or a visual picture He may give you. Wait on Him and expect Him to bring truth. His truth brings release from that lie.

If you continue to take every hurt and pain to Christ, lay them at His feet, and refuse to believe the lies, the food handcuffs will drop off you just like they did for Cathy. Come out of the eating closet. Exchange it for a prayer closet—a place filled with peace and rest.

Workbook Week 7

COMING OUT
(OF THE EATING CLOSET)

———— DAY 1 ————
Emotional Eating

In the next few pages we will look in greater detail at the important and surprisingly large role our emotions often play in our relationship with food. Before you begin, ask God to open your eyes to the truths you need to see, embrace, and live out. Ask Him for the courage to make any necessary changes.

LOOKING AT YOUR *LIFE*

Chapter 7 begins with some journal entries of a woman named Cathy. What situations in her life do you most relate to, and why?

_____

_____

Do others see you as an emotional person? How do you see yourself?

_____

_____

Some people bottle up all their emotions, sweeping them under the proverbial rug. Others go through life absolutely dominated by their changing feelings. What are the problems with each approach?

_____

_____

LEARNING A NEW WAY OF *LIFE*

The unique claim of Christianity is that Almighty God stepped out of eternity into time in the person of Jesus Christ (John 1:1, 14). What a jaw-dropping

"I stuffed away sad or emotional times by eating until I was emotionally numb. Now I've stopped medicating with food, and it's incredible to actually 'feel' my emotions—good and bad."
—Cathy, a Lose It for Life member.

truth—the Creator entering His own creation, to rescue us (Luke 19:10) and to show us what He is like (John 1:18)!

So what was Jesus like? What did He do? The Gospel writers record matter-of-factly that Jesus possessed and displayed a variety of human emotions:

- He wept (John 11:35).
- He got angry (Mark 3:5).
- He felt distressed and troubled (Mark 14:33).
- He was sorrowful (Matthew 26:37).
- He was joyful (Luke 10:21).
- He (apparently) got exasperated (Luke 9:41).
- He felt weary and tired (John 4:6; Mark 4:38).

If the perfect God-man felt all these things, what does that suggest to you about feelings?

_____

_____

_____

It is common for us to assume that good feelings and times are positive and should be pursued, while bad feelings and hard times should be avoided at all costs. Yet the Bible offers a different perspective on the "negative" unpleasant trials of life.

Read Romans 5:1–5. What surprises you about this passage? What are some good things that can come out of unpleasant experiences?

_____

_____

_____

Many people read, memorize, and discuss Romans 8:28. What does this verse suggest about the subject at hand?

_____

_____

_____

Sometimes we feel as if we'll be swept away by the force of our emotions. But God pledges His comfort, peace, and presence, no matter what.

Read two or three psalms (try any from Psalms 1–15). What emotions do you see expressed in these ancient Hebrew songs? What conclusions can we draw from this?

_____

_____

_____

_____

_____

_____

LOSING IT FOR *LIFE*

Read again what Cathy wrote:

> Imagine living your life numb. Never really experiencing true happiness, joy, sadness, etc. In this state, life just sort of passes you by while you exist. Sadly enough, this is how I have lived most of my life. . . . This was the way I protected myself from past hurts, humiliations, letdowns, and unforgiveness in my life. The good news is that with the Lord's constant guiding in this journey, I have made a U-turn. Let me tell you, it is an incredible thing to feel, to really live life experiencing the good and the not-so-good times. It is so much better than simply existing in a numb state, day after day after day.

Do you relate to Cathy's experience? Are you numb much of the time? What sense does it make to let ourselves feel—fully embrace—painful feelings? What is the danger if we don't?

_____

_____

_____

_____

Many overeaters are unaware that unidentified and unprocessed emotions are at the root of their hunger. Based on the twenty questions given in chapter 7, take the following self-test to see if you are an emotional eater.[2] Check all the boxes that apply.

☐ I think about food often or all the time.

☐ I eat to relieve tension, worry, or upset feelings.

☐ I eat when I am bored.

☐ I continue to eat after I feel full, sometimes to the point of feeling sick.

☐ I use eating to relieve anxiety.

☐ I eat without thinking.

☐ I feel I have to clean my plate.

☐ I eat in secret or hide food.

☐ I eat quickly, shoveling in the food.

☐ I feel guilty after I eat.

☐ I eat small portions in front of people, but go back for more food when people aren't around.

☐ I binge (eat large amounts of food in a short period of time).

☐ I seldom eat one serving; instead I eat the entire amount (for example, a bag of cookies or the entire half-gallon of ice cream).

☐ I feel out of control and impulsive when eating.

☐ I eat when I am not physically hungry.

☐ I lie to myself about how much I really eat.

☐ I have trouble tolerating negative feelings.

☐ I have impulse problems in other areas of my life (for example, shopping, gambling, sex, alcohol, pornography, or drugs).

☐ I have been on numerous diets over the years.

☐ I experience constant weight fluctuations.

If you checked a number of those boxes, you are probably an emotional eater. This means that nonphysical feelings often trigger your desire to eat. *When* you stop eating depends on *why* you are eating.

Is all this discussion of emotional eating a new thought to you? What do you think of the idea that food can be used as a comfort, a way of calming anxiety or numbing out trauma? How might a childhood of physical or sexual abuse, growing up in the home of an alcoholic or mentally ill parent, push someone in this direction?

_____

_____

_____

Emotional pain can lead us down the road to anxiety, depression, and eating problems if not handled well. It is our response to emotional pain that matters.

The authors tell about Dr. Paul Brand, a man who dedicated his life to helping people with leprosy. His discovery? Leprosy is disfiguring because its victims are unable to feel pain. His conclusion? Pain is God's warning signal to us that something is wrong. His commitment? Dr. Brand spent his life trying to find a way to give his patients the "gift of pain."

Have you ever thought of pain as a "gift"? What sort of hidden blessings might be lurking within and behind emotional pain?

_____

_____

_____

Do you mostly control your emotions or do they mostly control you? Why?

_____

_____

_____

What would you say to the person who looks disapprovingly at "all that feelings stuff" and says, "We're supposed to forget what lies behind and press on to what lies ahead. It does no good to dredge up the past. Besides, you can't change things that have already taken place"?

_____

_____

_____

We've seen that God can be trusted to understand us and help us. How can other people also come alongside us and walk with us through emotionally hard times? Write about a time when friends did this for you.

_____

_____

_____

— DAY 2 —
Identifying Feelings (Part 1)

In this chapter, we are focusing on eating as a response to negative feelings or emotional pain. Physical hunger is almost never the trigger for overeating. Overeating is typically a combustible combination of disturbing feelings and wrong thoughts, coupled with deeply ingrained behavior patterns and easily available food. We must learn: 1) how to identify the emotions associated with urges to overeat; 2) how to feel those emotions and manage them instead of allowing them to manage us; 3) how to work through emotional pain, grieve it, and allow God to transform it—and us.

LOOKING AT YOUR *LIFE*

Emotions aren't wrong or bad. What you do with an emotion is what counts. The work is to first acknowledge what emotion is triggering you.

Jot down a few details and/or recollections about each of the following. When was the last time you . . .

cried?

_____

got really furious?

_____

felt really scared?

_____

were overcome by anxiety?

_____

felt genuinely depressed?

_____

sensed deep envy in your heart?

_____

were filled with guilt or shame?

_____

What one emotion seems to keep popping up in your life more than others? What's your best guess as to what this is about?

_____

_____

LEARNING A NEW WAY OF *LIFE*

When you have the urge to eat, try to identify what you feel. This sounds simple but may not be if you were taught not to feel or even to acknowledge negative emotions like anger, pride, envy, and such. Yet negative emotions are part of our human condition and must be dealt with in a healthy and biblical way.

Many people are surprised when they realize how often emotions are named and discussed in the Bible. Spend a few minutes reading and thinking your way through the following passages and questions.

What do you think of the statement that *anger* is the most reported emotion tied to overeating? How, if at all, have you seen this in your experience?

_____

_____

_____

The Bible says, "Be angry, and do not sin" (Ephesians 4:26 NKJV). How is this possible?

_____

_____

If you struggle with clinical depression, there is nothing wrong with taking an antidepressant to help stabilize your mood and correct brain chemistry. You may need to see a doctor and/ or therapist to help with depression.

The authors say that many of us overeat when we are *fatigued*. They suggest, "If you are tired, rest is what you need." Do you see this habit in your life? Read the following scriptures that speak to the importance of rest. Then jot down the big idea of each passage.

Psalm 37:7

_____

_____

_____

Matthew 11:28–30

_____

_____

Psalm 43 is only five verses long, but it gives insight into the single best way to overcome feelings of *depression*. Ponder the passage for a few minutes. Why is food an inadequate answer to feelings of depression?

_____

_____

When we are *lonely*, why are we inclined to seek out food instead of the people who could help address our loneliness? What does Psalm 68:6 say about this? How can a spiritual family help in these times?

_____

_____

Guilt is only healthy when it relates to sin. We should feel guilty when we disobey God's Word. But once we confess that sin, it is gone and forgotten.

If you sometimes eat because of feelings of *insecurity*, how do the words of Jesus in John 10:27–30 give you new hope and confidence?

_____

_____

Do you struggle with feelings of *guilt* and *shame*? Why? How does Romans 8:1–2 speak to your situation?

_____

_____

LOSING IT FOR *LIFE*

What new insights have you discovered into why you sometimes overeat?

_____

_____

Let's get practical and make a plan. The next time you feel strong anger or anxiety or some other uncomfortable feeling, what specific steps can you take to avoid turning to food to numb your pain?

_____

_____

_____

_____

Shame often develops from a message that you are bad, weak, or unloved. Yet Jesus does not shame you or judge you by your weight or your failures.

Show your plan to two trusted friends. Ask for their honest feedback. Pray with them and ask them to pray faithfully for you. Ask them to be your safety net of accountability.

Try this. Listen to some praise CDs in your car or home stereo system. Really pay attention to the lyrics. Test the adage that praise is the antidote to feeling down. Record your experience here.

_____

_____

_____

_____

Here's another valuable project: Make a list of your strengths and weaknesses. Thank God for the things you are able to do well. Then ask God to help you with your weaknesses. By His Spirit, He is able to accomplish much, even with our limitations (Zechariah 4:6).

Identifying Feelings (Part 2)

This set of workbook lessons explores the various ways in which we often eat to combat or to numb troubling feelings. We're learning that food isn't the answer. It might give us a brief bit of comfort or distraction, but it doesn't address the deepest needs of our hearts.

If you are willing to take your hurts and pains to Christ and lay them at His feet, . . . if you will refuse to believe the lies of the evil one, the food handcuffs will drop off you.

LOOKING AT YOUR *LIFE*

As the *LIFL* book demonstrates, everyone has painful childhood memories—sad stories of betrayal or abandonment or abuse. The problem here is that when we suffer deep wounds as children, we simply don't have the vocabularies, life experience, opportunities, or tools to properly process these confusing events. Consequently, they lodge in our souls and become defining. After such episodes of deep hurt or loss, we typically form wrong conclusions about God, others, and ourselves. Even worse, we vow to do whatever it takes to avoid feeling pain again. The result is a life of running and hiding, feeling numb, and doing everything we can to avoid trusting God or others.

Can you relate? Does this summary ring true in your own experience?

_____

_____

Take a big step of faith, and list your top five hurts or disappointments. What events have most deeply marked you? (Note: the goal here is not to wallow in misery, but to uncover clues to the mystery of who you are and why you function as you do.)

1. _____

_____

2. _____
_____
3. _____
_____
4. _____
_____
5. _____
_____

LEARNING A NEW WAY OF *LIFE*

Before we look at some more emotional reasons people turn to food and end up overeating, consider this passage from the gospel of Luke. It's interesting and relevant because it occurs right at the beginning of Christ's ministry.

> When the devil had finished all this tempting, he left [Jesus] until an opportune time.
>
> Jesus returned to Galilee in the power of the Spirit, and news about him spread through the whole countryside. He was teaching in their synagogues, and everyone praised him.
>
> He went to Nazareth, where he had been brought up, and on the Sabbath day he went into the synagogue, as was his custom. He stood up to read, and the scroll of the prophet Isaiah was handed to him. Unrolling it, he found the place where it is written:
>
> > "The Spirit of the Lord is on me,
> > because he has anointed me
> > to proclaim good news to the poor.
> > He has sent me to proclaim freedom for the prisoners
> > and recovery of sight for the blind,
> > to set the oppressed free,
> > to proclaim the year of the Lord's favor."
>
> Then he rolled up the scroll, gave it back to the attendant and sat down. The eyes of everyone in the synagogue were fastened on him. He began by saying to them, "Today this scripture is fulfilled in your hearing." (Luke 4:13–21)

If you eat because you feel insecure, no amount of food will change that feeling. The only place you are truly secure is in your relationship with God.

What is significant about these phrases in the Isaiah passage that Jesus applied to Himself?

- "freedom for the prisoners"

_____

_____

- "recovery of sight for the blind"

_____

_____

- "set the oppressed free"

_____

_____

In what ways is food sometimes like a prison? How do we become oppressed by our eating habits and weight?

_____

_____

The *LIFL* book suggests that *jealousy* (comparing ourselves to others) can tempt us to eat when we're not really physically hungry. How so?

_____

_____

If you are one who eats when you are *happy*, what are some other ways you can celebrate (other than eating)?

_____

_____

Read the following passages that speak about *worry* or *fear*. What do you see in these verses that can help in your dieting?

Matthew 6:25–34

_____

_____

Philippians 4:6–7

_____

_____

What's the problem with being a nervous eater?

_____

_____

LOSING IT FOR *LIFE*

Spend a few minutes writing out responses to how emotions affect your eating habits. Then brainstorm some options.

Emotion	How This Prompts Me to Overeat	Some Options Instead of Food
Disappointment/Hurt		
Emptiness		
Procrastination		
Boredom		
Rejection		
Loss of Control		

With which of the above emotions do you seem to struggle most?

_____

_____

Write candidly about a vivid personal experience of rejection.

_____

_____

Eating is a great way to delay unpleasant tasks or waste time. But the task will still be there when you finish eating. It's best to tackle tough tasks head on.

When people continually hurt you or let you down, food can easily become a trusted friend. It is always available. It tastes good and satisfies for the moment. But no matter how many times we turn to food, the pain won't go away. The hurt stays buried beneath increasing layers of fat. The authors write:

> To be healed, you must face rejection. Feel it with all your soul. Pour out your heart to the Lord. Once you've allowed yourself to really feel the pain of rejection, pray and ask God to take it. Then ask Christ to speak His truth to you. You see, the enemy uses emotional pain to implant lies—that no one will want or love you; that people will only hurt you; that if only you were thinner . . . all lies!
>
> The truth is that there is Someone who will never reject you and is completely trustworthy. Your acceptance has nothing to do with your actions or your weight. Jesus unconditionally loves you because you are His. Know that Jesus Christ identifies with your pain. According to Isaiah 53, He was despised, rejected, and a man of sorrow. Because of His great love for you, He suffered the pain of rejection. On the cross, it was crucified once and for all. Once you allow His truth to soak your spirit, you can give up the pain of rejection and accept God's unfailing love.

Isn't it interesting that when we feel out of control, we eat out of control? You are not in control, so you might as well surrender to the One who is.

Comment about how this passage speaks to you, how it affects you. Does their advice seem crazy?

_____

_____

Remembering the words of Christ in Luke 4 about freedom, write a prayer expressing your desire to be delivered from the grips of emotional eating.

_____

_____

DAY 4
Expressing Your Feelings

So far we've seen that, like it or not, we are emotional creatures. All sorts of feelings permeate our souls. These feelings aren't inherently wrong, but if we're not careful, we can let them propel us in unhealthy directions. Much overeating is due to the fact that we fail to understand, identify, and process disturbing emotions. We substitute food for feeling our feelings.

After looking at the most common culprits behind emotional eating, now we want to spend a session coming to grips with how to express our feelings properly. In times of strong emotion, the answer isn't to *take food in* but to *get our feelings out*!

Once you've identified your feelings, you must learn to express them directly rather than medicating them with food.

LOOKING AT YOUR *LIFE*

How hard is it for you to put words to what you're feeling? Did you grow up in a home where this expression was encouraged?

_____

_____

_____

Can you name your emotions? From the following list, circle the words that best describe how you feel right now. What's stirring in you?

Tired	Anxious	Alive	Hopeless
Irritated	Rejected	Joyful	Worried
Lonely	Vulnerable	Confused	Peaceful
Bored	Fragile	Stressed	Disconnected
Frustrated	Sad	Depressed	Torn
Guilty	Ugly	Discouraged	Hopeful
Scared	Compassionate	Encouraged	Jealous

Describe a life in which you were no longer at the mercy of powerful emotional urges. What might that be like? Why would that be preferable to your current lifestyle? How specifically would your daily experience be different?

_____

_____

_____

LEARNING A NEW WAY OF _LIFE_

Determine if there is a need behind what you're feeling—for example, the need to be loved, accepted, approved of, or respected.

The Psalms are like a kind of textbook for learning how to process our feelings. Read Psalms 4–6. What do you observe? Does David seem like a guy who has difficulty admitting the struggles of his life and heart? Do you sense a hesitation in him to articulate the negative feelings he's experiencing? What's the implication for us?

_____

_____

_____

_____

See if you can list ten different ways feelings can be expressed. Which of these do you already do? Which would take some getting used to?

_____

_____

_____

Why do the authors place such emphasis on confession—that is, being honest about what is going on inside of you? (Hint: see Psalm 32:3.)

_____

_____

_____

What are the dangers and pitfalls of not being up front with others about our struggles, doubts, and failures? How does James 5:16 add to your understanding?

_____

_____

_____

What ingredients create an atmosphere in which confession is more likely among Christian friends?

_____

_____

_____

_____

What character qualities should we look for in a confessor/confidant/accountability partner?

_____

_____

_____

_____

By breaking our silence and speaking the truth about ourselves aloud to God and another person, we move out of the darkness and bring secrets into the light.

LOSING IT FOR _LIFE_

The authors say that _confession_ means that we:

____ submit ourselves to God's ways of handling secrets, respecting His desire for openness and vulnerability among His people

____ are willing to overcome our fear of rejection by revealing our failures to another person

____ reject our habit of self-protective secretiveness

____ admit to at least one other person that we have fallen short of God's best, including our character defects and judgment errors

____ have stopped trying to mask our true feelings

____ have chosen to humble ourselves before God and others

____ renounce our independence and admit that we need help from fellow believers

____ put our vague sense of guilt into written or spoken words and express the situation without making excuses

Go back through this list and put a check mark before the actions you have done or are willing to do. Leave empty the blanks in front of the action steps that you still need to take.

Why do some of the steps seem harder to you than others?

_____

_____

If you want to break free from emotional eating, you must confess the need that is not being met and be honest about what you truly feel. Honesty brings about authentic change.

Begin to develop the skill of healthily expressing your feelings. A good pattern to follow (until you get comfortable) is to say and/or pray the following:

God, I feel _____ *(name the emotion)*, I think because _____ *(describe the situation or event that may have triggered the feeling)*. But the truth about my situation is _____ *(remind yourself of pertinent facts and promises of God's Word)*. O Lord, renew my mind. Help me to see this situation through your eyes. Please give me the grace to cling to you. Grant me the courage to live by what you say is true, not by how I feel.

Try saying this prayer right now.

Why is it wise to have more than one person to talk with about your struggles?

_____

_____

_____

_____

God wants us to come to Him no matter what. Don't allow your losses and pain to turn you away from Him.

DAY 5
Reducing Stress

Stress can trigger overeating. If you remember from chapter 2, triggers (subtle or overt) always precede the urge to overeat. A trigger or cue can be a specific event or a person, or a feeling that arises from involvement in certain events or with certain people.

In this lesson we want to learn how to eliminate overeating triggers by reducing stress or avoiding certain events or people.

LOOKING AT YOUR *LIFE*

During the last year, check which of the following stressful events you've experienced.

____ death of a loved one	____ death of a personal dream
____ death of a friend	____ termination of a friendship
____ job loss	____ financial setback
____ change in jobs	____ lifestyle change
____ change in income	____ surgery/hospitalization
____ new home	____ tax troubles
____ new baby	____ big vacation
____ child moves out	____ holiday with family
____ change in marital status	____ death of a pet
____ new church	____ automobile accident
____ serious health issues	____ home remodeling
____ minor health issues	____ natural disaster (flooding, fire, etc.)
____ legal troubles	____ other
____ weight gain of more than 25 pounds	

NUMBER OF STRESSORS: ____

When a highly stressful period hits, put a time limit on the amount of time you'll give to thinking about it.

1–3	Pray for the rest of us—that we don't become envious!
4–8	(sigh) Welcome to life in a fallen world.
9 or more	Bless your heart, "Job"!

Think about the people in your life. Which individuals leave you feeling stressed and tense—maybe because they engage you in certain conversations or bring up old memories? What precisely do they do?

_____

_____

_____

What regular situations seem to get you agitated, so that you end up turning to food out of habit? Dissect those situations. What's really going on? What emotions do they stir within you?

_____

_____

_____

Another great stress reducer is exercise. There is nothing like a game of golf, tennis, or racquetball to get your mind off the pressure through physical exertion.

Use this chart to list the stressful triggers that upset you and lead to overeating. Put them in the appropriate column. You can easily see which ones to eliminate, reduce, or cope with in a different way. Look at this example:

Stress triggers to overeat	Can eliminate	Can reduce	Need new coping
Lunch partners overeat	X		
Uncle Jim and politics		X	
Fights with spouse			X
Dealing with mother			X

Stress triggers to overeat	Can eliminate	Can reduce	Need new coping

LEARNING A NEW WAY OF *LIFE*

Read Psalm 13. What clues do you see here about David's situation? How does he go about handling his stress?

_____

_____

_____

_____

Read Psalm 55. This is a lament of David in which he tells of betrayal at the hands of a close friend. What jumps out at you from this painful glimpse into David's "journal"? Was this an avoidable situation or one over which he had control?

_____

_____

_____

_____

What stresses in your life right now can't be eliminated? Instead of freaking out or bingeing on food, list some better options for handling this stressful situation.

_____

_____

_____

_____

Assertiveness is simply standing up for what you know to be true and holding your position. In order to be assertive you have to know what you want and then verbalize it. You can't be afraid to hurt people's feelings. When you set a boundary or tell someone no, he or she may get hurt, but that isn't your problem.

Have you ever journaled? Do you now? If not, what do you think about this discipline? How could a prayer journal help you?

_____

_____

LOSING IT FOR *LIFE*

Are you the kind of person who feels pressured to please everyone, so that you take on more responsibility than you should? Give some examples. What responsibilities have you taken on that are now burdensome and stressful?

_____

_____

How can learning to say no become an effective tool in overcoming stress?

_____

_____

If you grew up in the home of an alcoholic, addicted, abusive, or mentally ill parent, chances are you really don't know how to relax. Why? Because growing up in a household in which peoples' moods and actions were unpredictable creates tension in children. Those tense kids become tense adults who never learned how to relax. Relaxation wasn't safe. Your guard had to be up or you could get hurt.

When—in the last five years—have you felt the most deeply relaxed?

_____

_____

What are some ways you'd love to learn to relax—if only you could give yourself permission to do so?

_____

_____

Pain is not optional, but misery is. You can't always control pain, but you can do something about misery. If you are looking for a quick fix to emotional pain, find another book to read! We would rather you take this approach: "God's hand is upon me, and I am entering a process of healing—people to keep me accountable, support me, and confront me so I don't repeat the same mistakes along the way." Healing is often progressive because it requires changes in our character and actions. The way we cope with emotional pain must change if we decide to no longer eat our way through it.

Let's apply the RISE acronym to the issue of emotional eating.

REDUCE stress where and when you can; reduce eating in response to negative feelings and stress.

INCREASE confession—your ability to stand and confront negative feelings and tough issues.

SUBSTITUTE new ways—other than eating—to deal with painful emotions; substitute feeling for running from feelings.

ELIMINATE fear, stress whenever possible, feelings of rejection, and shame or hopelessness.

Keep a record of what you do when you become emotionally upset. You only have to record a few instances. Write down the event, the emotion, and how you behaved or what you did. For example:

Event: Received an upsetting phone call from my ex
Emotion: Very hurt
Reaction: Went to the refrigerator and opened the door to eat

Now, think of a new way to cope with that feeling. What could you substitute for eating? For example:

New behavior: Call a friend and let her pray with me

Here's another example:

Event: Heard someone gossip about me at church
Emotion: Anger
Reaction: Stopped for fries at fast-food restaurant
New behavior: Gently confront the person who did the gossiping

Make a list of ten behaviors you can substitute the next time you want to eat because of an intense emotion. Your list should include behaviors you can do while driving, at home, at work, and on the go. Post the list on your refrigerator and make a copy to take with you. Every time you are tempted to eat because you feel an unpleasant emotion, pull out your list and choose a new thing to do.

_____
_____
_____
_____
_____
_____
_____
_____
_____
_____

People who learn to respond to emotional pain without using food to numb themselves or to escape have a better and longer weight-loss maintenance record than those who only deal with eating and exercise. Both research and clinical experience support this idea. This work will be difficult because you'll be giving up a deeply ingrained way of coping. You may feel flooded with emotions that you haven't felt in a long time because eating has covered them up, but the rewards are well worth the effort. With God's help you can come out of the eating closet to a place of peace and rest.

8

Changing the Viewing

Did you see the reality television show called *Extreme Makeover*, which aired from 2002 to 2007? The concept of the show was this: Each week, the producers presented the viewing audience with two or more people who were extremely insecure about their looks. Because of their physical flaws, they lacked confidence, became introverts, or didn't fully engage in life. For years they had suffered teasing and insults concerning their appearances. Their stories touched viewers—we felt for them. Some of us could even relate to their emotional pain.

People wrote to the show and pitched their reasons for needing a makeover. When chosen, they reacted with delight, knowing they had basically won the makeover lottery—in the form of top plastic surgeons, dentists, eye surgeons, fashion experts, hair stylists, makeup artists, and personal trainers, all contributing to the extreme makeover. With a promise of life transformation in just six weeks, those chosen consented to going under the plastic surgery knife.

As they chose their new bodies, they could be sculpted to new proportions—breast implants, liposuction, a chin implant, face-lift, rhinoplasty, corrective eye surgery, even new dentures. If they wanted it, they got it!

As viewers watched these people anxiously go into surgery and then recovery, the emotional buildup began. Soon their lives were dramatically altered. We became voyeurs to the process. It was like watching a butterfly emerge from a cocoon, as the metamorphosis took approximately six weeks. At the end of that time, a limousine escorted the new person back to the reality of his or her life and family. And in true Hollywood fashion, the winner's coming-out party happened on a stage amid lights and cameras. The audience gasped with awe, applauded, cried, and hugged. The difference was dramatic and a testimony to the power of an extreme makeover.

All that to say, though we certainly feel sorrow for the emotional pain those chosen few endured because of their appearances, the message of the show was disconcerting. The solution proffered—that being thin and beautiful will fix life's problems—only added to the obsession our culture has with the body. Record numbers of people in bondage to eating disorders, as well as most Americans who are unhappy with their bodies, are embracing this message. If life's problems can be fixed with surgery, why shouldn't we all go under the knife? Pretty soon none of us will measure up!

The television show had the right idea but the wrong solution. The truth is, we all need an extreme makeover. If you struggle with negative self-image, the solution is surgery within the heart. The results last a lifetime, and the transformation that comes from being the bride of Christ is beyond any physical makeover one could ever experience. It is extreme, life changing, and affirming—"But we all, with unveiled face, beholding as in a mirror the glory of the Lord, are being transformed into the same image from glory to glory, just as by the Spirit of the Lord" (2 Corinthians 3:18 NKJV). Now that's an extreme makeover we want to support!

How does such a makeover happen? One important step in the process is the renewing of your mind, or, as we like to call it, *changing the viewing* in the way you think about yourself, God, and others. To start, let us address these three key areas.

Body Image

Whose image do you reflect? Should you try to meet society's warped standards of beauty and fitness, or should you be content with the body you were given while making every effort to be in good health? In Genesis 1:26–27, God explains that we are made in His image and reflect His likeness. He declared His created design "good," meaning that nothing about our bodies is a mistake. However, by not taking care of our bodies, we do harm. Eating too much food and not getting enough exercise are actually abuses against the human body that are a direct result of the human will. As a result, the body should not be viewed as the enemy in this weight-loss journey.

Identity

Your acceptance, security, and significance are to be found in Christ. If you look to any other source for your true identity, you'll be disappointed by the result. The root of all image problems is related to identity. Your identity must be fully secure in Christ. You are one of His and must not allow yourself to be defined otherwise.

Worth

God's love for you has nothing to do with your appearance or weight. You are His beautiful bride and are valued and esteemed *because of Him*, not because of the way you look. He looks at your heart and wants to capture it. You were bought with a price: the precious blood of the Lamb. Value is determined by how much someone is willing to pay for it. Christ obviously values you a great deal in that He gave His life for you.

Your perspective regarding your body, identity, and worth may require new focus as you meditate on God's Word and learn more specifically how God thinks about you. If you doubt these truths, then your mind is in need of renewal. As you make changes in eating and exercise, you must also focus on becoming a person of spiritual beauty—one who imitates Christ and desires to be like Him in mind, body, and spirit.

A NEW THOUGHT

When my (Dr. Linda's) daughter was young, she asked me an interesting question that really got me thinking. As she watched me step out of the shower and towel off the excess water one morning, she just stared at me. Thinking deeply (or as deep as a five-year-old can think), she asked, "Mom, will I get that crinkly stuff on your legs? It doesn't look too good."

I almost fell over. This tiny child was staring at my cellulite! And her conclusion was that it didn't look "too good." Well, I knew this was an important mother-daughter moment that could influence her feelings about her own body in years to come. So I calmly looked at my cellulite (that act in itself is a miracle) and explained, "You won't get this crinkly stuff on your legs until you are my age. And when you do, it's no big deal. It's just crinkly stuff." Part of me believed what I was saying, but the other part was screaming, "Oh really, no big deal? How long did you obsess over your thighs before you came to accept them?"[1]

Fortunately, by this point in my life, the cellulite wasn't a big deal. Years ago, my answer would have been different. I, like so many men and women, had to learn to make peace with my physical body. No matter what size we are, accepting our bodies is not easy to do in this culture.

We never measure up to the ideals plastered on billboards, magazines, commercials, and movies. And seeing images of perfection day in and day out does a number on our thinking. From Botox to cellulite creams, the message is that you can never be too thin, too fit, or too perfect. Yet it's time for all of us to think twice about these messages, because they have serious impact on our lives as well as others'.

One of the best sensations I (Steve) have ever had is the feeling of weightlessness experienced on a wild ride called the Fire Ball. In between the soaring up and plummeting down, something amazing happens. For about two seconds you are up and out of your seat and held into the contraption only by a harness. Literally, you are floating in a state of weightlessness. And what a feeling of freedom and joy that brings!

This is what I want for you. I want you to wake up in the morning and not have to drag yourself out of bed, not to have one thought about your weight or feeling about who you are relating to your weight. You would know your weight but it would not define you. You would not feel too heavy or too light or too anything. You would be able to relate without worrying about something being too big or bulging or even what others were thinking about your appearance. Your life would be something beyond weight, size, and comparison. You would be free. You would be weightless.

Negative body image is like a modern-day plague that continues to torment us. But it doesn't have to be. We can resist cultural prescriptions and renew our minds with biblical thought. Our bodies are the dwelling place of the Holy Spirit (1 Corinthians 3:16), literally, "holy temples"!

There is a healthy balance between body obsession and hating our bodies. Somewhere in the middle is acceptance and responsibility. The way we think about our bodies will be reflected externally. Proverbs 23:7 says, "For as he thinks in his heart, so is he" (NKJV). Hence, you are what you think! When a person hates his or her body, you can tell by the way he or she talks about it. Yet to hate your body is to reject the beautiful creation God has made in His image. Instead, you must accept your body, flaws and all, and take care for that holy temple. Five key steps to accepting your body are:

1. **Stop degrading your body**. "I am so fat. Who would want me?" "I'm ugly and undesirable." These kinds of statements are highly negative and lead to negative feelings. You would not say such things about a friend, and you shouldn't talk about yourself this way either. Become your best encourager

rather than worst critic. That voice would say, "You are overweight, but you're working on it."

2. **Stop putting life on hold because you don't like your body.** Dive in and do what you love to do. Feel good knowing that you are making every effort you can to change your weight, while accepting that your body is the Holy Spirit's temple no matter what and a reflection of God's likeness. Live in the present reality as you implement changes for the future.

3. **Think of good things to say about yourself.** You are more than your weight. Focus on the positive qualities you have outside of your physical size. We are not asking you to boast but to become more balanced and realistic. We all have good qualities that can be emphasized.

4. **Develop your own style and personality.** Not everyone judges you by your weight. Take a chance and reach out to others rather than hiding behind your weight. Let your true personality shine.

5. **Get your esteem from God.** *Self-esteem* is a misleading term. None of us can truly have esteem by looking to the *self*. The *self* is sinful, self-centered, and easily deceived. God esteems you just because He chose and loves you. You don't have to earn His esteem. You already have it. Remember, He values you so much that He gave His only Son to die for you.

Thoughts lead to feelings. Feelings lead to actions. Actions influence our perceptions, which then influence our thoughts. It's a vicious cycle. What we think affects how we feel, which in turn can prompt us to eat in response. Thus, many negative feelings can be avoided by changing the thought that prompts the feeling. If, for example, I feel sad because I purposefully think, *Nobody cares about me*, I can change my sad feeling by changing the thought to a more positive and realistic one—*God cares about me even when others don't*. Since this thought is reassuring and doesn't make me feel sad, I am unlikely to eat as a response to it.

If we apply the RISE formula to our thoughts, here are our goals:

Reduce negative thoughts and self-degrading statements.

Increase your awareness of God; increase esteem and acceptance of the body you were given.

Substitute positive thoughts for negative ones and a view of yourself that is not defined by your weight.

Eliminate thinking errors and lies.

RENEWING THE MIND

In this context, the word *renew* means a change of heart and life. It is work the Holy Spirit does in us. As we offer our bodies as a living sacrifice to God, we allow the Holy Spirit to radically work in our hearts and minds. Renewing the mind is different from positive thinking in that truth must be experienced from the One who is truth.

Whenever something negative or traumatic happens to us, the enemy uses those circumstances to implant a lie, because his plan is to deceive us about who God is. During times of emotional pain, he tries hard to seduce us away from God's truth and into a pit of darkness. If we don't know the truth, or we let our spiritual guard down, we can accept his lies in place of truth, just as Eve did.

So much of the pain and turmoil we feel today has to do with lies implanted from times when we experienced hurt and were wounded. Many of us continue to struggle with overeating because we believe a host of lies. We believe we are hopeless, that God doesn't care, that people are always letting us down. And though none of these statements is true, we adjust our reality to make them true.

While we are saved and our spirits are made new in Christ (2 Corinthians 5:17), our minds are still in need of renewal. Yet we cannot be free of the lies and distorted thinking on our own power. A renewed mind comes as we receive truth from Christ and deeply plant His Word in our hearts.

How many times have you known something to be true, such as, "God loves me and would never leave me," and yet you *feel* this isn't true? Your experience tells you that what you know to be true isn't true. And here is the great disconnect: we can know truth in our heads but not have it connect to our hearts. We need an experience of truth to make it real to us and connect our heads and hearts. That's where prayer comes in. When you know your heart says one thing and your head says another, ask Christ to speak His truth to you. Read His Word and ask Him to penetrate it deep into your mind and soul. Look at the Gospels. Do you notice that Jesus healed (an experience) and then spoke to the person (cognitive)? The Truth gave truth, both experientially and cognitively.

Identify the lies that create your emotional pain. Lies can come to us by the words of others, by our own perceptions, or during times of hurt and trauma. Once you identify a lie, ask Christ to speak His truth. Here's an example: An obese woman struggled with urges to binge regularly. In counseling, she discussed times she was prevented from having food as a form of punishment when she was a child. The lie she believed was that she would never get enough food. Thus she binged because she was afraid food would not be available. And though she knew in her head that this wasn't true, she prayed and asked God to show her His truth. She described hearing Christ tell her that He always has enough of what she needs. She read scriptures that reminded her of this truth and meditated on them. As soon as she did this, that lie no longer had power over her. Experientially, she knew her needs would be met.

In another case, a man was deeply hurt over the rejection from his wife when she divorced him. As a result, he began to think he was unlovable. Those in the adult singles' group at his church encouraged him to join the group. He did and found people willing to accept him and spend time with him. His experience with this group of believers countered his earlier belief. *If these people can accept me, and I know God accepts me, maybe I'm not unlovable.* The power of the lie was broken through the development of a new community. His overeating diminished when he was no longer eating out of feelings of rejection.

Perhaps the biggest lie we tell ourselves is that all we can do about our problem is to pray to God to get rid of it. And though this might be true, and you can pray that prayer, the answer is often going to require more than waiting for God. Or God may choose not to take away this burden, which is often the case.

Whether or not you have a life of meaning and purpose or stagnation and death is quite often dependent on what we are willing to change. We wait for God to do what God is waiting for us to do. Why? Because God wants to build our character, and the way He does that is by sticking with us through a struggle, gently supporting our efforts if they are honorable and glorify Him.

TAKE THE NEGATIVE THOUGHT CAPTIVE

In 2 Corinthians 10:5 we are told to take our thoughts captive. "We use our powerful God-tools for smashing warped philosophies, tearing down barriers erected against the truth of God, fitting every loose thought and emotion and impulse into the structure of life shaped by Christ" (MSG).

If you grew up in a home in which you were constantly criticized, negative thoughts have been deeply ingrained. Don't worry. You can renew your mind with the help of God and others.

To apply this scripture, we must be aware of what we are thinking. Once we realize the thought is negative, self-degrading, or untrue, we should stop the thought. To stop a thought, pretend you are grabbing it out of the air. You have now taken it captive. You say, "I've got you, thought. Now what am I going to do with you?" Hopefully, you will smash it or replace it with a thought that is true, one that fits a life shaped by Christ.

Here's an example of this principle in action. The thought occurs: *I just ate all those cookies. I am so bad.* The latter part of that thought must be stopped. Grab it and replace it with God's truth by saying, "I am not bad. Christ is in me, and though I am tempted and do sin, when this happens I ask for forgiveness and move on. I wish I hadn't eaten all those cookies, but it's not the end of the world. I can regain control right now with God's help. Lord, give me the self-control I need right now."

In order to Lose It for Life, you have to gain control of your thoughts. And with practice, you can do this. Sometimes it helps to put a rubber band on your wrist and snap it every time you tell yourself a negative thought or lie. The mild pain is a simple reminder to grab the negative thought. Until you do something like this, you may not realize how many times a day negative thoughts race through your mind. Like spam mail on a computer, the thoughts just show up and keep on coming. As with e-mail, the trick is to not click on the thoughts to open them. Instead, delete them instantly and avoid giving negative thoughts a foothold in your mind, because they are the messages of Satan, not God.

KEEP A THOUGHT RECORD

A tool that is often used to help people get in touch with their thoughts is the Dysfunctional Thought Record (DTR).[2] This is a simple chart laid out as follows (see Appendix F):

Dysfunctional Thought Record					
Date	Situation	Emotion / Intensity	Automatic Thought	Rational Response / Intensity	Outcome
3–20	Overate	Disgust / 80%	I am a loser	I blew it but I can get back on track / 10%	

Here's how you use the chart. You record the date and briefly describe the situation. Next write down what emotion you felt and rate its intensity from 0 to 100 percent in terms of emotional intensity. Then record the automatic thought that came into your mind. Once you identify the automatic thought and write it down, try to think of a more rational and true thought and write it down. Then rate your emotion again. It should be less intense.

Keeping this chart will help you recognize the thoughts that cue your emotions. And you can review your thoughts and write alternative ways to think about the situation. For example, let's use the situation of overeating. The emotion recorded is *disgust* and you gave it an 80 percent rating, which means you felt it intensely. Your automatic thought was, *I am a loser.* The more rational response or truth is, *I blew it but can get back on track. It was only ten cookies. I am weak in my own power, but with Christ I can do all things.* You re-rate your emotion to 10 percent.

Eventually, you'll be able to do this exercise in your head. The purpose is to expose the automatic, negative thoughts and replace them with more rational alternative thoughts that are consistent with biblical truth.

THE ANSWER FOR ANXIOUS THOUGHTS

"I am just anxious; I'm not thinking anything." Wrong! You have thoughts behind those anxious feelings. The feelings may be so intense that you aren't aware of the self-talk that preceded your anxiety, but such talk is behind most anxious feelings. Remember, your thoughts impact your feelings.

Most anxious people think, *What if . . . ?* We suggest you change the "What if . . ." to "So what" to reduce anxiety. Does this sound easy? It's not. Anxious thoughts are automatic for people with anxiety problems. A person may *feel* anxious and yet be unaware of preceding thoughts. The first step is to identify your thought before the anxious feeling occurs, although the thought won't always be obvious. For example, Pat sat in a meeting with several of his superiors. He was nervous about his presentation and flashed back to a time early on in his career when he botched a presentation. These thoughts started running through Pat's head: *What if I mess up again? I could get fired. I will embarrass myself.* The more Pat allowed himself to think these thoughts, the more anxious he became. By the time he stood up to give his presentation, he was close to panic. Had this man used his self-talk in a positive way, he might have warded off anxiety. *I may have messed up early on in my career, but now I'm much more experienced. I've done these presentations many times with good outcomes. I have every reason to believe these people will like what I have to say and be impressed.*

Notice how the first self-talk creates or reinforces anxious feelings while the second example dismisses anxious thoughts and builds confidence. Self-talk is that powerful. When lies and negative thoughts become frequent and a regular part of your thinking, they create and sustain anxiety, which is often responded to by overeating. Anxious people think in ways that perpetuate anxiety. Review this checklist and find out if you think like an anxious person.

Am I Anxious?

☐ **It's going to be a catastrophe!** You think of the most extreme negative consequences possible, and assume they're going to happen. Disaster will hit, whether it's in the form of an event or personal humiliation and embarrassment.

☐ **It's personal!** Whatever happens around you is somehow personally relevant to you and will most likely happen to you next. For example, if there is a fire in the city, your house is next.

☐ **It could happen!** Here's why. You magnify the one part of the issue that could create a problem and ignore the nonthreatening parts. For example, you forget the words to the song you've practiced multiple times. Even though it's unlikely, since you've never forgotten the words during practice before, you tell yourself it could happen.

☐ **It doesn't matter what else is going on; I see danger.** You ignore the context of a problem and choose to focus on the one thing that could be dangerous or problematic. For example, your daughter could fall off the swing even though the grass is soft, the swing almost touches the ground, and she loves to be outside. Anxious thinkers focus on the possibility of falling off the swing even though the likelihood of harm is slight.

☐ **I can tell this is trouble!** At any sign of trouble, you immediately jump to conclusions. For example, air turbulence means the plane is crashing. Or a tightness in your chest means you are dying from a heart attack. A call from the school means your child is in trouble.

☐ **I can't. I don't have what it takes. I won't be able to do it.** You believe nothing will change and you can't meet the challenge. You have given up before starting and aren't asking God to help you overcome your weakness. Though you can't do something in your own power, God can do all things through you if you allow His power to be made known.

☐ **It will happen again.** Because something happened once, you assume it will happen again.

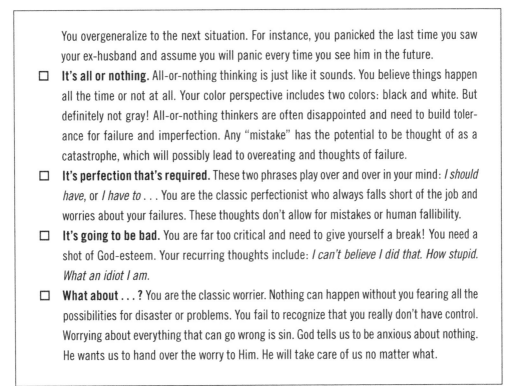

You overgeneralize to the next situation. For instance, you panicked the last time you saw your ex-husband and assume you will panic every time you see him in the future.

☐ **It's all or nothing.** All-or-nothing thinking is just like it sounds. You believe things happen all the time or not at all. Your color perspective includes two colors: black and white. But definitely not gray! All-or-nothing thinkers are often disappointed and need to build tolerance for failure and imperfection. Any "mistake" has the potential to be thought of as a catastrophe, which will possibly lead to overeating and thoughts of failure.

☐ **It's perfection that's required.** These two phrases play over and over in your mind: *I should have,* or *I have to . . .* You are the classic perfectionist who always falls short of the job and worries about your failures. These thoughts don't allow for mistakes or human fallibility.

☐ **It's going to be bad.** You are far too critical and need to give yourself a break! You need a shot of God-esteem. Your recurring thoughts include: *I can't believe I did that. How stupid. What an idiot I am.*

☐ **What about . . . ?** You are the classic worrier. Nothing can happen without you fearing all the possibilities for disaster or problems. You fail to recognize that you really don't have control. Worrying about everything that can go wrong is sin. God tells us to be anxious about nothing. He wants us to hand over the worry to Him. He will take care of us no matter what.

If you relate to these statements, you need to change out your thoughts. Write down positive statements that will counter the negative ones, and use scriptures to back up your new positions. For example, instead of thinking, *I can't do that because it's too scary,* tell yourself, *It looks scary but I can meet a new challenge. The worst possible thing that can happen is that I'll feel scared for a moment and then it will pass. And if I make it through, I will have accomplished something new.*

After you've written down positive statements to replace your negative thoughts, meditate on the truth. Here's a powerful scripture you can always use: "I can do all this through him who gives me strength" (Philippians 4:13). The next time you feel anxious, stop and ask yourself what thought is making you feel worried. Chances are it's a negative thought that needs changing.

Acknowledging the possibility of danger in a situation does not necessarily make you an anxious person. You may be a realist. But if your focus is constantly on the possible harm, or the one factor that could go wrong, or whether you did the right thing, you are an anxious thinker. Anxious thinking makes anxious people, but by changing your thoughts, you can lessen your anxiety and even the feelings that result from the thought.

CHANGING THE ATTITUDE

It's 5:30 a.m. The alarm goes off and Rita rolls out of bed. Exhausted from the night before, Rita forces her body to head to the shower. As she towels off, her daily fight with anxiety begins. Every morning she spends four hours getting ready for work. Every hair must be perfectly in place and her makeup impeccable.

Rita worries that people will reject her if she appears less than perfect. Even though she knows her thoughts and behaviors are irrational, she can't stop herself from performing the lengthy routine.

Worry is Rita's constant companion. It helps her prepare for unpredictable moments in life. Her greatest fear is that she will somehow be rejected for the way she looks. To change this irrational behavior, Rita had to be convinced that her worry was unproductive and not helping her control anything. In fact, the worry was controlling her. It was time to say good-bye to her lifelong friend—worry.

In order to stop worrying, she had to change her attitude by embracing two ideas. First, her sacrifice of time and energy was not worth the small amount of control she thought she gained, because uncertainty is part of the world in which we live. People can reject her for all sorts of reasons, including her weight. So rather than avoid this uncertainty, Rita needed to accept it as a part of her life.

Second, Rita needed to accept that this type of comfort is overrated. All of Rita's hours of makeup application were directed at making her feel more comfortable with her physical appearance. Now comfort could no longer be the goal. Instead, she had to get comfortable with discomfort. She could learn to live with it, even if sometimes it was difficult or might feel lousy. But she needed to tolerate "lousy" and get past it.

When Rita allowed herself to feel discomfort, we applauded her and welcomed her to the human race. And we encouraged her to stay with the race and not run away from it! So every day, she was to wake up and recite this message:

Worry is unproductive. I can't predict how life will go today and that is okay. Discomfort will come, but it will also pass. I can live with uncertainty and change because God is in control, and He promises He won't give me anything I can't handle.

As Rita developed a new attitude about worry, her anxiety lifted. Gradually she cut down her morning routine to a reasonable time. To her amazement, it didn't seem to make any difference to her coworkers. When something felt out of Rita's control, she would check her thoughts by telling herself, "This is normal. Life is unpredictable. God will give me the grace to deal with it." Of course, the side effect was that Rita had more control over her eating.

CONTAIN STRESSFUL THOUGHTS

Stress can originate from your thoughts. Two good strategies to help with stressful thoughts are visualizing and meditation. We are not talking about repeating mantras or engaging in transcendental meditation, so please stay with us. Christians can meditate and visualize. The Bible even directs us to do so: "Whatever is true, whatever is noble, whatever is right, whatever is pure, whatever is lovely, whatever is admirable—if anything is excellent or praiseworthy—think about such things" (Philippians 4:8).

All you do is focus your mind on what brings you peace and a sense of well-being. Think about God's intense love for you and dedicate some time to Him. When we pray and spend time with our heavenly Father, we feel better and less stressed. This Dad has promised to take care of us and meet our needs. If that reality doesn't lessen your stress, nothing will!

Another tactic is to visualize yourself in a quiet, peaceful place. This is calming. Some people like to imagine themselves resting on a sunny beach with a gentle breeze, the smell of the ocean, clear skies, and water all present in their imagination. Other people find a mountain cabin in the snow to be a quiet, calming place.

Others imagine basking eternally in the presence of Christ. I (Dr. Linda) like to read Revelation 21 and picture the New Jerusalem based on the visual description John gives in that chapter—the gates, the angels, the gems, but mostly the glory of God that will shine and illuminate the city! It doesn't matter what scene you choose, as long as you think of something peaceful and try to engage all your senses in the scene. If you succeed, your anxious thoughts will melt as you settle into a place of peace.

True peace comes from having a personal relationship with Jesus Christ. One of His promises is to keep us in perfect peace if we keep our minds fixed on Him (Isaiah 26:3). God is the author of peace and serenity. Think about Him and His goodness, love, and all that He has done for you and will do as we approach His eternal presence.

A renewed mind is a mind that agrees with God. God is incapable of having bad motivations toward us, and yet we often attribute these to God. In Him, there is no darkness. When we know His character, His promises, and we believe who He says He is, we cannot think of God as bad or unloving. The key is intimacy with Him. The more you know Him, the more you trust and believe that He is truth. And the more time you spend with Him, the more you experience His truth.

In 2 Corinthians 1:8–9, Paul affirms that God brings comfort in the midst of trouble:

> We don't want you in the dark, friends, about how hard it was when all this came down on us in Asia province. It was so bad we didn't think we were going to make it. We felt like we'd been sent to death row; that it was all over for us. As it turned out, it was the best thing that could have happened. Instead of trusting in our own strength or wits to get out of it, we were forced to trust God totally—not a bad idea since he's the God who raises the dead! (MSG)

As you engage in the process to Lose It for Life, you will hit bumps along the way related to how you think. Sometimes we think too much! It is easy to question God in times of difficulty. We can grow impatient and allow the enemy to gain ground in our thoughts. But God wants to teach us to depend on Him all the time as we renew our minds with His truth and know that He is powerful and able to accomplish much in us if we submit to His plan.

Workbook Week 8

CHANGING THE VIEWING

DAY 1

Extreme Makeover

Our culture is obsessed with makeovers. Popular television shows document how people and houses undergo quick renovations. And, at least on the surface, the before-and-after differences *are* dramatic.

Our goal in this lesson is to focus on a deeper kind of makeover—one that starts in the heart and becomes a foundation for true, lasting change.

LOOKING AT YOUR *LIFE*

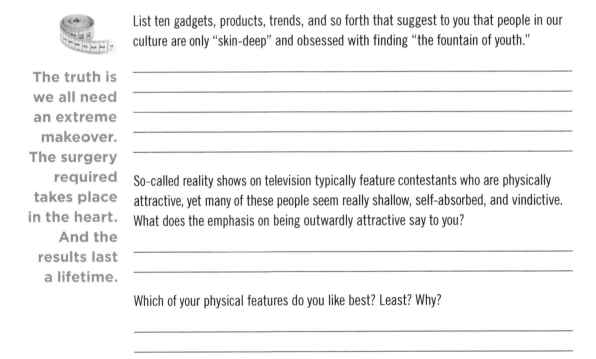

List ten gadgets, products, trends, and so forth that suggest to you that people in our culture are only "skin-deep" and obsessed with finding "the fountain of youth."

The truth is we all need an extreme makeover. The surgery required takes place in the heart. And the results last a lifetime.

_____

_____

_____

_____

_____

So-called reality shows on television typically feature contestants who are physically attractive, yet many of these people seem really shallow, self-absorbed, and vindictive. What does the emphasis on being outwardly attractive say to you?

_____

_____

Which of your physical features do you like best? Least? Why?

_____

_____

The world's foremost plastic surgeon calls you and says, "I'll perform any cosmetic procedure you desire, for free." How would you react? What kind of cosmetic alteration would you choose?

_____

_____

_____

Do you think television network executives would ever be interested in making a reality series about a group of Lose It for Life people deciding to lose weight? Why or why not? What features/underlying principles of LIFL might scare away the Hollywood crowd?

_____

_____

LEARNING A NEW WAY OF *LIFE*

Speaking on behalf of those who know Jesus Christ by faith, the apostle Paul wrote, "And we all, who with unveiled faces contemplate the Lord's glory, are being transformed into his image with ever-increasing glory, which comes from the Lord, who is the Spirit." (2 Corinthians 3:18).

What kind of transformation is this talking about? Put it into your own words.

_____

_____

_____

Read the following passages and jot down your thoughts after each one. Ask, "What does this say about God? About me? About how to change? What promise is here? What command?"

Anyone who belongs to Christ has become a new person. The old life is gone; a new life has begun! (2 Corinthians 5:17 NLT)

_____

_____

Just as we are now like the earthly man, we will someday be like the heavenly man. (1 Corinthians 15:49 NLT)

_____

_____

Dear friends, now we are children of God, and what we will be has not yet been made known. But we know that when Christ appears, we shall be like him, for we shall see him as he is. (1 John 3:2)

_____

_____

What kind of makeover is God after? What kind of differences does He want to see in us?

_____

_____

How can deep change (insights, renovations at the soul level, and so forth) result in change at the surface level of your life (eating habits, weight, and others)?

_____

_____

_____

Don't allow others to define you. Your identity must be fully secure in Christ.

LOSING IT FOR _LIFE_

We need a deeper kind of makeover, the kind that originates in the soul and that lasts longer than a Botox injection or a face-lift. One important step in the process is changing the way we think. Let's focus first on our _body image_.

Read Genesis 1:26–27 and Psalm 139. What is the message of these passages?

_____

_____

Whose image do you reflect? Should you try to meet society's warped, ever-morphing standards of beauty and fitness, or should you be content with the body you were given, making every effort to be in good health?

_____

_____

Can we ever get comfortable and okay—really and truly okay—with flawed bodies? How?

_____

_____

Think for a few moments about your _identity_. Write ten short phrases or one-word descriptions to answer the questions: "Who am I—really? What makes me significant?"

_____

_____

What would you say to the insecure teenager who is desperately relying on friends, looks, or talents to give him or her a sense of identity and significance? What's the flaw in this approach?

_____

_____

Now, let's focus on the subject of _personal worth_. We're not speaking here of net worth (as in money), but of worth in the sense of "where do I find value?" How would you answer the thoughtless person who insensitively says, "You're worthless—overweight, ugly, and unloved. No one will _ever_ care for you!"?

_____

_____

How do you know such a cruel remark is a total lie?

_____

_____

Read through the following list of practices that can aid you in this lifelong process of reprogramming your mind. How can these help you think and live in a way that honors God and brings joy? Write out your responses.

- Meditating on God's Word

_____

- Eating healthily

_____

- Exercising consistently

_____

- Doing realistic self-appraisals that involve more than just physical appearance

_____

- Focusing on becoming a person who is attractive internally

_____

- Learning to accept your body and what can't be changed

_____

- Refusing to compare yourself with others; understanding that's God's plans and designs for each person are unique

_____

_____

What is one big take-away truth you got from this lesson? How do you intend to put it into practice immediately?

_____

_____

_____

We will never measure up to the perfect bodies plastered on billboards or parading around on TV. It's time for all of us to think twice about these messages because they impact our lives in hugely negative ways.

DAY 2
Achieving Weightlessness

Negative body image is a modern-day plague tormenting many of us. But this doesn't have to be. One of the stated goals of Lose It for Life is to achieve a state of "weightlessness."

LOOKING AT YOUR *LIFE*

How do you explain our culture's obsession with the human body? Why the relentless focus?

_____

_____

_____

What people do you know who really like their bodies and are content with the way they look?

_____

_____

_____

What about you? Write five words or phrases that describe how you honestly feel about your body.

_____

_____

_____

There is a healthy balance between body obsession and hating our bodies. Somewhere in the middle is acceptance and responsibility.

LEARNING A NEW WAY OF *LIFE*

In Lose It for Life lingo, "weightlessness" means you are no longer defined by your weight. How do you think someone gets to this place?

_____

_____

_____

The Bible says, "Don't you know that you yourselves are God's temple and that God's Spirit dwells in your midst? If anyone destroys God's temple, God will destroy that person; for God's temple is sacred, and you together are that temple" (1 Corinthians 3:16–17). How can this truth alter the way we *view* our bodies? How can it affect the way we *treat* our bodies?

_____

_____

_____

Spend a few minutes pondering this ancient truth: "For as he thinks in his heart, so is he" (Proverbs 23:7 NKJV). What does this verse have to say to those who view their bodies with contempt?

_____

_____

Think about the following people and situations:

- the overweight person who loudly and constantly jokes about how "fat" he or she is
- the young girl with the beautiful body who, because of emotional emptiness, gives herself sexually to every young man who comes along
- the individuals who make it their lifelong goal to look just like someone famous
- the people who spend hours daily pumping iron and admiring their mirrored, muscled images

- the heavy person who has a garage full of unused exercise equipment bought impulsively
- the hyperkinetic young woman who exercises obsessively out of fear of gaining weight
- the anorexic model who is told she's a "cow" because her weight "ballooned" from 105 to 112 pounds

What common threads do you see in these behaviors?

_____

_____

_____

Which of these do you find the most understandable? The most bizarre? Why?

_____

_____

_____

LOSING IT FOR *LIFE*

Give yourself a much-needed break! *Accept your body*, flaws and all, and care for it as the holy temple it is.

Why is it important to stop making degrading statements about how you look?

_____

_____

_____

The authors say, "Become your best encourager rather than your worst critic. That voice would say, 'You are overweight, but you're working on it.'"

Is being kind to yourself difficult for you? Why?

_____

_____

_____

Some people put their lives "on hold" until they are more comfortable with their bodies. What are the pitfalls of that kind of thinking?

_____

_____

Name three or four positive qualities you have. Why is this sometimes hard to do?

_____

_____

In what ways can a person's weight or "oversized" body become a kind of mask?

_____

_____

Our minds easily doubt God and can be deceived. Therefore we are to take each thought captive (2 Corinthians 10:5) and renew our minds with God's truth (Romans 12:2).

The authors write, "*Self-esteem* is a misleading term. None of us can truly have esteem by looking to the *self*. The *self* is sinful, self-centered, and easily deceived. God esteems you just because He chose and loves you. You don't have to earn His esteem. You already have it. Remember, He values you so much that He gave His only Son to die for you."

Do you agree with their assessment? Why or why not?

_____

_____

What truth or reminder in this lesson means the most to you and why?

_____

_____

DAY 3
Renewing the Mind

In this lesson, we want to look closely at the way we think. Consider this: Thoughts lead to feelings. Feelings lead to actions. Actions influence our perceptions that then influence our thoughts. It's a vicious cycle. What we think affects how we feel. And we eat in response to our feelings.

The bottom line? How and what we think—about life, God, ourselves, food—is crucial!

LOOKING AT YOUR *LIFE*

Feelings are prompted by thoughts. For example, if you feel angry, it's because an angry thought preceded that feeling.

Give some examples from your own life from the last couple of days. Do a little soul-searching and record your thoughts below.

I found myself feeling . . .   **because (consciously or unconsciously) I was thinking . . .**

(Ex: Depressed   "I'll always be overweight and I'll never get married.")

_____

_____

_____

Everyone engages in some kind of self-talk. That's where we say things to ourselves (or about ourselves), either out loud or internally. For example, a runner on the verge of exhaustion might say, "C'mon—keep going. You can do this!" A person who spills chili in his or her lap might blurt out through clenched teeth, "You idiot!"

Why do we do this self-talk? Where do you suppose we learned it? Why are some people so negative in what they say to themselves, while others are upbeat and positive?

_____

_____

_____

What about you? Describe your own self-talk habits. What kinds of remarks or statements do you find yourself speaking to yourself?

_____

_____

_____

Put yourself in each of the following situations and try to imagine what you would think, feel, and say.

If I . . .	I'd think . . .	I'd probably feel . . .	I'd likely say to myself . . .
Didn't get invited to an office party	Ex: They don't like me because I'm fat.	Embarrassed and angry	"When are you going to get off your butt and lose some weight?"
Heard someone make a "fat joke"			
Discovered I couldn't fit in a new outfit			
Strained a muscle trying to exercise			
Gave in to the urge to eat a candy bar			

If I . . .	I'd think . . .	I'd probably feel . . .	I'd likely say to myself . . .
Were assigned to work with a good-looking, thin person			

LEARNING A NEW WAY OF *LIFE*

To paraphrase the noted author C. S. Lewis, people tend to make one of two mistakes in thinking about Satan, the evil one. Either they don't believe he is real, or they think they see demons behind every bush. Neither mind-set is accurate. Jesus stated matter-of-factly: "The devil . . . was a murderer from the beginning, not holding to the truth, for there is no truth in him. When he lies, he speaks his native language, for he is a liar and the father of lies" (John 8:44).

How did Jesus view Satan? If the devil isn't real, what are we to conclude about Jesus?

_____

_____

_____

_____

Revelation 12:10 calls the devil "the accuser." First Peter 5:8 warns, "Stay alert! Watch out for your great enemy, the devil. He prowls around like a roaring lion, looking for someone to devour" (NLT). From these descriptions, what conclusions can you draw about Satan? Is he benign?

_____

_____

_____

Read Ephesians 6:10–18. Notice that verse 16 says, "Take up the shield of faith, with which you can extinguish all the flaming arrows of the evil one." What do you think that phrase "flaming arrows" means? Is it possible that some of our persistent negative thoughts about ourselves might actually be whispered lies from the evil one?

God knows and understands our thoughts. "You know my sitting down and rising up; You understand my thought afar off" (Psalm 139:2 NKJV).

Whenever something negative or traumatic happens to us, you can be sure the enemy uses that situation to implant a lie and get us to doubt God's goodness.

LOSING IT FOR *LIFE*

The New Testament book of Romans is often regarded as the most comprehensive yet concise presentation of the Christian faith ever penned. Bible scholars note that the first eleven chapters of Paul's masterpiece are devoted to *what Christians should believe*, while the final five chapters focus on *how Christians should behave*.

Right at the hinge point between Paul's descriptions of right thinking and right living is this amazing verse: "Don't copy the behavior and customs of this world, but let God transform you into a new person by changing the way you think. Then you will learn to know God's will for you, which is good and pleasing and perfect" (Romans 12:2 NLT).

Older Bible translations refer to this process of changing the way we think as "renewing our minds." What does it mean to "renew" something?

_____

_____

_____

How do we renew our *minds*—begin to change the way we think, so that it ends up changing the way we live?

_____

_____

_____

Meditate for a few minutes on these verses:

> "For My thoughts are not your thoughts,
> Nor are your ways, My ways," says the LORD.
> "For as the heavens are higher than the earth,
> So are My ways higher than your ways,
> And My thoughts than your thoughts." (Isaiah 55:8–9 NKJV)

The authors note that many times we become aware of a false way of thinking. We identify it (for example, "I realize I've been feeling all alone, . . . that no one cares for me") and perhaps we even know in our heads the truth of God ("Yet Jesus promised in Matthew 28 that He would never fail or leave His followers"). Still, sometimes, the truth isn't "real" to us. It doesn't seem at home in our hearts.

What is the solution to this kind of disconnect? How do we get the truth of God to take root deeply in our souls?

_____

_____

_____

_____

No amount of self-effort can make someone think differently. A renewed mind comes as we receive truth from God's Word.

The authors suggest the following practices and habits for beginning the lifelong process of "deprogramming and reprogramming" our minds. Think about each one and jot down why you think it is a valuable act.

- When you discover your heart is saying one thing and your head another, pray and ask Christ to speak His truth to you. Read His Word and ask Him to penetrate it deep into your mind and soul.

_____

_____

_____

- Skim the Gospels. Notice that Jesus typically touched and healed broken bodies and souls (an experience) while also speaking truth to hurting and confused minds (cognitive). Why are both aspects important?

_____

_____

_____

The word *renew* means a change of heart and life. It is work the Holy Spirit does in us.

- Identify the lies that create emotional pain. Lies come to us by the words of others, by our own wrong perceptions, or by the evil one during times of hurt and trauma. Once you identify a lie, ask Christ to speak His truth.

_____

_____

_____

In conclusion, let's apply our RISE formula to our thought lives. Here are the goals:

REDUCE negative thoughts and self-degrading statements.

What specifically do you need to do on this front?

_____

_____

_____

INCREASE your awareness of God-esteem and acceptance of the body you were given.

List two practical ways you can do this, this week.

_____

_____

_____

SUBSTITUTE positive thoughts for negative ones; substitute a view of yourself that is defined by God, not by your weight.

What new biblical truths are helping you form a more accurate identity?

_____

_____

_____

ELIMINATE thinking errors and lies.

How has this lesson helped you identify any wrong thoughts or unhealthy patterns of self-talk?

_____

_____

_____

DAY 4

Taking Negative
Thoughts Captive

In order to Lose It for Life, you have to learn to identify negative and extreme thoughts, stop them from running rampant in your mind, and replace them with thoughts that are true and reflect who you are in Christ. That is the focus of this workbook lesson.

LOOKING AT YOUR *LIFE*

When you were growing up, were your parents more optimistic or pessimistic?

_____

_____

_____

If your parents were critical or harsh, how did this contribute to your self-view?

_____

_____

_____

Describe your thought processes and mental habits by checking all that apply:

____ I'm definitely scatterbrained.

____ I have a mind like a steel trap; I remember most everything.

____ My mind is always racing, juggling a zillion different things.

___ No matter how crazy life gets, I am able to turn my brain off and just relax.

___ I have a disciplined mind.

___ I often have a different perspective on things, a different way of solving problems.

___ I'm an outside-the-box thinker.

___ Friends joke that I'm spacey or an airhead.

___ People tell me I think too deeply, too much.

___ The truth is I try not to think too much.

___ It's hard for me to organize and articulate my thoughts.

___ I daydream and fantasize a lot.

How do you typically respond when people ask, "What's on your mind?" or "A penny for your thoughts"?

_____

_____

_____

How much do you engage in self-talk? When life gets challenging or stressful what kinds of thoughts run through your mind? Are they mostly supportive and positive, or discouraging and negative?

_____

_____

_____

When you're not at work or on duty at home, where does your mind go? What kinds of daydreams do you have? Why?

_____

_____

_____

Why does it matter what we think?

_____

_____

_____

"Since, then, you have been raised with Christ, set your hearts on things above, where Christ is, seated at the right hand of God. Set your minds on things above, not on earthly things" (Colossians 3:1–2).

LEARNING A NEW WAY OF *LIFE*

Second Corinthians 10:4–5 tells us to take our thoughts captive: "The weapons we fight with are not the weapons of the world. On the contrary, they have divine power to demolish strongholds. We demolish arguments and every pretension that sets itself up against the knowledge of God, and we take captive every thought to make it obedient to Christ."

The Message paraphrase puts it this way: "We use our powerful God-tools for smashing warped philosophies, tearing down barriers erected against the truth of God, fitting every loose thought and emotion and impulse into the structure of life shaped by Christ."

What does it mean to "take thoughts captive"? Why is this important?

_____

_____

_____

Once we realize a thought is negative, self-degrading, or untrue, we must move to stop the thought. To stop a thought, pretend you are grabbing it out of the air and taking it captive.

Picture your mind as the vital control center of your whole life. Now, picture inside your mind a shadowy and strong group of untrue, destructive thoughts and attitudes and conclusions—sort of mental terrorists. These bogus ways of thinking are loose inside your mind. Their goal? To wreak havoc. They want to get you to act in wrong ways by getting you to believe wrong ideas about God, the world, yourself, others, and so forth. Our only hope is to be alert and to begin the deliberate task of identifying, arresting, and replacing every one of these dangerous thoughts. If we don't, a full and rich life will elude us. If we don't, tragedy awaits.

Read Philippians 4:8. Why is this command so crucial?

_____

_____

Give some examples of some common wrong, negative, or degrading statements you find yourself saying to or about yourself. Then write out some positive, encouraging statements that need to be substituted.

A Thought That Needs to Be Replaced	**The Truth That Needs to Be Embraced**
1. Ex: *I just ate all those cookies. I am so bad.*	1. *I am not bad, because Christ is in me. I am tempted and sometimes sin, but when I do, I ask forgiveness and move on. I wish I hadn't eaten all those cookies, but it's not the end of the world. I can regain control with God's help. Lord, give me the self-control I need right now.*
2. _____ _____ _____ _____	2. _____ _____ _____ _____
3. _____ _____ _____ _____	3. _____ _____ _____ _____
4. _____ _____ _____ _____	4. _____ _____ _____ _____
5. _____ _____ _____ _____	5. _____ _____ _____ _____

LOSING IT FOR *LIFE*

The authors say, "Sometimes it helps to put a rubber band on your wrist and snap it every time you tell yourself a negative thought or a lie. The mild pain is a simple reminder to grab the negative thought."

Do you think this would be an effective tool for change for you? Why or why not?

_____

_____

_____

What of the following is more common in your mind, and why?

- negative thoughts (pessimism)
- false beliefs (thoughts contrary to what God says is true)
- self-degrading sentences (condemning attacks on your own character or actions)

_____

_____

_____

In Appendix F, the authors recommend that you keep a Dysfunctional Thought Record (a chart designed to help people get in touch with their conscious and not-so-conscious thoughts). Simply record the date, briefly describe the situation, record what emotion you felt, and rate its intensity from 0 to 100 percent in terms of how intense that emotion felt. Next, record the automatic thought that came into your mind. Once you identify the thought and write it down, then try to think of a true thought and write that thought down. Then re-rate your emotion—it should be less intense. It might look like this:

Dysfunctional Thought Record					
Date	Situation	Emotion / Intensity	Automatic Thought	Rational Response / Intensity	Outcome
3–20	Overate	Disgust / 80%	I am a loser	I blew it but I can get back on track / 10%	

Ex: The situation was overeating. The emotion you record was *disgust* and you gave it an 80 percent rating, which means you felt it intensely. Your automatic thought was, *I am a loser.* The more rational response or truth is, *I blew it but can get back on track. It was only ten cookies. I am weak in my own power, but with Christ I can do all things.* Letting that truth sink in brings peace, so you re-rate your emotion to 10 percent.

Keeping such a chart will help you begin to recognize the thoughts that trigger your emotions. You can review your thoughts and write alternative ways to think about situations.

What is anxious thinking? Is this a recurring problem for you? How does negative self-talk make things worse?

_____

_____

_____

List a couple of events, meetings, appointments, or situations coming up in the next few days that make you feel anxious. Spend a few minutes trying to uncover the thoughts (or negative self-talk) behind your nervous feeling. Now go back and put a more positive, more truthful spin on things.

_____

_____

_____

Review the following anxious-thought checklist, and see if you think like an anxious person.

Anxious thinking makes anxious people. Learn to take those thoughts captive and turn your thinking around.

ANXIOUS-THOUGHT CHECKLIST

- ☐ I immediately think in terms of the worst-case scenario.
- ☐ I am convinced I'm the next victim of every tragedy or illness.
- ☐ I focus on an unlikely problem, ignoring all the opposing data that suggests success.
- ☐ I interpret things in their worst possible light.
- ☐ I automatically believe nothing will change and I can't meet the challenge, so I just give up.

☐   I assume because something happened once, it will happen again.

☐   I believe things happen all the time or not at all.

☐   I am the classic perfectionist who doesn't allow for mistakes or human fallibility.

☐   I am extremely critical of myself and need to give myself a break!

☐   I am the classic "what if" worrier, who sees only possibilities for disaster or problems.

If you checked even a few of these statements, it's past time to change your thoughts. Think of the biggest challenge you are facing over the next month. First, write down your honest thoughts (even if they're negative) about that situation. Next, write down some positive, Scripture-based statements (like Philippians 4:13) to counter your anxious, negative thinking.

A New Attitude

In the last four lessons, we explored a number of life-changing truths. We've also proposed some exercises that—if practiced faithfully over time—can lead to a new way of thinking and living. In this lesson we want to tie up loose ends and make "renewing our mind" a regular, ongoing part of our lives.

LOOKING AT YOUR *LIFE*

Sometimes life comes crashing down, and changes that we didn't want or expect are forced on us. Other times we choose to make changes. Which kind of change is harder? Give some examples of each from your own life.

_____

_____

_____

_____

Name a few helpful practices that are a part of your daily routine (for example, *flossing my teeth*). How and why did you develop this habit? How long did it take for you to make this a regular activity? How do you maintain the discipline to keep at it?

_____

_____

_____

_____

Why does the word *discipline* or the phrase *disciplining ourselves* have a nasty connotation to most people?

"Worry is unproductive. I can't predict how life will go today and that is okay. I can live with uncertainty and change. God promises He won't give me anything I can't handle." (One lifelong worrier's new morning self-talk routine)

_____

_____

_____

As we've been examining the ways we think and the kinds of ideas and beliefs that drive us, what surprises you most? What have you learned about yourself?

_____

_____

_____

_____

LEARNING A NEW WAY OF *LIFE*

In chapter 8, we meet Rita, a woman controlled by worry. Find her brief story and review it. What about her experience speaks to you most powerfully?

_____

_____

_____

"I have chosen the way of faithfulness; I have set my heart on your laws" (Psalm 119:30).

Read Matthew 4:1–11, the biblical account of Christ's temptation. Theologically, this is a profound passage with infinite implications that make our finite brains dizzy. Practically, it can be argued this is a simple battle over what's true. In what ways do we fight the same sort of battle and face the same sort of choices every day?

_____

_____

_____

What can we learn here about the evil one?

_____

_____

What can we learn from Christ in watching how He handles the tempter?

_____

_____

_____

In many of the apostle Paul's New Testament letters, he goes to great lengths laying out what Christians should believe, before telling them what they should do. Why do you think he does this?

_____

_____

_____

Spend a few minutes pondering these passages that speak about the importance and the power of God's Word:

> How can a young person stay on the path of purity? By living according to your word. . . . I have hidden your word in my heart that I might not sin against you. (Psalm 119:9, 11)

> Your word is a lamp for my feet, a light on my path. (Psalm 119:105)

> All Scripture is God-breathed and is useful for teaching, rebuking, correcting and training in righteousness, so that the servant of God may be thoroughly equipped for every good work. (2 Timothy 3:16–17)

According to these verses, what benefits do we get from knowing and following God's Word?

_____

_____

_____

Is it possible to live a healthy, productive, and fulfilling life apart from a deep knowledge of the truth of God? Why or why not?

Meditation is focusing your mind on things that bring peace and a sense of well-being. Think about God's intense love for you. Our God has promised to take care of us and meet all our needs. If that doesn't lessen your stress, nothing will.

_____

_____

_____

LOSING IT FOR _LIFE_

Noting that much stress originates from our own thought lives, the LIFL authors propose two strategies to help with stressful thoughts: (1) visualizing peaceful scenes and (2) meditating.

What is your immediate reaction to these suggestions?

_____

_____

_____

What does Philippians 4:8 suggest about meditation?

_____

_____

_____

_____

What is the promise of Isaiah 26:3? What guarantees peace?

_____

_____

_____

The authors suggest that when you feel stressed and tense, you can:

. . . visualize yourself in a quiet, peaceful place. This is calming. Some people like to imagine themselves resting on a sunny beach with a gentle breeze, the smell of the ocean, clear skies, and water all present in their imagination. Other people find a mountain cabin in the snow to be a quiet, calming place.

Others imagine basking eternally in the presence of Christ. I (Dr. Linda) like to read Revelation 21 and picture the New Jerusalem based on the visual description John gives in that chapter—the gates, the angels, the gems, but mostly the glory of God that will shine and illuminate the city! It doesn't matter what scene you choose, as long as you think of something peaceful and try to engage all your senses in the scene. If you succeed, your anxious thoughts will melt as you settle into a place of peace.

How might this practice change your mind-set and outlook in everyday life?

_____

_____

_____

Since God is the source of ultimate peace and serenity, how can thinking about Him (His goodness, His love, what He has done for you, the hope of His eternal presence, and so forth), bring about deep changes in our overall state of mind?

_____

_____

_____

We serve a God who raises the dead. Certainly He can resurrect our lives from defeat to new life with meaning and purpose.

As you engage in the Lose It for Life process, be prepared! You will hit bumps along the way related to how you think. It is easy to question God in times of difficulty, and it is easy to grow impatient and allow the enemy to gain ground in our thoughts. But God wants to teach us to depend on Him all the time, to renew our minds with His truth, and to know that He is powerful and able to accomplish much in us if we submit to His plan.

Write out a short prayer to God summarizing all you are learning, thinking, feeling, and hoping. Ask Him to give you victory in the battle to renew your mind.

_____

_____

_____

9

Changing the Doing

Ever noticed how good intentions don't always bring success? The reality is that action is required to achieve goals. Knowing what we know about eating, exercising, and losing weight, we often try to will ourselves to do what is "right" and stay on our plan. Yet too often, we find ourselves doing what is wrong.

Faith is the belief or confidence that God will do all He says He will do. As we read God's Word and implant it deep into our hearts, action must follow what we read and hear. James confirms this in his epistle (1:22–25):

> Don't fool yourself into thinking that you are a listener when you are anything but, letting the Word go in one ear and out the other. Act on what you hear! Those who hear and don't act are like those who glance in the mirror, walk away, and two minutes later have no idea who they are, what they look like. But whoever catches a glimpse of the revealed counsel of God—the free life!—even out of the corner of his eye, and sticks with it, is no distracted scatterbrain but a man or woman of action. That person will find delight and affirmation in the action. (MSG)

Don't you want to be that person who finds delight and affirmation in action? With the Holy Spirit operating in your life, you are empowered to do those things you know to be true. Even if you have a history of weight-loss failure, it's time to look forward and begin applying action to your decision to Lose It for Life. There is no time like the present to begin. God has already given you what you need to overcome. When you confess Christ as your Savior, the Holy Spirit takes up residence in you. It is His presence that empowers each of us to overcome.

TOOLS FOR CHANGE

Change is a process that involves multiple steps. Below is an outline of six steps necessary to bring change to your life.

Illumination

When you see the need for change, you have reached illumination. It is, to be precise, your lightbulb moment—the point at which you finally understand your situation in a whole new way. As Ephesians 5:8 says, "You groped your way through that murk once, but no longer. You're out in the open now. The bright light of Christ makes your way plain. So no more stumbling around. Get on with it!" (MSG). Hopefully at this point in the program, your weaknesses have come to light and you are ready to get on with it.

Inspiration

Once you see the need for change, you must be inspired to make necessary changes. Ask God for His help and guidance. Change may be needed in several areas of your life—eating, exercise, dealing with your emotions, or how you think and act. Also ask God for the courage to change and be transformed into what is God's best for you. See what you can become and become motivated by the vision.

Examination

As we are inspired to make changes, we must take a good, hard look at how we measure up to God's standards. Socrates once said, "The unexamined life is not worth living." We couldn't agree more. How does your life measure up to God's standards? Do you imitate Christ in all you do? Are you living a holy life? Are you obedient to the Word? Whatever your answers are to these questions, the good news is you can begin today to evaluate your life according to God's Word. No one is perfect, but after examining your life closely, you should be more inclined to want to live in obedience to God's Word.

Motivation

Are you motivated to be used by God and to know His purposes for your life? When you understand that the life God has for you is beyond what you could even imagine, you have reached the step of motivation. Walking in His truth and staying obedient to His Word are your secret weapons to developing a purpose-driven life. God doesn't want you immobilized by your weight. Ask the Holy Spirit to fill you so full of Him that something beyond yourself will happen.

The more we seek the kingdom of God and all His righteousness first, the more used of God we will be. Colossians 3:12 tells us how to "dress" for this type of success— "So, chosen by God for this new life of love, dress in the wardrobe God picked out for you: compassion, kindness, humility, quiet strength, discipline" (MSG).

If you have struggled with motivation for years, perhaps it is time to realize that you just don't have the ability to motivate yourself. But you can reach out to someone else; you can bring people around you to help coach you and provide you with the motivation you do not possess on your own. This is what God has in mind when we surround ourselves with a body of believers.

Determination

No matter what you've been through already, don't give up. If you fall down and blow it, get up and try again. God gives us second chances. He wants us to succeed. With Christ, all things are possible. Stay in the fight and keep reaching for the prize.

All the people I know who have lost weight and kept it off have had a tremendous amount of determination. They just won't give up. If their weight plateaus, they just keep doing what they have been doing while making minor changes that eventually result in a return of weight loss. For them, there is no excuse good enough to give up, so they persevere. And the longer they stay determined, the stronger their transformation becomes.

Realization

Supernatural things can happen. Persevere until change comes, and be of good courage. You are a champion because of God's ability to change people. Your life matters and God has plans for you. James 1:12 says, "Blessed is the one who perseveres under trial because, having stood the test, that person will receive the crown of life that the Lord has promised to those who love him."

CONTINUE TO RISE ABOVE THE CHALLENGES

You will want to review the RISE formula from each chapter and make changes in your eating and exercise habits, as well as how you deal with your emotions and thinking. Spiritually, the more you press into God and depend on Him, the better you'll do as you Lose It for Life.

Let's revisit our RISE formula again in terms of behavior:

Reduce eating in response to social cues.
Increase the number of changes you make. Start small and add more as you are able.
Substitute forgiveness for any bitterness or unresolved misdeed; substitute new behaviors for eating.
Eliminate eating for the wrong reasons.

Reduce

Another type of cue besides those based on emotions or feelings that often triggers overeating is a social cue. One of the most common social triggers is the television commercial. Visually, TV commercials stimulate our desire to eat. The best way to handle commercials, especially late at night when you are tired and your defenses are down, is to use the remote to click past the commercials. Don't watch them and you won't be drawn in by the trigger. And certainly don't watch food channels or cooking shows! Both can trigger a desire to overeat.

Another common social cue that triggers eating is driving in the car. If you are used to downing Big Gulps, eating candy bars, or running by the drive-thru for a quick pick-me-up snack, you have conditioned yourself to eat in the car. Food billboards can also stimulate the urge to eat. This association of the car with eating must be broken. We know the concept sounds impossible, but the best way to do this is not to eat in the car at all, even though eating in the car is almost an American way of life! However, if you stop doing this, you'll not only reduce your calorie intake but also have a cleaner car. Relegate all eating to the kitchen table.

What about the movies? Do you have to have that buttered popcorn to watch a movie? We hear your emphatic *yes*—because a movie just wouldn't be a movie without popcorn or the supersized Junior Mints, right? Surprise! Movies can be very enjoyable without the snacks. Drink a full glass of water before you go, and eat a low-calorie snack so the sight and smell of all those goodies won't be so tempting. The association between eating and watching movies needs to be broken, which requires that you unlearn that behavior.

Parties, celebrations, and other special occasions like weddings, birthdays, and showers are also social events that cue overeating. If you are asked to bring food to an event, bring something healthy you can snack on, and park your body close to that snack food. Otherwise, use the same strategy as you did for the movies—drink water and eat a small snack before you go to the event. Focus on the conversation and the people who are attending. You can hold a glass of punch or diet drink in one hand for a long time while you are busy making conversation and interacting with new people.

If you are anxious at social events, practice deep breathing and relaxation techniques (see Appendix E). Don't use food to calm your anxiety. Again, this is a habit you can break.

You may want to look around your workplace. Are there places in that setting that trigger eating? How about the coffeepot? It can be a place of gathering and snacking. We've worked in several offices in which doughnuts, cake, cookies, and all sorts of goodies are placed by the coffeepot. Naturally, when you go for that cup of java, you are faced with added temptation. You may have to skip the informal chatting in the coffee room and socialize by the water fountain instead.

If a physical space triggers you to eat, change the space. For some of you, this means cleaning out your desks. Hidden in many of those desk drawers are bags of candy and other snack items that you grab when work gets boring or you just need a break.

Grocery shopping can be a tempting activity for overeating, especially if you shop hungry. The best way to avoid this quandary is to eat before you shop, which also helps cut down on buying impulse items. In addition, dietitians frequently recommend that you shop the outside ring of grocery stores where the fresh produce is located. Avoid the cookie aisle and prepackaged foods that are high in trans fat.

Another problem can be cooking. For many of you, cooking means tasting and sampling an entire portion before the food is ever served. You must break that habit while cooking. The smell of food cues you to want to eat, but the extra calories add up. So ask someone else to taste the stew if you think it may need more salt. If you have to stir the pot, do so, but then immediately put down the spoon before you can sample it. And during cleanup, don't eat the leftovers on people's plates.

Become comfortable throwing food away in spite of what your mother told you about the starving people in Africa. To our knowledge, no food from your plate has ever been sent to Africa! It's okay. Throw it away! One final word on cooking: don't cook the things you love that are hard to resist. Your family can survive without your award-winning chocolate cake if having it around trips you up. Remember, you are setting up your environment for success.

As mentioned before, the sight of leftovers can cue the desire to eat, which is why we suggested using foil wrap for leftover foods. When you don't see what the dish is, it isn't as tempting to eat it. Our sight and smell often trigger an urge to overeat. When this happens, we have to decide if we are responding to true physical hunger. For example, whenever I (Dr. Linda) see pies and pastries, I'm ready to eat them whether I'm hungry or not. In part, this is because I grew up with a mother, grandmother, and aunts who all could have been professional pastry chefs. Their desserts are truly out of this world. Just the sight of those desserts brings back great family memories and fun in the kitchen. But if I ate dessert every time I was triggered, I'd weigh a lot more than I do. So when I see a pie sitting on the kitchen counter, I have to ask myself if I'm really hungry or not. Or I have to cut down on my meal in order to enjoy a dessert from time to time. I don't deprive myself, but I also don't indulge every time I see or smell the pastry coming.

Try to think of which social situations or cues trigger you to overeat. Then plan ahead of time how you will handle that situation. Problem solving is actually a useful skill for making life changes because it forces you to anticipate a situation and have a plan. I (Dr. Linda) have worked with several professional chefs who spend their days around food and cooking. Together, we had to plan ways for them to make it through the workday without overeating. First, they wrote down their eating habits while preparing food so we could spot the problem times and items. Then we developed a behavioral plan to ward off overeating. Strategies like keeping a fresh bowl of fruit by their preparation area, drinking lots of water, taking breaks in which they could relax and think, and identifying the type of hunger they experienced (emotional or physical) were all elements of the plan that we implemented.

Increase

Many changes have been suggested—perhaps more than you feel comfortable with. Don't worry. No one expects you to make all the changes at once. In fact, it's a good idea to begin this transformation with a small change. Choose one thing you can do differently for a month and begin by making that change. For example, if you have been a total couch potato, decide to walk five minutes, three times a week. Do that for a month and it will become part of your routine.

Then, add another small change. Perhaps every time you reach to eat out of a need for comfort, you instead choose something from your behavior substitution list (see chapter 7) and make yourself do that instead. Make that one behavior change your goal for a month. Keep adding changes as you are able. Eventually these small changes will add up. Remember, if you took years to put on the weight, you need to give yourself time to take it off.

Substitute

As you surrender your life to God, another action becomes necessary: forgiveness. Throughout the Word, Jesus is very specific about our need to forgive. "If you forgive other people when they sin against you, your heavenly Father will also forgive you" (Matthew 6:14). This is stated as a contingency, meaning we have an active part to accomplish as well as the action of our heavenly Father forgiving us.

Forgiveness, when empowered by God's Spirit, is a process of detaching painful events from our emotional responses to them, thus facilitating the process of healing. When we forgive, we recognize our own failures and are humbled. To forgive and to receive forgiveness are gracious acts of love. These acts have supernatural power to change both the life of the forgiven and the one who forgives. When you look at how God has forgiven you, it moves you to find a way to forgive others even if they have deeply hurt you. Only the cross of Christ makes forgiveness possible.

Forgiveness is inextricably interwoven into Christian salvation. Jesus clearly taught that unless we forgive others, our heavenly Father cannot forgive us. At first glance, this may appear to be a rigid and rigorous principle, but it is God's means of extending His grace to everyone. When we refuse to forgive, we play "god" in the lives of others and pass our judgment onto them. This interferes with the process of grace Jesus Christ initiated at the cross. Forgiveness means:

- we hand back our rights to God (the rights we usurped from Him) and invite Him to be in charge.
- we obey Jesus' instructions to forgive, and in turn we can be forgiven.
- we no longer energize ourselves with rage or hatred over events or feelings from the past.
- we stop trying to change other people and ask God to do it.
- we begin a process of restitution to right whatever wrongs we may have caused.

Forgiveness can be difficult—almost impossible—for those who have been abused physically, sexually, or even spiritually. It is never easy or instant; it may in fact take years to complete. However, if forgiveness isn't rendered, the injured person remains trapped in the abuse of the past where they endlessly relive the offenses done against them. Our yesterdays must be put in the past so we can fully enjoy today.

The forgiveness process also involves making things right with those we have wounded. This may require us to write letters or make phone calls, to repay debts, or to make amends or otherwise do our part in making wrongs as right as possible. This, of course, can result in enormous spiritual blessings, both for others and for ourselves. Sometimes it is difficult to face a person or speak with him or her on the phone. In such instances, a letter like this one may be the right choice:

Dear Bob,

You may be surprised to be hearing from me, but I have been doing some soul-searching lately. You came to mind and I realized I could have done things differently regarding _____.

I hope you will forgive me. I am making changes in my life so I won't repeat the same mistakes. I hope you are doing well and that God is blessing you.

Sincerely,

It is amazing what a simple letter like that can do to lower the barriers between two people. You will be surprised by the letters you get back and amazed at how ready people are to forgive.

Eliminate

Your goal should be to eat for nourishment and the enjoyment of meals. It's up to you to discover the other functions eating has served in your life. For example, does eating calm you, relax you, numb you, boost your mood, or fill your time? Whatever the function eating has served, you will need to make a change and do something different.

There is an old saying in therapy—if you take something away, replace it with something else or the patient will just substitute another problem-behavior in its place. Many of you can already attest to the truth of this. Perhaps you stopped overeating but began to overspend. Or you stopped overeating and replaced it with another addiction. Obviously, we don't want you to trade addictions or substitute other compulsive behaviors for overeating.

Get at the root of your overeating and resolve it. This may require counseling or additional support to make changes. Don't underestimate the fact that change is difficult. To succeed, we all need the help of family or friends as well as God. Don't be an island determined to do this all alone. Let others come alongside and encourage you. Humble yourself before the Lord and acknowledge your need of Him, and He will lift you up.

Often it is painful to change our behavior. When we have been wronged, it is so much easier to break off all contact and not have a relationship with the person. Yet this isn't what God asks us to do. We must move beyond our hurt and seek forgiveness, as Christ forgave us. If you struggle with this very difficult task, consider this prayer your official starting point:

Dear Lord,

You have commanded me to forgive others, just as You have forgiven me through the sacrifice of Your Son, Jesus. I choose to obey You, even though this is not easy for me. You listed all of my sins. Then You nailed them to the cross so that Jesus' blood could pay for them. Help me to release this account to You and not to seek justice for my sake. Help me to trust that You are just and will carry out Your will.

Yet, while I transfer this account to You, wounds still remain as a result of this wrong. As I obey You by releasing this person from my debt, I pray You will heal the hurts they have caused me. Help me to trust that You are willing and able to redeem me from the wrongs that have been done against me. If thoughts of revenge recur, I pray You will help me to continually release this person's account to You. Amen.

God sees your heart and knows if you are sincere. He will help you move through the process of forgiveness if you desire to do so. It may help to make a list of those grudges and offenses you have held on to and would like to release. Then take each item and pray, asking the Lord to forgive you or the person who hurt you.

Releasing these burdens is powerful in the battle to lose weight and keep it off. This is not a step you can skip and still succeed. Take the time, examine your heart, and ask God to show you if there is hidden resentment or judgment. Seek release today.

Workbook Week 9

CHANGING THE DOING

DAY 1
Acting in the Truth

Throughout the Lose It for Life program, we've been encouraging lifestyle changes. In this set of workbook lessons, we want to reinforce the need to make changes not only in the way you think and feel but also in the way you *behave*.

LOOKING AT YOUR *LIFE*

How many diet or exercise books have you bought in your lifetime? How many have you actually read and tried to follow? How many are on your shelves or by your bedside?

_____

_____

A few years ago, an athletic company saw sales skyrocket with an ad campaign built around the catchphrase "Just Do It." In what ways is this simple philosophy good and helpful? In what ways is it not helpful?

Good intentions don't bring success. Action is required.

_____

_____

What are some right behaviors you have no problem doing?

_____

_____

What are some good and wise actions or habits you have to force yourself to do? Why?

_____

_____

For most people who battle with their weight, is the problem a lack of *information* or a lack of *application*? What about for you? Explain.

_____

_____

LEARNING A NEW WAY OF *LIFE*

Read this Scripture passage from the apostle Paul that discusses the difficulty of knowing the truth and acting in the truth:

> What I don't understand about myself is that I decide one way, but then I act another, doing things I absolutely despise. So if I can't be trusted to figure out what is best for myself and then do it, it becomes obvious that God's command is necessary. But I need something more! For if I know the law but still can't keep it, and if the power of sin within me keeps sabotaging my best intentions, I obviously need help! I realize that I don't have what it takes. I can will it, but I can't do it. I decide to do good, but I don't really do it; I decide not to do bad, but then I do it anyway. My decisions, such as they are, don't result in actions. Something has gone wrong deep within me and gets the better of me every time. (Romans 7:15–20 MSG)

Do you relate to Paul's honest admission? Pick a recurring temptation in your life and record a bit of your own recent struggle.

_____

_____

How does a person move beyond good intentions to disciplined action and, ultimately, success?

_____

_____

What's the difference between trying really hard (good intentions, human willpower) and trusting God (faith)?

_____

_____

Knowing what we know about eating, exercising, and losing weight, we often try to will ourselves to do right and stay on our plan. Too often, we find ourselves doing what Paul says—the very things we say we won't do. We need something more.

Read Romans 10:17. What does it offer to this study?

_____

_____

Discuss your own current "intake" of the message of the Word of God.

_____

_____

God has already given you what you need to overcome. With the Holy Spirit operating in your life, you are empowered to do those things you know to be true.

Speaking of the need for action rooted in faith, the apostle James warned:

Don't fool yourself into thinking that you are a listener when you are anything but, letting the Word go in one ear and out the other. Act on what you hear! Those who hear and don't act are like those who glance in the mirror, walk away, and two minutes later have no idea who they are, what they look like. But whoever catches a glimpse of the revealed counsel of God—the free life!—even out of the corner of his eye, and sticks with it, is no distracted scatterbrain but a man or woman of action. That person will find delight and affirmation in the action. (James 1:22–25 MSG)

What action is called for here?

_____

_____

What is promised to the person who takes decisive action?

_____

_____

LOSING IT FOR *LIFE*

As we saw above, we build a stronger faith in God by getting into His Word—or more precisely, by letting His Word get into us. Some ways God's truth can take root and bear fruit in our lives include:

- hearing the Word preached (listening and taking notes)
- reading the Bible
- participating in small group Bible study
- studying the Bible for ourselves
- memorizing Bible passages
- meditating on Scripture (mulling it over in our minds, reflecting upon its meaning and implications)

In which of these activities do you engage regularly?

_____

_____

_____

Which ones do you not do? Why?

_____

_____

Which ones do you want to learn how to do?

_____

_____

_____

Answer the following questions by writing "Yes" or "No."

____ Do you have a Lose It for Life support team?
____ Do you have daily contact with your support team?
____ Do you rely on your support team—calling them in times of weakness, etc.?
____ Are you gut-level honest with your support team about your deep struggles and even your failures?

___ Have you given your support team permission to ask you hard questions and tell you hard truths?

___ Do you listen to your support team?

___ When all is said and done, are you submitted to your support team (that is, would you follow their collective advice even if you didn't feel like it or want to)?

Even if you've had a history of weight-loss failure, it's time to look forward and begin applying action to what you've read.

The more "no" answers you wrote, the less your chances of success. (See Proverbs 27:17.)

What's the truth or reminder you are taking away from this lesson?

_____

_____

Write a prayer expressing your need for God to work in you to "will and to act in order to fulfill his good purpose" (Philippians 2:13).

_____

_____

DAY 2

Tools for Change

Change is a process that involves multiple steps. In this lesson we will look at some helpful tools that—if used properly and consistently—can make your goal of Losing It for Life a reality.

LOOKING AT YOUR *LIFE*

Thinking back over the last five years, what technology, insight, or learned skill has resulted in the greatest positive change in your life?

_____

_____

Overwhelmed? Don't worry. No one expects you to make all the changes at once.

What's the most helpful tool you own and use regularly? Why is it such a favorite of yours?

_____

_____

What tool or gadget or gizmo do you *not* have that you feel certain would make your life better, easier, or richer? Why?

_____

_____

Play counselor for a moment to people desirous of change. A smoker friend asks, "How can I stop?" What counsel would you give?

_____

_____

A family member in financial distress sighs, "We need a miracle . . ." What advice would you offer?

_____

_____

A colleague at work laments the moral condition of our nation and wonders aloud, "Will things ever change?" What do you say in response?

_____

_____

_____

LEARNING A NEW WAY OF _LIFE_

Chapter 9 of _Lose It for Life_ suggests six steps that can be tools for change. Based on the discussion of these concepts from the book, write a brief definition or description of each:

Illumination

_____

> **Motivation comes when you understand that the life God has for you is beyond what you could even imagine. God doesn't want you immobilized by your weight.**

Inspiration

_____

Examination

_____

Motivation

_____

Determination

_____

Realization

_____

Ephesians 5:8 says:

You groped your way through that murk once, but no longer. You're out in the open now. The bright light of Christ makes your way plain. So no more stumbling around. Get on with it! (MSG)

What does this verse tell us about the concept of *illumination*?

_____

_____

The apostle Paul warned:

Don't become so well-adjusted to your culture that you fit into it without even thinking. Instead, fix your attention on God. You'll be changed from the inside out. Readily recognize what he wants from you, and quickly respond to it. Unlike the culture around you, always dragging you down to its level of immaturity, God brings the best out of you, develops well-formed maturity in you. (Romans 12:2 MSG)

What does this verse suggest about the source of *inspiration*?

_____

_____

Read Psalm 139:23–24. What do these verses say about the process of *examination*?

_____

_____

_____

In what ways is taking a hard look at one's true condition terrifying? Why is this scary step so crucial?

_____

_____

_____

How can comparing ourselves with others be demotivating?

_____

_____

LOSING IT FOR _LIFE_

If you fall down and blow it, get up and try again. God gives us second chances. He wants us to succeed.

If _illumination_ means seeing the need for change, describe the illumination that has taken place in your life so far in the LIFL program.

_____

_____

What is your current _inspiration_ level? How would you say God has worked and is working within you to prompt long-term lifestyle changes?

_____

_____

Socrates said, "The unexamined life is not worth living." How and when do you regularly assess yourself—your heart, your motives, your attitudes, and your actions?

_____

_____

Other than God's Word, what other sources of feedback help you know where you are and how you're progressing?

_____

_____

Colossians 3:12 tells us how to dress for success: "So, chosen by God for this new life of love, dress in the wardrobe God picked out for you: compassion, kindness, humility, quiet strength, discipline" (MSG). How does a person do this? What role does the Spirit of God play in this process?

_____

_____

_____

How can these internal qualities or tools make a difference in your external appearance?

_____

_____

_____

Luke 18 tells about Jesus encountering a desperate blind man and asking him an amazing question: "What do you want me to do for you?" Imagine yourself at Jesus' feet and hearing Him ask you the same thing. Dream big. Don't be superficial and ask just for a thin physique. What do you want—really want—in your deep heart? How would you like Him to transform who you are?

_____

_____

_____

Illumination, inspiration, examination, motivation, determination, and realization. Take some time to pray these tools of change into your life. Talk to God about each one.

— DAY 3 —

You Can Do It!

The goal of this short lesson is to bolster our faith and our resolve by helping us remember the limitless power and grace and goodness of our God.

LOOKING AT YOUR *LIFE*

With Christ, all things are possible. Stay in the fight and keep reaching for the prize.

What is your greatest accomplishment in life—your proudest achievement? How did you do it?

_____

_____

What lessons did this experience teach you?

_____

_____

What positive, upbeat people do you admire and like to be around?

_____

_____

_____

How did they develop such a positive, can-do attitude?

_____

_____

_____

What's the difference between faith that can move mountains and everyday positive thinking that doesn't necessarily involve God?

_____

_____

_____

It's been said, "If you have a little God, you'll have big problems. But if you have a big God, you'll have little problems." Why is one's view of God so important in life?

_____

_____

_____

LEARNING A NEW WAY OF _LIFE_

James 1:12 says, "Anyone who meets a testing challenge head-on and manages to stick it out is mighty fortunate. For such persons loyally in love with God, the reward is life and more life" (MSG).

What rewards await the person who drops fifty pounds?

_____

_____

What rewards await the person who drops fifty pounds and who also undergoes radical changes in the way he or she thinks about God, self, food, and exercise?

_____

_____

Ephesians 3:20 reminds us, "God can do anything, you know—far more than you could ever imagine or guess or request in your wildest dreams! He does it not by pushing us around but by working within us, his Spirit deeply and gently within us" (MSG).

Spend a few minutes meditating on these Bible passages:

Is anything too hard for the LORD? (Genesis 18:14)

Ah, Sovereign LORD, you have made the heavens and the earth by your great power and outstretched arm. Nothing is too hard for you. (Jeremiah 32:17)

"I am the LORD, the God of all mankind. Is anything too hard for me?" (Jeremiah 32:27)

"Truly I tell you, if you have faith as small as a mustard seed, you can say to this mountain, 'Move from here to there' and it will move. Nothing will be impossible for you." (Matthew 17:20)

Jesus replied, "What is impossible with man is possible with God." (Luke 18:27)

Jot down your observations and insights from these verses.

_____

_____

A wise old saint once said, "Expect great things from God; attempt great things for God." What great things would you love to see God do *in* you?

_____

_____

_____

What "impossible" things would you love to see God do *through* you?

_____

_____

Supernatural things can happen. Persevere until change comes.

LOSING IT FOR *LIFE*

When Jesus began his public ministry at age thirty, he went to the synagogue in his hometown of Nazareth (Luke 4:16–21). He read a passage from Isaiah 61:1–2, in essence saying that his ministry would involve these activities:

The Spirit of the Sovereign LORD is on me,
    because the LORD has anointed me to proclaim good news to the poor.
He has sent me to bind up the brokenhearted,
    to proclaim freedom for the captives
    and release from darkness for the prisoners,
    to proclaim the year of the LORD's favor.

Look at the phrases that Jesus quoted. What do you need him to do in your life?

_____

_____

The issue really isn't how much faith we have; it's who or what we have our faith in. How has your trust in God's character and power grown during your LIFL experience?

_____

_____

Assorted voices (internal and external) call out to us each day—mocking us, discouraging us, and trying to dampen our faith. What negative voices ring out loudest in your ears?

_____

_____

What can you do to stand strong on the truth of God's Word in a noisy world filled with lies?

_____

_____

Food in Social Settings?

Previously we talked about eating in response to specific *emotions* such as anger, boredom, guilt, and others, as well as eating triggered by specific negative *thoughts* (for example, "I am a loser," "I might as well eat because nothing I do ever succeeds anyway," This is too difficult," and so forth). In this lesson, we want to examine another cue that triggers overeating: the social cue.

LOOKING AT YOUR *LIFE*

When you're on a trip or vacation, what restaurants do you stop at most and why?

_____

_____

How susceptible are you to food advertisements on television? When did a billboard or commercial prompt you to head straight for a restaurant?

_____

_____

Do you tend to eat more when you are alone, or when you're in a public setting where there is a lot of food? Why?

_____

_____

Rank the following social food settings/scenarios from 1 to 10, with 1 = "the least tempting" and 10 = "an almost certain overeating disaster."

____ You go in the break room at work, and a grateful client or supplier has sent over a giant cookie basket.

____ At a small group social, the host's dining room table is overflowing with rich, fatty finger foods.

____ The church has a big potluck dinner with tables filled with delicious foods and desserts.

____ It's late night—you're restless, and a commercial for your favorite fast-food restaurant (which is only half a mile from your house) comes on TV.

____ The whole family is sitting down to a sumptuous Thanksgiving feast with all your holiday favorites.

____ Your coworkers ask you to lunch, and they choose your favorite pizza buffet.

____ You realize you need to run to the grocery store—and you are also *starving*!

____ At a kid's birthday party in a popular fast-food restaurant, you notice your child's "kiddie meal" has been all but ignored, leaving you staring at a tray full of tempting fries, cheeseburger, and chocolate shake to boot!

____ A lavish wedding reception features several tables of exotic seafood dishes you don't normally get to sample.

____ Visiting friends insist that you keep all the leftover yummies from a spontaneous cookout/pitch-in dinner.

LEARNING A NEW WAY OF *LIFE*

Upon rebuilding the walls of Jerusalem, Governor Nehemiah had Ezra the scribe come and read the law of God, while the Levites explained its meaning to the Jewish people. Upon hearing God's Word, the people were convicted about their sin and failure to live as they should. They were weeping as they listened. But then Nehemiah said, "Go and enjoy choice food and sweet drinks, and send some to those who have nothing prepared. This day is holy to our Lord. Do not grieve, for the joy of the LORD is your strength" (Nehemiah 8:10).

What does this event suggest about eating and celebrating together with others?

_____

_____

Social cues are triggers in your living or working environment that increase your likelihood of overeating.

The authors say, "The best way to handle commercials, especially late at night when you are tired and your defenses are down, is to use the remote to click past the commercials. Don't watch them and you won't be drawn in by the trigger. And certainly don't watch food channels or cooking shows! Both can trigger a desire to overeat."

Has this food commercial trigger been a problem for you? How so?

_____

_____

Proverbs 19:20 says: "Listen to advice and accept discipline, and at the end you will be counted among the wise." Read the following tidbits of advice and discipline from chapter 9 of *Lose It for Life*. Then jot down your initial honest responses to each.

1. "This association of the car with eating must be broken. We know the concept sounds impossible, but the best way to do this is not to eat in the car at all. . . . Relegate all eating to the kitchen table."

_____

_____

2. "Movies can be very enjoyable without the snacks. Drink a full glass of water before you go, and eat a low-calorie snack so the sight and smell of all those goodies won't be so tempting. The association between eating and watching movies needs to be broken, which requires that you unlearn that behavior."

_____

_____

3. "If you are asked to bring food to an event, bring something healthy you can snack on, and park your body close to that snack food. . . . You can hold a glass of punch or diet drink in one hand for a long time while you are busy making conversation and interacting with new people."

_____

_____

4. "Look around your workplace. Are there places in that setting
   that trigger eating? How about the coffeepot? It can be a place of
   gathering and snacking. . . . You may have to skip the informal
   chatting in the coffee room and socialize by the water fountain
   instead."

_____

_____

5. "Eat before you [grocery] shop, which also helps cut down
   on buying impulse items. . . . Avoid the cookie aisle and
   prepackaged foods that are high in trans fat."

_____

_____

6. "You must break [the habit of tasting and eating] while
   cooking. . . . Ask someone else to taste the stew if you think it
   may need more salt. If you have to stir the pot, do so, but then
   immediately put down the spoon before you can sample it. . . .
   And during cleanup, don't eat the leftovers on people's plates."

_____

_____

7. "[Use] foil wrap for leftover foods. When you don't see what the
   dish is, it isn't as tempting to eat it."

_____

_____

Proverbs 21:5 says, "The plans of the diligent lead to profit as surely as haste leads to
poverty." How, specifically and practically, can advance planning help you avoid overeating
in social situations?

_____

_____

_____

What would it be like and how might it work if you planned the next day's menu (or approved eating list) each night before you went to bed?

_____

_____

LOSING IT FOR *LIFE*

No one can make all these changes at once. It's a good idea to begin with something small. What one thing will you choose to do differently for a month? Write down that commitment, and begin by making that change.

_____

_____

Try to think which social situations or cues trigger you to overeat. Then problem-solve ahead of time how you will handle that situation.

Research experts tell us that it takes three weeks to a month to learn a new habit and make it a part of our routine. Theoretically, then, someone serious about making lifestyle eating and exercise changes could develop *twelve new habits a year.*

What twelve small changes would you like to see in your life? Be specific. Write them down.

_____

_____

_____

_____

_____

_____

Now look into the future and imagine how these new lifestyle patterns could add up to make your life experience richer. Record your hopes and dreams here.

_____

_____

_____

_____

Remember, make one small behavior change your goal for each month. Keep adding changes as you are able. If you fail, cut yourself a break. Keep plodding. Eventually these small changes will add up. If you took years to put on the weight, give yourself time to take it off.

Usually if you take something away, you need to replace it with something else. Otherwise most of us will merely substitute another problem-behavior in its place. (For example, maybe you have stopped overeating but now notice you're beginning to overspend.)

When has this kind of problem substitution been the case with you?

_____

_____

Your goal is to eat for nourishment and the enjoyment of meals. It is up to you to discover the other illegitimate functions that eating has served in your life. Some of those wrong functions are using food to calm yourself, to relax, to numb you, to boost your mood, to fill time, or something similar.

What specific healthy and appropriate actions have you begun to make a part of your life to address these emotional needs?

_____

_____

DAY 5

Forgiveness

In this last lesson for chapter 9, we want to examine the important role of forgiveness in an all-around healthy, God-honoring lifestyle.

LOOKING AT YOUR *LIFE*

What is the greatest example of human forgiveness you have ever seen?

_____

_____

Other than God, what person would you say has had to forgive you most? Why?

_____

_____

Change is difficult. We all need the help of others and God. Don't be an island determined to do this alone.

LEARNING A NEW WAY OF *LIFE*

Jesus said, "For if you forgive other people when they sin against you, your heavenly Father will also forgive you. But if you do not forgive others their sins, your Father will not forgive your sins" (Matthew 6:14–15).

What do you think Jesus' words imply?

_____

_____

How does Psalm 66:18 add to your understanding of this passage?

_____

_____

On what occasions did an unforgiving spirit of bitterness toward another person short-circuit the power of God in your life or make Him seem distant?

_____

_____

The authors write, "Forgiveness can be difficult—almost impossible—for those who have been abused physically, sexually, or even spiritually. It is never easy or instant; it may in fact take years to complete. However, if forgiveness isn't rendered, the injured person remains trapped in the abuse of the past where they endlessly relive the offenses done against them. Our yesterdays must be put in the past so we can fully enjoy today."

Express your honest reaction to this statement.

_____

_____

Jesus said, "Therefore, if you are offering your gift at the altar and there remember that your brother or sister has something against you, leave your gift there in front of the altar. First go and be reconciled to them; then come and offer your gift" (Matthew 5:23–24). In other words, the forgiveness process also involves making things right with those we have wounded. This may require us to write letters or make phone calls, to repay debts, to make amends, or otherwise to do our part in making wrongs as right as possible. This, of course, can result in enormous spiritual blessings, both to others and to us.

What people do you need to seek out in order to ask forgiveness? Who did you wrong and how did you wrong them? Be specific. How and when is God urging you to contact them?

_____

_____

Forgiveness, when empowered by God's Spirit, is a process of detaching painful events from our emotional responses to them, thus facilitating the process of healing.

Hebrews 12:15 reiterates the need to forgive everyone and anyone who has hurt you: "Make sure no one gets left out of God's generosity. Keep a sharp eye out for weeds of bitter discontent. A thistle or two gone to seed can ruin a whole garden in no time" (MSG).

What are some consequences of becoming bitter and harboring resentment?

_____

_____

LOSING IT FOR *LIFE*

Forgiveness means:

- handing back our rights to God (the rights we usurped from Him) and inviting Him to be in charge
- asking for forgiveness and making restitution for the damage we've done
- no longer energizing ourselves with rage or hatred
- not trying to change other people, but asking God to do it
- stepping out of the past and into the present
- accepting the pardon of the cross for others as well as for ourselves
- obeying Jesus' instructions to forgive so that we can be forgiven

"Make allowance for each other's faults, and forgive anyone who offends you. Remember, the Lord forgave you, so you must forgive others" (Colossians 3:13 NLT).

Which of the above actions do you find the most difficult to do? Why?

_____

_____

Is forgiveness more an emotional state or an act of the will? Why?

_____

_____

If you are aware of anyone toward whom you feel intense rage or strong bitterness, what do you intend to do? Why is it imperative that you forgive?

_____

_____

The authors recommend the following prayer:

Dear Lord,

You have commanded me to forgive others, just as You have forgiven me through the sacrifice of Your Son, Jesus. I choose to obey You, even though this is not easy for me. You listed all of my sins. Then You nailed them to the cross so that Jesus' blood could pay for them. Help me to release this account to You and not seek justice for my sake. Help me to trust that You are just and will carry out Your will.

Yet, while I transfer this account to You, wounds still remain as a result of this wrong. As I obey You by releasing this person from my debt, I pray You will heal the hurts they have caused me. Help me to trust that You are willing and able to redeem me from the wrongs that have been done against me. If thoughts of revenge recur, I pray You will help me continually release this person's account to You. Amen.

Is this a prayer that you need to pray? Make a list here of any slights, grudges, and offenses you have held on to and would like to release. Then pray about each item, asking the Lord to forgive you (or someone who hurt you) on each point of your list.

_____

_____

_____

_____

In summary, revisit the RISE acronym again. In terms of behavior, we need to:

REDUCE eating in response to social cues.

INCREASE the number of changes you make. Start small and add more as you are able.

SUBSTITUTE forgiveness for any unforgiveness or unresolved misdeed; substitute new behaviors for eating.

ELIMINATE eating for the wrong reasons.

Part Three

A LIFELONG JOURNEY

If we live our lives without meaning or purpose and become self-obsessed, we've missed what God can do. Don't you want God to take your years of struggle with weight problems and transform it all for His glory? If that is your desire, then you will emerge from this experience stronger and better, and you will be able to help others along the way.

Stay in the race. Press on to the mark. Don't give up. God's desire is that we all push ourselves to do our best in the race of life. We have to train—read the Word, pray, worship, and develop intimacy with God. Then we develop endurance, the ability to stay in the race no matter how difficult things become. Push yourself in your relationship with Him. Go a little deeper—more faith, more dependence, less of you (physically and emotionally), and more of Him.

Friends, training is hard work, but the payoff feels so good. We are all in training for the eternal. What we do today matters. And we don't have to wait until the race is over to receive rewards. God has set up stations of blessings along the way to encourage us to keep going.

When we train for anything, we must keep our minds fixed on the goal. Know where you are heading and keep your mind fixed on getting there. Will you endure the hardships around you? Will you be faithful to the end? Can God count on you? Or will you give up and complain that life is just too hard? We pray you stay in the race no matter how difficult it becomes.

Father,

For everyone who feels like giving up, for everyone who thinks they can't go on, give them a revelation of Your love and help. You desire them to go the distance. Your reward is great, both today and eternally. Help us to keep our eyes fixed on You and the final prize. Give us the strength to endure when we think we can't. More than anything, give us Your presence. Connect us with those who will encourage and share in the race with us until the end—and may we be strengthened through the love of Jesus Christ. Amen.

10

Community—
The Connection Cornerstone

American Christianity is influenced by the culture in which it operates. We live in a society known for placing value on independence, self-sufficiency, and what is called "rugged individualism." Historically, autonomy, individual drive, and self-motivation have been admired characteristics, yet this is not the biblical practice suggested for the body of Christ.

Relationship is characteristic of the Godhead—God is three in one. The Trinity enjoys fellowship. Relationship has existed from the beginning of time. Since the beginning of creation, God knew it was good for a man to have a helper, which is why He created woman.

While God's triune relationship is often mysterious to our human understanding, we do know that God so loved the world that He sent His only Son Jesus to die and take the sins of the world for our redemption (John 3:16). Out of love, God found a way to relate to us through His Son. While on earth, Jesus was highly relational as He communed with His Father, chose disciples, spent time with sinners, and even gave of His time to play with children.

A central message of Jesus' teaching was for us to live in unity with one another. When Jesus returned to the Father, the Holy Spirit was sent as Comforter. If we explore the beginnings of church history in the book of Acts, we find a record of how Christianity was practiced under the power of the Holy Spirit. As the church developed and spread, believers learned to live together, sharing freely with one another while maintaining meaningful fellowship. Even in the face of strong personalities and differences, the church found a way to listen and to submit to one another in Christian love. Because of the dedication of this early church in fasting and in prayer, people were released to do incredible miracles and extraordinary acts. Through the power of the Holy Spirit and the unity and love practiced in community, believers were healed. Now delivered, we must resist spiritual oppression. In Christian community, we learn to love, heal, and live together as one body.

Lose It for Life believes strongly in the connections made in Christian community. We need each other. As we encourage one another and lift each other up in prayer, we move forward in the Christian life in ways not possible as a lone sojourner. Relationships are important in order to meet our needs for intimacy and support, but also to grow and avoid relapse.

RISE TO THE CHALLENGE

In order to RISE above the challenges, we need connection and community. Add these goals to your program:

Reduce negative relationships that sabotage your success.

Increase connection with others, social skills, and community.

Substitute the healing of community and connection for the belief that you must go it alone.

Eliminate the lone-ranger mentality and toxic relationships that undermine your success.

FIGHT DISCONNECTION

When we are obsessed with food and weight, we often hide while feeling outcast and alienated from others. Embarrassed by what we weigh and feeling out of control, many of us feel like second-class citizens and pull back from active involvement with others. Instead of being our true selves, we do things to please others and hope they never see who we really are for fear they won't like us. Maybe you've been bullied or rejected because of your weight. Consequently, you've pulled back from others in fear of more of the same. People who grow up in overly critical homes or homes in which they were teased about their weight often try to hide within social situations rather than connect.

Food obsessions involve time and energy that take you away from other activities. When you are overweight, you leave early, come late, sit by yourself, and refuse to share certain parts of yourself with others. There is an assumption that once the weight is gone, you'll become a social butterfly. However, Cathy found out that "flying solo" wasn't a good idea.

March 15, 2004—I wish I could say that after losing 119 pounds all my food issues are finally behind me. I guess somewhere in my imagination I believed that if I ever lost this much weight again I would surely be floating from social event to social event never desiring to eat junk food or binge again. It was going to be great! I guess this is a good time for a reality check! I was so wrong.

The truth is that some days now are just as hard as the first day I began this journey. There are days I make poor choices and fall off the wagon and, as crazy as it sounds, there are days I am tempted to go back to my old habits. Changing patterns and habits is hard. Maturing and dying to self is hard.

But letting go of God's hand is detrimental. I've noticed that just when I think I have this whole food addiction thing licked—and I start flying solo—I tend to crash. But the Lord has been so faithful. He knows my heart. As I cry out to Him to help me change, He always provides a way of escape for me. How wonderful to have a Daddy who loves me this much.

I am beginning to understand that this will never be an easy feat. Good health— emotional, spiritual, and physical—does not just happen. It is truly a gift from God. We must do our part and allow Him to do His part. It's a journey taken one day at a time.

—Cathy

When someone loses as much weight as Cathy did, one of the most common expectations is that life will be dramatically different. This is particularly true from a social perspective. There are assumptions that when the weight is gone, the dates will be many and the whole outlook will be different, including being able to socially engage for the first time. It will be magical, or so the person thinks!

Then the weight comes off and reality hits. *Where are all those new party invitations? Why isn't the healthy, trim me getting invited out?* The disappointment is that all this effort has not resulted in a new and exciting social life. Why? Because losing weight doesn't necessarily change who you are inside!

When you spend your life as an overweight person, you learn to feel uneasy in social situations and avoid and withdraw. There is work to be done on the inside of the person too—to build confidence and to be put in new social situations. This means taking new risks, which is never easy. A person can still struggle with major insecurities even when his or her body looks healthier. So part of the work of losing it for life is to venture into the uncertain and unpredictable world of people and relationships.

YOU NEED THE BODY

It helps to remember the source of your true worth. Jesus Christ says you are already accepted, loved, and special. Other people may not always be so positive and affirming. However, there are those people who will be, and you must find them and make a connection. You need their support and encouragement.

One reason people struggle even when they know their relationship with Christ is vital to success is that they are not connected to a community of fellow believers. No matter how successful you are at doing this program, you need connections with people who can help when you feel down or want to give in and give up. As one woman who was losing weight confided,

> People are always asking me for advice. I don't want to give advice! I'm still dealing with weight loss myself. Yes, I've had some success, but I'm still working on issues and prefer to talk to those who are struggling. I don't want to "help" everyone else in the way I used to. That was my old pattern and it took me away from doing what I needed to do to help myself. I think I can most help by being honest and saying this isn't easy, but that one day at a time, I'm making it.

When you are the consummate giver and never expect to receive in a relationship, you tend to attract needy people who can suck you dry. And then, guess what? You feel empty and use food to fill that void again. This woman knew she needed others to help her and wasn't in a position to be their expert. Community is so important in this journey because it links you with support and encouragement for these moments of difficulty. In the body of Christ, when you feel strong, you encourage another. When you are down, another person encourages you. This give-and-take is the basis for healthy relationships.

Revisit Social Skills

When you begin to take risks socially, you must also take a hard look at your social skills. Maybe you need to be more assertive, learn how to initiate conversation, or demonstrate a new interest in others. Weight loss will boost your confidence, but it won't teach you social skills.

If you've spent a lifetime hiding and you come out of the eating closet, you may have to practice new skills. So today, make it your goal to approach someone you would like to get to know better. Find out an interest he or she has and begin to ask about it. Broaden your own interests now that you aren't so obsessed with food and eating. Try a new activity and see how it feels. Certainly it will feel a little scary at first. That's okay. It gets easier the more you do it. If you aren't invited to the party, bring the party to you! That's right. You throw a party and ask people to come. If you are tired of no social life, create one. Start small. Ask a few old friends to come and include one or two new ones. Don't make the focus of the party food or drink (time to let go of that crutch). Instead, have a structured activity, like playing board games. Then relax, laugh, and enjoy the fun. The more you practice doing things that are uncomfortable, the easier they will become.

Don't Alienate Yourself

Overeating can keep us from the very people we need support from. In addition to shame, fear, and embarrassment, or thinking we lack good social skills, we can stay isolated because of pride. We convince ourselves that needing others is too painful or is weakness. We really don't need people to help us in life because we've bought the American idealism of doing it on our own. We have to gut it out, and our failure to do so is because we lack willpower, not because we need others along the way.

In some cases, our lack of experience with healthy relationships keeps us from trying. Growing up alone and isolated, we see no benefit in relationships. Our experience only brought hurt. Or in cases where relationship may have started out strong, we were betrayed or disappointed. People cannot be trusted. In the end, you believe you will be rejected.

Many of us just give up on relationships and fail to make the distinction between the benefits of healthy relationships and the needy and overly dependent relationships in which we may be entwined. The former are healthy; the latter are toxic. Because we fail to define who we are outside of our weight, we lack appropriate boundaries within our relationships and self-care. We want people to fill those empty places, even when we know this isn't healthy. So we pull away altogether, deciding we are too needy and too messed up for this relationship.

Yet even with all our reasons for pulling back and protecting ourselves from hurt or pain, we still desire connection. We were created to relate to God and others. It is in relationships that we grow and learn about ourselves. Through our experiences with others, we define how we think and feel. Attachment is a basic need that never goes away but longs to be met. And while we try to meet that need through eating, the need is never satisfied.

The need for connection is not unhealthy, but how you meet that need can be. In God's kingdom, nobody is more important than the next. You aren't less because you weigh more. We approach each other with humility and must have the courage to be open to what we can receive from others. Yes, we can be rejected, but we can also find people who will accept and love us no matter what we weigh or how many times we fail. If we don't allow bad relationships to derail our efforts, we can have meaningful connections and our needs will be met.

Healthy relationships include loving God, ourselves, and others. We don't love with a puffed-up sense of importance. We love because God loves us and has purpose and meaning for our lives. As we surrender to that purpose and plan, we purposefully connect with others to accomplish what we can't accomplish alone. Connection brings healing and healing brings joy.

When we are willing to be open, transparent, and vulnerable to others, we break free of the isolation that keeps us hidden in the dark. We feel God's love because we aren't moving in pretense. We learn to accept who we are because we are in process. We ask for healing so we can grow and give to others and find rest.

FOOD, MARRIAGE, AND FIDELITY

In some marriages, weight creates a sense of protection. We referred early on to the idea that being heavy can protect you from your own sexual impulses or the impulses of others.[1] People who aren't sure they can resist sexual temptations may stay heavy as a way to control their impulsivity. Also, the fear of feeling sexually attractive makes some people uncomfortable, in part because they aren't certain they can control their impulses.

How many times have you or someone you know complained that the necessary support for weight loss was lacking? Those around us and in our intimate relationships can actually sabotage our efforts. For example, the best way to prevent your spouse from losing weight is to demand that he or she do so. After years of working with couples, this fact is certain: when a spouse demands weight loss, weight loss undergoes a death sentence. Why? Because there is something about a demand that says you don't accept the partner as he or she is. Acceptance is instead conditioned on the basis of weight. A demand to look different is often accompanied by criticism and comparisons, which usually signal deeper issues in a relationship that must be addressed.

Another interesting observation is the number of husbands who seem to sabotage their wives' efforts to lose weight. In some cases, husbands worry that their wives' thinner appearances will make them more vulnerable to other men. In other cases, if one spouse takes responsibility for a weight problem, there may be the expectation that the other spouse will tackle a specific problem, like anger, drinking, or gambling. We have also seen cases of sabotage because spouses are unwilling to have their routines and eating habits altered for the sake of their partner's healthy desire to lose weight.

I (Dr. Linda) remember one woman I worked with whose husband brought home candy almost every day despite the fact that she was paying me to help her lose weight. Repeatedly, she asked him to stop bringing candy into the house. Yet he never stopped. At my request, he came to a counseling session. I discovered that he was worried that he would be asked to make changes in his own life if his wife overcame her weight problem. And while he didn't like the fact that his wife was significantly overweight, he preferred to keep life the way it was—with the pressure off. He later admitted that he felt inadequate to make changes in his own life and secretly did not want his wife to succeed because he would feel more like a failure.

Weight-loss efforts can also be sabotaged because you've spent your entire life playing the victim. While this isn't a role you probably desire, it may be a familiar one. To move out of the victim position would mean forgiving people and making other changes. Giving up anything you know well to move into the unknown is always a bit unsettling, but the gains are certainly worth a bit of anxiety. A lack of trust is at the root of this problem. You must trust that being obedient to God's Word, as well as forgiving others' wrongs and extending grace, will turn out to be beneficial to you and others in the long run. As we discussed in the last chapter, don't allow bitterness to prevent you from moving forward.

Spousal support and the support of families and intimate others is very important when it comes to losing weight.[2] Talk about your goals with loved ones before you begin any program. Discuss whether there are hidden fears or relationship concerns about your losing weight. Then work together as much as possible. The best situation is when your intimate relationships can be part of your support system.

EMBRACE COMMUNITY

If you decide to be more vulnerable and open your life up to others, recognize that it won't be easy or a positive experience 100 percent of the time. You'll have times of frustration and you'll learn who can handle your openness and who cannot. There are people who are not trustworthy, and you must be discerning about who you will open up to. Yet be careful how you do this! Paul addresses how we are to behave with one another in Romans 14:1–9:

> Welcome with open arms fellow believers who don't see things the way you do. And don't jump all over them every time they do or say something you don't agree with—even when it seems that they are strong on opinions but weak in the faith department. Remember, they have their own history to deal with. Treat them gently.
>
> For instance, a person who has been around for a while might well be convinced that he can eat anything on the table, while another, with a different background, might assume all Christians should be vegetarians and eat accordingly. But since both are guests at Christ's table, wouldn't it be terribly rude if they fell to criticizing what the other ate or didn't eat? God, after all, invited them both to the table. Do you have any business crossing people off the guest list or interfering with God's welcome? If there are corrections to be made or manners to be learned, God can handle that without your help.
>
> Or, say, one person thinks that some days should be set aside as holy and another thinks that each day is pretty much like any other. There are good reasons either way. So, each person is free to follow the convictions of conscience.
>
> What's important in all this is that if you keep a holy day, keep it for God's sake; if you eat meat, eat it to the glory of God and thank God for prime rib; if you're a vegetarian, eat vegetables to the glory of God and thank God for broccoli. None of us are permitted to insist on our own way in these matters. It's God we are answerable to—all the way from life to death and everything in between—not each other. That's why Jesus lived and died and then lived again: so that he could be our Master across the entire range of life and death, and free us from the petty tyrannies of each other. (MSG)

If we allow Jesus to be our Master who can "free us from the petty tyrannies of each other," dynamic things will happen. We all have differences that can divide us if we let them. However, we are called to unity and we should work out our differences in Christian love and maturity. The unity that results will create an atmosphere for healing. Make it your goal to find people with whom you can be authentic, and whom you can trust to maintain confidences and to pray with you. Work on your differences with others and learn to live in Christian love.

Relationships are work because they often act as mirrors to our problems. In intimacy, we see our weaknesses and need for God's help. As we grow, we become aware of our separateness, but also our need for each other. As we learn to define who we are, set boundaries, deal with conflict, and manage differences, we grow if we stay connected to others in the process.

What should we look for when it comes to building relationships with one another? Ephesians 4:2 says, "Be completely humble and gentle; be patient, bearing with one another in love." We are to pursue community with one another and be patient and humble in the process.

Jesus recognized the need for community in His darkest hour. He took His disciples with Him to pray as He faced the biggest challenge of His earthly life—the cross. As He hung on the cross, He thought of others and even welcomed a thief into Paradise! He also arranged for John, the beloved, to care for His mother. And in those last moments before His death, He cried out from a sense of estrangement, "My God, my God, why have you forsaken me?" (Matthew 27:46). For a brief moment, He felt abandoned by the Father and became a curse for us, as Paul reminds us in Galatians.

Jesus is all about community. He tells us that people will know us by our love (John 13:35) and that we are to love one another. When you face any difficult change or trial in your life, support and community make the difference in your ability to survive and come through the trial. Seek wise counsel from those who can help you. Be responsive to your pastors and leaders who will provide spiritual accountability. Take advantage of counselors and therapists who can help you sort out the complexity of weight loss as it applies to you and your specific life. Be persistent and have the courage to be open in relationships with others.

As you seek a more intimate connection with God through your church, you may find that you redefine your weight problem as a fruit problem. Fruit is the visible part of our lives that others can see. Galatians 5:22–23 describes what builds healthy relationships in our lives: "But the fruit of the [Holy] Spirit [the work which His presence within accomplishes] is love, joy (gladness), peace, patience (an even temper, forbearance), kindness, goodness (benevolence), faithfulness, gentleness (meekness, humility), self-control (self-restraint, continence). Against such things there is no law [that can bring a charge]" (AMP).

Do you evidence the fruit of the Spirit is in you when it comes to dealing with other people? As you submit yourself to God's growing and pruning process, ask Him to put you with others who are committed to bearing this type of fruit also. Healthy communities bear this kind of fruit. Look for it.

All praise to the God and Father of our Master, Jesus the Messiah! Father of all mercy! God of all healing counsel! He comes alongside us when we go through hard times, and before you know it, he brings us alongside someone else who is going through hard times so that we can be there for that person just as God was there for us.

—2 Corinthians 1:3–4 (MSG)

What fabulous verses! God comes alongside us when we go through difficulty. That in and of itself is reassuring, but there is even more—God will use us to help someone else who is going through a hard time as well. In God's economy, nothing is ever wasted, not even pain!

We can never know God's plans or His gain from our loss, unless we give Him our misery and allow Him to transform it into a mission for our lives. Once our loss and pain point us to God's grace, we can also lead others into His grace. In doing so, we partner with God as He accomplishes His purposes. After we emerge from our own despair, become transparent, and candidly share our victories, we will be in a position to share our struggles and God's power to overcome, attracting others into His grace.

God's church is our earthly home. Embrace the love and support He has instituted for you and build on that connection for life.

Workbook Week 10

COMMUNITY—
THE CONNECTION
CORNERSTONE

— DAY 1 —
The Miracle and Mystery of Community

In healthy Christian community we learn to love and be loved, to serve and be served, and to celebrate and be celebrated. In Christian community, we find acceptance, grace, and healing. In Christian community, we hear the truth spoken firmly yet gently, and we learn how to live a new life together. It's no wonder that Lose It for Life believes strongly in the connections made in Christian community. In fact, we do not believe it's possible to live successfully or enjoyably apart from the miracle and mystery of true Christian fellowship.

Here's how to apply the RISE acronym to building community:

We live in a society that values independence, autonomy, and self-sufficiency.

Reduce negative relationships that sabotage your success.
Increase connection with others, social skills, and community.
Subsitute the healing of community and connection for the belief that you must go it alone.
Eliminate the lone-ranger mentality and toxic relationships that undermine your success.

That's what these next five lessons are about.

LOOKING AT YOUR *LIFE*

Think back to the closest friendships you ever enjoyed. Maybe it was kids in your neighborhood, a high school team you once played on, a Boy or Girl Scout troop, a

416

collection of roommates, sorority sisters in college, or a small group at church. What made this group of folks and the friendships you enjoyed so meaningful?

_____

_____

_____

Think back to the best church you've ever been a part of. What made it so special?

_____

_____

_____

In your own words, define *community*. Then describe your personal experience of community (whether good or bad) at this point in your life.

_____

_____

_____

LEARNING A NEW WAY OF *LIFE*

Autonomy, individual drive, and self-motivation are admired characteristics in our culture; that is, do it your own way, succeed by your own power. But are these qualities in keeping with the way the body of Christ is designed to function?

Read Genesis 1:26. What do you observe about God in this verse?

_____

_____

The authors say, "Relationship is characteristic of the Godhead—God is three in one. The Trinity enjoys fellowship. Relationship has existed from the beginning of time."

In your own words, expand on this idea of God—Father, Son, and Holy Spirit—being in community.

_____

_____

Jesus was highly relational. He communed with His heavenly Father, lived and traveled with His disciples, and spent time with all kinds of people.

If it's true that we are dependent creatures made in the image of a God who exists "in relationship," what does this suggest about our own needs for community?

_____

_____

_____

Read Acts 2:42–47. Describe the daily lifestyle of the early church. How was their Christian experience different from that of many modern-day churches?

_____

_____

_____

The authors argue:

If we explore the beginnings of church history in the book of Acts, we find a record of how Christianity was practiced under the power of the Holy Spirit. As the church developed and spread, believers learned to live together, sharing freely with one another while maintaining meaningful fellowship. Even in the face of strong personalities and differences, the church found a way to listen and to submit to one another in Christian love. . . . Through the power of the Holy Spirit and the unity and love practiced in community, believers were healed.

When have you been part of a close-knit fellowship of believers where people cared deeply for one another and actually "did life together" as the early church did? Describe that experience.

_____

_____

LOSING IT FOR _LIFE_

The New Testament lists a number of attitudes and actions that should mark the lifestyles and interactions of Christians. Here are a few:

"A new command I give you: Love one another. As I have loved you, so you must love one another. By this everyone will know that you are my disciples, if you love one another." (John 13:34–35)

Honor one another above yourselves. (Romans 12:10)

Live in harmony with one another. (Romans 12:16)

Therefore let us stop passing judgment on one another. (Romans 14:13)

Accept one another, then, just as Christ accepted you, in order to bring praise to God. (Romans 15:7)

I appeal to you, brothers and sisters, in the name of our Lord Jesus Christ, that all of you agree with one another in what you say and that there be no divisions among you, but that you be perfectly united in mind and thought. (1 Corinthians 1:10)

Be kind and compassionate to one another, forgiving each other, just as in Christ God forgave you. (Ephesians 4:32)

In what specific ways does living by these "one another" commands build healthier, happier community?

_____

_____

How effectively does your church live by these commands?

_____

_____

Go back through the list and grade yourself. Which of these "one anothers" are you faithful to put into practice on a regular basis?

_____

_____

_____

Which of these commands have you been guilty of neglecting? In what areas do you need improvement?

_____

_____

Relationships are necessary to meet our needs for intimacy and to help us grow and avoid relapse into old, unhealthy lifestyle habits.

What new thing did you learn about community from this lesson? Or what old truth were you reminded to put into practice today?

_____

_____

_____

Overeating Versus Community

Perhaps you've never thought about it, but overeating and weight problems can disconnect us from one another. In this lesson we want to explore how unhealthy eating habits often contribute to dysfunctional relationships, and, on the other hand, how healthy eating habits can be encouraged by functional relationships/community.

LOOKING AT YOUR *LIFE*

How do you feel when overweight people are made fun of on television programs or by comedians?

_____

_____

If you have ever been made to feel like a social outcast because of your weight, what happened in your heart? How did the experience alter the way you related to people?

_____

_____

If you have ever been bullied or verbally abused because of your weight, write some candid memories of those experiences.

_____

_____

When we are obsessed with food and weight, we often hide or pull back from active involvement with others.

What people have accepted you with no strings attached—fully and completely, despite your weight or appearance?

_____

_____

What can you do to express your appreciation to those folks?

_____

_____

LEARNING A NEW WAY OF _LIFE_

Take a few minutes to read through the entire prayer that Jesus prayed in John 17. Then focus on this excerpt:

> My prayer is not for [the twelve apostles] alone. I pray also for those who will believe in me through their message [Christians down through the centuries—including us!], that all of them may be one, Father, just as you are in me and I am in you. May they also be in us so that the world may believe that you have sent me. I have given them the glory that you gave me, that they may be one as we are one—I in them and you in me—so that they may be brought to complete unity. Then the world will know that you sent me and have loved them even as you have loved me. (John 17:20–23)

How would you summarize the main point of Jesus' prayer? What is it that He wants for the world? For His followers?

_____

_____

How do you think our enemy, the devil, might view Christian unity and healthy community?

_____

_____

When we pull back from others and remain isolated and alone because of our weight (or for any other reason), how do you think God feels about it?

_____

_____

Consider these situations and offer your assessment, based on what you just studied.

Situation . . .	What God might think/feel	How Satan probably reacts
You resist an invitation to a ski party at the lake because of your weight.		
You take lunch early and eat by yourself in your car rather than with colleagues.		
You tell yourself you'll become more socialble when you drop about fifty pounds.		
You drop out of a small group because someone told a "fat" joke.		
You come late to social events and leave early if food is involved.		

Look again at Romans 15:7. This verse stresses the importance of accepting others. What other important fact does it reveal about Christ? How does that truth help us build a healthier self-image?

_____

_____

Regardless of what you weigh, it's up to you to push yourself out there in the unpredictable world of relationships.

The authors point out that when someone loses a large amount of weight, one of the common expectations is that life will be dramatically better. The reasoning goes like this: *When I lose weight, I'll get lots of invitations and everything will be different. Socially, I'll become outgoing and active.*

But then, they point out, the weight comes off and reality hits. *Where are all those new party invitations? Why don't people see the new me and invite me out?*

This happens because an overweight person learns to feel uneasy in social situations. He or she develops deeply ingrained habits of hiding, avoiding, and withdrawing. Just because a person's body is getting thinner doesn't mean that his or her heart is now oozing with courage and confidence. Losing weight does not automatically result in losing fears of rejection. We still have to take social and relational risks.

React to this statement: "A person can still struggle with major insecurities even when his or her body looks healthier."

_____

_____

_____

LOSING IT FOR *LIFE*

How can and should you respond to people who are not positive and affirming?

_____

_____

How does knowing—deep in your soul—that Christ accepts and loves you unconditionally make a difference in your effort to become healthier physically, emotionally, socially, and spiritually?

_____

_____

On whom can you count for faithful support and encouragement?

_____

_____

_____

The authors observe, "When you are the consummate giver and never expect to receive in a relationship, you tend to attract needy people who can suck you dry. And then, guess what? You feel empty and use food to fill that void again." Have you experienced this in your life? Explain.

_____

_____

Do you feel comfortable "needing" others? Are you more at ease giving or taking?

_____

_____

In Day 1 you read through several New Testament "one another" commands (guidelines for healthy community). Here are a few more to ponder and put into practice:

> [Speak] to one another with psalms, hymns, and songs from the Spirit. (Ephesians 5:19)

> Submit to one another out of reverence for Christ. (Ephesians 5:21)

> Therefore encourage one another and build each other up, just as in fact you are doing. (1 Thessalonians 5:11)

> And let us consider how we may spur one another on toward love and good deeds. (Hebrews 10:24)

> Offer hospitality to one another without grumbling. (1 Peter 4:9)

> All of you, clothe yourselves with humility toward one another, because, "God opposes the proud but shows favor to the humble." (1 Peter 5:5)

Community is so important. When you feel strong, you encourage others. When you are down, others support you. This reciprocal give-and-take is part of healthy relationships.

How can living out these commands and associating with others who hold these values make a difference in losing it for life?

_____

_____

DAY 3
Social Skills

Weight loss may boost your confidence in how you look, but it won't teach you how to interact with others. In this lesson we'll focus on social skills—changing for the better the way you interact with others.

LOOKING AT YOUR *LIFE*

Social skills must be practiced. If you've spent a lifetime hiding, you may have to practice new skills.

How sociable are you? How good are your skills at relating to others? Rate yourself on a continuum of 1–10 in the following areas.

1= low (I need improvement); 10 = high (I do this really well)

	1	2	3	4	5	6	7	8	9	10
Smiling at others										
Making eye contact										
Feeling at ease around people										
Taking the initiative to speak										
Making conversation										
Making others feel comfortable										
Making others feel cared for										
Making people feel included										
Listening										
Drawing people out										
Showing hospitality										
Showing compassion										
Being assertive										

Gathering people   _____

Displaying a sense of humor   _____

What areas received your lowest marks? Why did you give yourself these low scores?

_____

_____

Who do you know that displays ease and grace in social settings? What do you think is their secret?

_____

_____

LEARNING A NEW WAY OF _LIFE_

Reflect on the following Scripture passages:

> Do to others as you would have them do to you. (Luke 6:31)

> Do nothing out of selfish ambition or vain conceit. Rather, in humility value others above yourselves, not looking to your own interests but each of you to the interests of the others. In your relationships with one another, have the same mindset as Christ Jesus. (Philippians 2:3–5)

> Be devoted to one another in love. Honor one another above yourselves. (Romans 12:10)

What do these verses suggest about the way we are called by God to relate to others?

_____

_____

Why is hanging back and avoiding others not an option for those who claim to be followers of Christ?

_____

_____

_____

If you are tired of no social life, then begin to create one.

After reading chapter 10, imagine that a reclusive friend of yours says, "Look—I'm just shy. That's the way I am and the way I've always been. I can't help that. God made me with this personality. I feel like all this emphasis on social skills is an attempt to make me become something I'm not." What would you say? Is this a legitimate argument?

_____

_____

Just the thought of doing something new (for example, taking social risks) can be nerve-wracking. If you are anxious about taking some new risks, think about Jesus' words: "Peace I leave with you; my peace I give you. I do not give to you as the world gives. Do not let your hearts be troubled and do not be afraid" (John 14:27). How does this promise help you?

_____

_____

How do we access this supernatural peace and banish our fears of rejection?

_____

_____

LOSING IT FOR _LIFE_

The _LIFL_ book suggests a few practical ways to get out there mixing and mingling with others. One suggestion: "Today, make it your goal to approach someone you would like to get to know better. Find out an interest he or she has and begin to ask about it."

Jot down your honest reaction to that recommendation.

_____

_____

How much do the following beliefs or attitudes contribute to your own reluctance to engage others?

	A LOT	SOME	BARELY AT ALL
I have nothing to offer.			
I'm ugly and unworthy.			
I'm afraid of rejection.			
I never know what to do or say.			
I'm okay. I really don't need others.			
I've been hurt before—never again.			
People are fickle/untrustworthy.			
I'll just embarrass myself.			
People take advantage of me.			
I feel awkward and just freeze up.			

Which of these attitudes do you want to begin working on? What's your specific plan to address this area of needed change?

_____

_____

In the book we read: "Yet even with all our reasons for pulling back and protecting ourselves from hurt or pain, we still desire connection. We were created to relate to God and others. It is in relationships we grow and learn about ourselves. Through our experiences with others, we define how we think and feel. Attachment is a basic need that never goes away but longs to be met. And while we try to meet that need through eating, the need is never satisfied."

What are your comments, thoughts, and responses to this idea? How do you handle the ambivalence of wanting connection and fearing it?

_____

_____

Relationships contain risks, but they also contain rewards. How can we overcome our fear of the former so that we boldly pursue the latter?

_____

_____

When we are willing to be open, transparent, and vulnerable with others, we break the isolation that has kept us hidden and in the dark.

Think about the relationships in your life right now. Do you need more? Do you want deeper connection with others? Or do you want to stay on the same path you're on?

_____

_____

Remember, you are on a certain life trajectory. In other words, your current habits and ways of thinking and relating have you pointed in a certain direction that leads to a final destination.

As you fast-forward your life, is that destination the place you really want to end up? Or would you like a different outcome?

_____

_____

It's pretty basic. The only way to end up in a different place is to go in a new direction. That means making little changes today.

What social interaction changes do you intend to make beginning today? (Be specific: "I'm going to walk over to Debbie's cubicle at work, smile, and tell her good morning." Or "I'm going to ask Debbie if she wants to go with me to lunch.") Make your list in this space. Write at least three clear, measurable, achievable social goals.

_____

_____

_____

_____

Sabotage!

Weight-loss efforts can also be sabotaged because you've spent your life being a "victim." To move out of the victim role means forgiving people and making changes.

How many times have you (or someone you know) complained that you lacked any real support for weight loss? It's a fact: those around us and in our intimate relationships can actually block or sabotage our efforts! That's the focus of this lesson.

LOOKING AT YOUR *LIFE*

If you are married, have you ever felt that your spouse was unsupportive of your attempts to lose weight? What do you think might be the reason?

_____

_____

_____

The authors write, "In some cases, husbands worry that their wives' thinner appearances will make them more vulnerable to other men. In other cases, if one spouse takes responsibility for a weight problem, there may be the expectation that the other spouse will tackle a specific problem like anger, drinking, or gambling." Do these worries seem like a legitimate possibility?

_____

_____

What has happened when you have tried to get your spouse to go on a diet, to exercise, or to lose weight with you?

_____

_____

When has a spouse/boyfriend or girlfriend/parent ever demanded that you lose weight? How did that make you feel?

_____

_____

How do you typically respond when people *demand* a certain behavior from you?

_____

_____

_____

LEARNING A NEW WAY OF *LIFE*

Whenever we begin to change, it affects everyone around us. People are used to the old you. But now you're eating differently, exercising regularly, processing your "stuff," changing your attitudes. You're becoming more honest, more vulnerable, and more outgoing. All these things are good and God-honoring, but that doesn't mean your LIFL experience will always be easy and positive. You'll have times of frustration and you'll learn who can handle your new way of thinking and living and who cannot.

Avoiding these new conflicts means either avoiding people altogether—*not* an option, as we've already seen—or learning better how to cultivate good relationships and live in harmony with those who don't always agree with you.

Consider this passage from Romans 14 that touches on that very subject:

Welcome with open arms fellow believers who don't see things the way you do. And don't jump all over them every time they do or say something you don't agree with—even when it seems that they are strong on opinions but weak in the faith department. Remember, they have their own history to deal with. Treat them gently.

For instance, a person who has been around for a while might well be convinced that he can eat anything on the table, while another, with a different background, might assume all Christians should be vegetarians and eat accordingly. But since both are guests at Christ's table, wouldn't it be terribly rude if they fell to criticizing what the other ate or didn't eat? God, after all, invited them both to the table. Do you have any business crossing people off the guest list or interfering with God's welcome? If there are corrections to be made or manners to be learned, God can handle that without your help.

Or, say, one person thinks that some days should be set aside as holy and another thinks that each day is pretty much like any other. There are good reasons either way. So, each person is free to follow the convictions of conscience. What's important in all this is that if you keep a holy day, keep it for God's sake; if you eat meat, eat it to the glory of God and thank God for prime rib; if you're a vegetarian, eat vegetables to the glory of God and thank God for broccoli.

None of us are permitted to insist on our own way in these matters. It's God we are answerable to—all the way from life to death and everything in between—not each other. That's why Jesus lived and died and then lived again: so that he could be our Master across the entire range of life and death, and free us from the petty tyrannies of each other. (MSG)

How do Paul's words of counsel speak to your LIFL experience?

_____

_____

Relationships make the difference in your ability to survive and come through trials. Have the courage to stay in relationships with others.

How exactly does Jesus "free us from the petty tyrannies of each other"? Give examples from your own life.

_____

_____

Ephesians 4:2 says, "Be completely humble and gentle; be patient, bearing with one another in love." How would compliance with this command make a tangible difference in your closest relationships?

_____

_____

You can't change others, but you can—with God's help—change your own attitudes and behavior. If you are guilty of pride and harshness and impatience, what do you need to do to correct things?

_____

_____

The authors argue that relationships are work because they often act as mirrors to our own problems. It's when we're close to others that we most vividly see our own shortcomings and our need for God's help. As we mature, we become aware of our uniqueness and also our need for others. We learn to define who we are, set boundaries, deal with conflict, and appreciate and manage differences, *but only so long as we stay connected to others in the process.*

What do you like about this observation? What about it is difficult for you?

_____

_____

LOSING IT FOR *LIFE*

Studies show that spousal support and the support of families and other friends is very important when it comes to losing weight.[3]

Did you have any good, substantive discussions of your goals with others before beginning the LIFL program?

_____

_____

It may be helpful now to think through or discuss with someone your hidden fears or concerns about your losing weight. (Remember: the best situation is when your intimate relationships can be part of your support system!)

Galatians 5:22–23 describes the things that build healthy relationships in our lives: "But the fruit of the [Holy] Spirit [the work which His presence within accomplishes] is love, joy (gladness), peace, patience (an even temper, forbearance), kindness, goodness (benevolence), faithfulness, gentleness (meekness, humility), self-control (self-restraint, continence). Against such things there is no law [that can bring a charge]" (AMP).

What evidence of the fruit of the Holy Spirit do you see in your current dealings with other people?

_____

_____

_____

_____

Articles posted on the LIFL website can help you get started and encourage you to keep "losing and moving for life."

LIFL counselors online at the LIFL website (www.LoseItForLife.com) can be a helpful resource, and will offer ongoing support. You can ask them questions anytime. Ongoing interaction and accountability may be just what are needed to get you moving forward for life!

Have you accessed this help on the web? How about the message board on the LIFL website? Or have you visited the online community in the chat room to talk about your victories and struggles? In what ways can this support help in your journey?

_____

_____

_____

What do you think of the suggestion of taking some social risks and starting your own LIFL group? Think about it—you could gather together some friends or fellow strugglers and form a support group in your community. Use this book and print additional materials from the LIFL online community to use in a group setting. Groups are great ways to encourage one another and hold each other accountable. What's holding you back? What steps can you take to starting a group?

_____

_____

—— DAY 5 ——
Trading Your Pain
for His Purposes

The Bible says that God comes alongside us when we go through difficulty. That in and of itself is reassuring, but there is even more—God wants to use us to help others who are going through a hard time. In God's economy, nothing is ever wasted, not even our pain. In this final lesson from Week 10, we'll do a quick study of what's involved in trading our pain for God's purposes.

LOOKING AT YOUR *LIFE*

When you were a child, what was your favorite fairy tale? What did you like about it?

_____

_____

Why are fairy tales so popular?

_____

_____

_____

_____

In what ways is real life *different* from fairy tales? In what ways is it *similar*?

_____

_____

_____

The Christian gospel brings a profound promise of evil being transformed into eternal good, weakness into strength, and tragedy into triumph.

Is "happily ever after" a foolish dream? Or for the Christian, is it the way God works?

_____

_____

_____

_____

What tough or even tragic incidents can you remember in your life that ultimately led to something good?

_____

_____

_____

LEARNING A NEW WAY OF _LIFE_

What is your typical reaction to hard or unpleasant trials? (Check all that apply.)

____ I pout.

____ I cry.

____ I scream and yell.

____ I eat.

____ I look for distractions.

____ I throw things.

____ I curse.

____ I thank God.

____ I trust that God has his reasons.

____ I clam up.

____ I pray.

____ I complain.

____ I get angry.

____ I laugh (so that I don't cry).

____ I try not to think about it.

____ I quote my favorite Bible verses.

____ I call my friends.

____ Other (specify): _____

Second Corinthians 1:3–4 says, "All praise to the God and Father of our Master, Jesus the Messiah! Father of all mercy! God of all healing counsel! He comes alongside us when we go through hard times, and before you know it, he brings us alongside someone else who is going through hard times so that we can be there for that person just as God was there for us" (MSG).

What does this passage promise?

_____

_____

Share a personal example for each of the following truths about trials:

- "We can never know God's plans or His gain from our loss, unless we give Him our misery and allow Him to transform it into a mission for our lives."

_____

- "Once our loss and pain point us to God's grace, we can also lead others into His grace."

_____

_____

In 2 Corinthians 4:16–17 we read, "Therefore we do not lose heart. Though outwardly we are wasting away, yet inwardly we are being renewed day by day. For our light and momentary troubles are achieving for us an eternal glory that far outweighs them all."

What different perspective does this passage offer regarding difficulties and trials?

_____

_____

God's ultimate goal for us is nothing less than total transformation. Second Corinthians 3:18 says, "We are transfigured much like the Messiah, our lives gradually becoming brighter and more beautiful as God enters our lives and we become like him" (MSG).

Don't you want God to take your years of struggle with weight problems and transform it all for His glory? If so, you will emerge from this experience stronger and more able to help others along the way.

Look at the following "Transformation Report Card." Grade yourself with A–F.

___ Learning how to forgive others (and doing it!)

___ Loving others unselfishly and deeply

___ Being honest with God and others about who I am

___ Becoming aware of my spiritual gifts

___ Carrying the message of spiritual transformation to others

___ Reaching out in compassion to those facing similar struggles to our own

___ Surrendering to the truth that God is working all things together for good

___ Seeking to apply past pain to positive purposes

___ No longer saying, "Why me, Lord?" but saying instead, "What do you want me to learn and do here?"

___ Being a giver instead of a taker

___ Learning to listen rather than always needing to be heard

___ Allowing humbling experiences to give me a servant's heart

___ Investing my spiritual gifts in the lives of others

LOSING IT FOR *LIFE*

Training is hard work, but the payoff feels so good. We are all in training for the eternal, and what we do today matters.

How does serious, sometimes agonizing training help athletes? How can serious spiritual training help us?

_____

_____

_____

What happens if we give up at the first signs of difficulty?

_____

_____

_____

What practical steps can we take to become tougher and more resilient in the face of tough times?

_____

_____

_____

List six things (biblical truths, people, goals, etc.) that you can lean on this next month to help you stay in the Lose It for Life race.

_____

_____

_____

_____

_____

Here's a prayer for endurance. If it expresses your desire, voice it to God. Or write your own prayer.

Heavenly Father,

When I feel like giving up, when I think I can't go on, give me strong reminders of Your love and help. You desire for me to go the distance. Your reward is great, both today and eternally. Help me to keep my eyes fixed on You and the final prize. Give me the strength to endure when I think I can't. Amen.

11

Pressing On—Keeping It Off

Grant me the serenity to accept things I cannot change, the courage to change the things I can, and the wisdom to know the difference. Amen.

By now you know that losing it for life is not something you do quickly. Rather, you are engaged in an ongoing transformation that comes through connection and community and practicing what you know works: exercising and eating healthily. It is possible to lose weight and keep it off. However, the journey required to make necessary changes isn't easy and doesn't end with losing the amount of weight desired.

We can know what to do, do it, and still slip back into old patterns of behavior, thinking, and feeling. In fact, John 6:66 reminds us that we can know the truth and still turn from it. Whenever you deal with a chronic problem like weight loss and maintenance, you have to be willing to do whatever it takes to avoid relapse. Planning is key to preventing relapse. You have to begin recovery and follow through or you place yourself at risk for relapse.

Relapse is more than a "slip" or return to overeating. An overeating episode is preceded by a process—one that generally involves a predictable progression that gradually moves you further and further away from doing what you know worked in the first place until, ultimately, you lose control. You revert to old patterns. For example, your thoughts focus on failure, your feelings on disgust and self-hate, and your actions on giving up or responding to unhealthy guilt in an unhealthy manner. All of these instances will bring you back to feeling failed and hopeless.

Yet if you can recognize the signs of relapse early, you will know when you are entering dangerous waters and choose to get back on track. If you can assess your situation and be watchful of the warning signs, you can avoid relapse.

THE SIGNS OF RELAPSE

1. Dishonesty

Feeling: You feel victimized and entitled.

Thinking: You're not at fault; the reasons for overeating are rational.

Action: You lie and present a false self once again hidden under the protection of fat.

2. Negative self-centeredness and pity

Feeling: You feel sorry for yourself; you revert to the victim position.

Thinking: You feel the world is against you, owes you, and revolves around you; you are resentful, defensive, and overly sensitive.

Action: You can do anything you want to do because nothing is helpful.

3. Low frustration tolerance

Feeling: You feel irritation, excitement, impatience, dissatisfaction.

Thinking: You need it now. People aren't acting right. This is taking too much time.

Action: You experience impulsivity and arguments.

4. Anxiety

Feeling: You feel pressured and worried; you feel strained, a lack of confidence, and free-floating fear.

Thinking: You are confused and indecisive.

Action: You are paralyzed; you have no plan to follow.

5. Grandiosity

Feeling: You feel overconfident, powerful, and arrogant.

Thinking: You're the exception to the rule. You've got it made. You'll show them. You need to be the center of attention.

Action: You play counselor with others, impress others with accomplishments, need to have the best; you act like a martyr; you are generous to a fault.

6. Perfectionism

Feeling: You feel guilt over never doing enough; you are constantly driven to do more.

Thinking: Nothing is ever correct. You must make up for past mistakes.

Action: You are cut off from others.

7. There-and-then living (opposite of here-and-now living)

Feeling: You feel fear of the future, regret of the past, resentment.

Thinking: You experience wishful thinking, fantasy; "If only . . ."

Action: You live according to "shoulds" rather than needs; your needs are not met in the present.

8. Defiance

Feeling: You feel inner conflict.

Thinking: No one knows but you.

Action: You run from help and experience destructive expression of feelings, open rebellion.

9. Isolation

Feeling: You feel boredom, loneliness; "I don't belong."

Thinking: You don't need anyone. You can do it yourself. No one cares.

Action: You experience withdrawal and reject help.

THE PHASES OF RELAPSE

Because relapse is not just one episode of overeating but a gradual process that builds over time, you should also be aware of the phases of relapse. If you note similarities between yourself and any of these descriptions, make immediate changes to compensate.

Complacency

Complacency is the first phase of relapse and begins when you stop doing what you know helps. This can happen because you get bored with your plan, drop your plan, become tired of making changes, feel upset or overwhelmed with all the changes required, or begin to believe you don't have the same needs that led you to surrender in the first place.

Giving up weight and food obsession involves moving into unfamiliar territory where weight no longer protects you from attention, intimacy, and vulnerability. It can also mean creating instant space from others, relieving sexual tension, and providing new excuses. While you can intellectually know these are all good things to give up, you have to be willing to stay the course when these issues are confronted.

You may stop going to counseling or support groups or activities that keep you connected and accountable to others and begin to think you don't need any more help. Or you may become too involved with others and not set appropriate boundaries. As a result, you can become lost in the needs of others and lose sight of your own.

Negative thinking can take hold in which you deny negative emotions such as fear and live in a fantasy world. There you daydream, set unrealistic expectations, intellectualize, engage in naval gazing, become easily angered and dissatisfied, and begin to obsess about food and weight as you entertain wishful thoughts and stop doing what has led you to lose the weight in the first place.

Confusion

Next, confusion sets in. You begin to doubt that anything works or will make a difference. You become double-minded. The issues related to losing weight and the lifestyle changes needed are doubted as you settle back into thinking you don't need to do all that is required. Perhaps your weight problems weren't that problematic and all this change isn't necessary. Doubt is the main thought—doubt about the depths of your difficulties or the need for recovery, help, or ongoing support.

You find yourself disconnecting from your support system and from people to whom you have been accountable. Self-doubt and low self-esteem occupy your thoughts. More expectations turn into "false hopes." Problem solving becomes difficult and you give in to living for the moment. Your plan goes by the wayside. This leads to irrational and inconsistent behavior.

Compromise

As complacency and confusion grow, you begin to engage in behaviors that set you up for problems once again. Overeating creeps back in and you rationalize, "It was only this one time; I'll be okay." And you return to old patterns of thinking and acting, using food to comfort and to fill emotional needs once again. Food, weight, and eating occupy your day as you think about the next meal or what you will eat in the next hour. You give in to impulsive eating, seeking momentary relief from this new life stress. The weight gain starts to creep back up.

Thoughts of apprehension and "if only . . ." statements fill your head. Giving in to the moment leads to an attitude of not caring when it comes to food and eating. You give up your routine with exercise and meal planning, rationalizing that action in spite of your obvious need.

Your emotional states intensify, especially anger and dissatisfaction, because you are not dealing with life head on and are instead allowing negativity, blame, dishonesty, and other destructive emotions to grow.

Because you are unwilling to confront the issues related to overeating and refuse to take responsibility, you further separate yourself from your support system and those who will lovingly hold you accountable. You are back to thinking your own effort and self-will will prevail when you decide to get serious again.

Catastrophe

Any feeling of control over the food is gone and you are bingeing, overeating, and overindulging once again. And since you have "blown it," why care? There are no attempts to limit what you eat, when, and how much. Sedentary once again, you feel physically sluggish, emotionally drained and overwhelmed, depressed, anxious, and disconnected from others. Thus, you engage in more risk and irresponsible behavior with food and your eating. The main feeling at this stage is helplessness and hopelessness. You are in trouble and have gained a significant amount of weight back, and there is no end in sight to that state of being.

PROTECTION FROM RELAPSE

In order to prevent relapse, you want to establish a system of protection. This system should include the following components:

An Exercise Plan

Exercise isn't something you do to lose weight and then quit; it promotes health, enhances your sense of well-being, and is a form of stress reduction. It is a natural form of stimulating the body and also providing relaxation. When you exercise, you feel you've accomplished something. We recommend trying to involve your entire family in exercise as a way to make it easier to do. For example, learn a new sport together, go on after-dinner walks, or take up a new hobby like dancing or hiking. Exercise and physical activity are essential to a healthy lifestyle and must be a part of your regular, daily routine.

Nutrition

Changes in your eating habits must also become habit in order to prevent relapse. Remember to eat foods high in protein and low in sugar in order to rebuild tissue and stabilize your blood sugar and moods. Reduce your fat intake, especially trans fats. Keep your eating habits healthy by only eating at the table; eating smaller, more frequent meals during the day; and eliminating high-sugar sodas and caffeine. These changes are about living a healthy lifestyle—not just dieting and losing weight. Make good nutrition a lifelong change.

Rest and Relaxation

Both must be scheduled. Take scheduled time-outs and regularly practice relaxation methods such as deep breathing and deep muscle relaxation. Work on keeping your body de-stressed. Stress leads to overeating for so many people. Work hard but learn to play and rest as well.

Think Lifestyle

The overall goal of making changes is to have them become part of your lifestyle. Everything you've learned and are applying to your life will become part of who you are and a lasting change. Losing weight for life is about thinking with a long-term perspective and making choices that will give your body good health.

Keep Growing

We must continue to grow and mature as we make it our goal to imitate Christ in all we do. You may need counseling and support groups to help move you forward in this area. Interaction with the church community provides numerous opportunities to grow: cell groups, prayer groups, seminars, classes, and other activities are opportunities for you to spiritually grow and mature. Take advantage of all the materials and planned meetings designed to help you develop a deeper walk with God.

Spiritual maturity does not come about in isolation. Becoming part of a church community is essential to your growth as a person. As we interact with others, we have numerous opportunities to practice being like Christ and loving one another. In addition, others can mentor us in Christian maturity and help keep us accountable.

Living One Day at a Time

The changes you are making and the personal growth and maturity that come with accepting responsibility for your health and well-being are best lived out one day at a time. It's easy to become overwhelmed, stressed, and discontented, so stay focused on today. Ask God to give you the grace you need to meet each day's challenges.

Avoid thinking in an "If only . . ." fashion; it is not compatible with surrender and reflects an attitude of discontent while also being a form of fantasy thinking. Look to the past to learn from your mistakes, but don't stay there in unhealthy guilt! There is forgiveness for what is confessed and past. Remember that how you live today sets your course for the future, so live well!

Accept Accountability

In order to be accountable, you cannot hide from the truth. Confess your sins and do not hide from hidden abuses or fantasies. All of us need spiritual support and thus need to find those who can support us in prayer, give and receive comfort, and share encouragement. You can benefit greatly from the experience of others. Stay teachable and keep a humble spirit. Accept advice and learn to listen. Take seriously Proverbs 15:22: "Plans fail for lack of counsel, but with many advisers they succeed."

Rely on God

Though it may sound like a cliché, God does have a plan and purpose for your life. He doesn't necessarily reveal those plans moment by moment, but God wants us to trust Him and take Him at His word. Nothing is too hard for God. "Jesus looked at them and said, 'With man this is impossible, but not with God; all things are possible with God'" (Mark 10:27). What an incredible statement from God's mouth!

Now believe it and act on its truth. Even though we know God is never late or early, waiting for His perfect timing requires patience and faith. He sees the big picture and intimate details of your life. His plans for you are good, but you must trust in His promises.

Spiritual Disciplines

It is absolutely essential to your spiritual growth and health to practice the spiritual disciplines of prayer, worship, confession, Bible study, giving, fasting, submission, service, and forgiving. Scripture is our one reliable source of truth and instructs us on the life that will bring satisfaction and victory. Intercession and confession bring us into communion with our Father. Praise and worship take us into the presence of God. In His presence there is joy and healing. We live in a time of great spiritual warfare, one in which the enemy of our souls will contest our spiritual progress at every turn. We must live godly lives and develop as God has instructed according to His will.

PROTECT THE SPIRITUAL GAINS MADE

The Christian gospel brings a profound message about earthly evil being transformed into eternal good: weakness into strength, tragedy into triumph, loss into gain, mortality into immortality, death into life. These concepts might be superficially discounted as theological abstractions, except that they translate into inescapable, day-by-day "miracles" that are clearly evident in the lives of Christian believers throughout the world.

The cosmic turning point in the transformation of evil-to-good is the death and resurrection of Jesus Christ. We activate this process in our lives through faith in God's Son, through hope in His good and loving character, and through relinquishment of our lives to His flawless will.

The process of surrendering to God's love and authority is a lifelong process. By the time we have made our way through the process of spiritual transformation, we know we need other Christians to help us stay on the right path. Without them, we are likely to return to patterns of secrecy, sin, and sickness. Yet when we place ourselves in a position of accountability to others, we invite their scrutiny.

At first this goes against our natural bent and seems like an invasion of our privacy, but accountability to others is an invaluable means of preventing a recurrence of sinful behavior. The removal of secrets from our lives was essential to our healing; now we need to introduce spiritual disciplines in our lives so that we are not entrapped by either overconfidence or a return to secret sins.

Paul wrote, "We must live decent lives for all to see. . . . Clothe yourself with the presence of the Lord Jesus Christ. And don't let yourself think about ways to indulge your evil desires" (Romans 13:13–14 NLT). We are able to remain "decent" only because God is with us, upholding us, and giving us new life. By continually surrendering to His will and through ongoing and honest accountability to trustworthy individuals, we are transformed. Yet we must never forget where we came from and how we got where we are, just as 2 Peter 1:5–9 urges us:

> So don't lose a minute in building on what you've been given, complementing your basic faith with good character, spiritual understanding, alert discipline, passionate patience, reverent wonder, warm friendliness, and generous love, each dimension fitting into and developing the others. With these qualities active and growing in your lives, no grass

will grow under your feet; no day will pass without its reward as you mature in your experience of our Master Jesus. Without these qualities you can't see what's right before you, oblivious that your old sinful life has been wiped off the books. (MSG)

Scripture indicates that human willfulness is at odds with God's plan for His people. He created us to be entirely dependent upon Him. We must continue to repent of our sins and to return to His ways. He wants us to communicate with Him in prayer. He also has indicated in His description of the multidimensional body of Christ (1 Corinthians 12; Romans 12) that we are meant to be dependent on other Christians. Our sinful nature will always tell us that we can handle life quite well on our own. However, God's Word and painful experiences remind us that we can't. Preservation is a key to spiritual renewal and transformation, which means we:

- establish boundaries to prevent a return to sick, sinful behaviors
- continue to forgive and be forgiven, including ourselves when we slip
- remain accountable to others and keep their confidences in turn
- choose to be part of a godly community
- practice the spiritual disciplines on a daily basis
- develop with God's help a deep and godly character
- continue the process of surrender—day by day, year by year

Friends, there is reason to be hopeful about this journey. While we all struggle with difficulty and pain, we can learn to surrender our all to God. He wants us to succeed in this journey, because to do so means to find freedom in Christ and a release from the bondage of overeating. But only with God's leading can you Lose It for Life and stay on this journey. To Him be the glory!

Workbook Week 11

PRESSING ON—
KEEPING IT OFF

---- **DAY 1** ----
The Danger of Relapse

By now you know that Losing It for Life is not something you do quickly or halfheartedly. You are engaged in a lifelong, 24/7, comprehensive, external and internal transformation. Always lurking is the danger of losing heart, losing your way, retreating. How to guard against that possibility is the focus of these final lessons.

LOOKING AT YOUR *LIFE*

Take a self-inventory test. Check all the following statements that are true of you.

___ I like to visit the places I lived as a child.
___ I go to reunions (class, family, and others) whenever I can.
___ People say I am nostalgic.
___ I actually watch my old home videos from time to time.
___ I enjoy television reruns.
___ I tell lots of stories from my childhood.
___ I often fail to learn from my mistakes.
___ I prefer music from my younger days.
___ I watch my favorite movies over and over.
___ I pull out old picture albums periodically and enjoy looking back.
___ I think about the past as much or more as I think about the future.

What, if anything, does this exercise reveal about yourself?

_____

_____

_____

Describe three life events you'd love to go back and experience again.

_____

_____

_____

Describe three experiences you'd rather not repeat—*ever.*

_____

_____

_____

The authors remind us that we can know what to do and be doing it, yet still slip back into old patterns of behavior, thinking, and feeling. What are your biggest fears about your weight loss and keeping it off?

_____

_____

_____

LEARNING A NEW WAY OF *LIFE*

Writing about his struggle to know and serve Christ, the apostle Paul described his resolve to keep pressing ahead and not give up:

> Not that I have already obtained all this, or have already arrived at my goal, but I press on to take hold of that for which Christ Jesus took hold of me. Brothers and sisters, I do not consider myself yet to have taken hold of it. But one thing I do: Forgetting what is behind and straining toward what is ahead, I press on toward the goal to win the prize for which God has called me heavenward in Christ Jesus. (Philippians 3:12–14)

Go through that passage carefully and circle the verbs. What kind of action do they describe?

_____

_____

Whenever you deal with a chronic problem like weight loss, you have to be willing to do whatever it takes to avoid relapse.

Of all the disciples chosen by Christ, Peter seemed the most solid and the most dependable. He even earned the name "Rock." It was Peter, speaking for all the rest, who confidently and correctly answered the ultimate question about Jesus' true identity. "You are the Messiah," he declared, "the Son of the living God" (Matthew 16:16).

Then, after three years of listening to Jesus and following Him, after hearing life-changing words and witnessing jaw-dropping miracles, Peter received a sobering warning from the Lord about failing and falling (Luke 22:31–34). Peter was shocked—even wounded. He protested loudly. "Not me!" he insisted. "Never!"

Read Luke 22:54–62. What does Peter's experience teach you?

_____

_____

How have you recently wrestled with having good intentions but not keeping them?

_____

_____

LOSING IT FOR *LIFE*

Relapse is more than a "slip" or return to overeating. It involves a predictable progression until, ultimately, you revert to old patterns.

Good intentions are not enough against great temptations. Planning is key to preventing relapse. You have to begin recovery and follow through, or you place yourself at risk for relapse. We want you to be successful losing weight and keeping it off. So let's concentrate on preventing relapse.

Define *relapse* in your own terms.

_____

_____

What's the difference between "slipping" in the area of eating and a full-fledged relapse?

_____

_____

Describe a "driftwood" approach to eating/weight loss/exercise/etc.

_____

_____

Describe a "piloted sailboat" approach to eating/weight loss/exercise/etc.

_____

_____

What time of day, or what day of the week, or in what situations are you most tempted to give up and say, "I'm just gonna live my comfortable old life"?

_____

_____

How much do feelings of failure, self-disgust, or hopelessness contribute to people's relapsing into old patterns? What do you think is the solution to these negative thoughts and feelings?

_____

_____

Identify one or two helpful conclusions from this lesson that you can tuck away in your mental "Relapse Response Kit."

_____

_____

_____

DAY 2
Signs of Relapse

If you can recognize the signs of relapse early, you will know when you are moving into dangerous waters and you can choose to get back on track.

Planning is key to preventing relapse.

LOOKING AT YOUR *LIFE*

Relate the idea of recognizing early warning signs to other areas of your life. Look at the following areas. What specific early warning signs might you see that would prompt you to take action . . .

- where your child's academic performance is involved?

_____

_____

- where your vehicle is concerned?

_____

_____

_____

- with regard to your financial condition?

_____

_____

_____

- regarding the health of your marriage?

_____

_____

_____

- in the area of your own medical health?

_____

_____

_____

- concerning a parent's ability to live independently?

_____

_____

What safeguards do you have in place to alert you to potential trouble in your LIFL journey? (For example, "My scales—when my weight hits _____ lbs., I know something is wrong.")

_____

_____

_____

LEARNING A NEW WAY OF *LIFE*

Many people who followed Jesus for a while found His teachings too difficult to put into practice and eventually stopped following Him. They came face-to-face with ultimate truth and turned away.

What do you think prompts reasonably smart people to reject the very things that can rescue them?

_____

_____

The apostle Paul urged, "If you think you are standing strong, be careful not to fall" (1 Corinthians 10:12 NLT). In what ways is this verse timeless advice for many areas of life?

Each new struggle or obstacle presents us with a choice: We can cave in and quit. Or we can lean hard into God, letting Him fill us with new strength.

_____

_____

When things are going well, why do we tend to drop our guards and become vulnerable to failure? Cite examples of this from your life (not necessarily pertaining to weight loss).

_____

_____

Read the following warnings from Scripture:

And pray in the Spirit on all occasions with all kinds of prayers and requests. With this in mind, be alert and always keep on praying for all the Lord's people. (Ephesians 6:18)

So then, let us not be like others, who are asleep, but let us be awake and sober. (1 Thessalonians 5:6)

Be alert and of sober mind. Your enemy the devil prowls around like a roaring lion looking for someone to devour. (1 Peter 5:8)

How do these truths apply to your LIFL program?

_____

_____

LOSING IT FOR _LIFE_

Based on much research and experience, we've identified common thoughts, feelings, and behaviors that are warning signs for relapse. Read through the chart; then work through the accompanying questions.

When I start *feeling* . . .	I begin *thinking* . . .	What I *do* is . . .	I *become* . . .
Victimized and entitled	Not my fault; others are to blame	Lie and present a false self	Dishonest
Sorry for myself; resentful and depressed	The world owes me and revolves around me	Anything I want; have a pity party	Negative, self-centered
Irritated, impatient, dissatisfied	"I need it *now* . . . this is taking too long."	Get impulsive and argue a lot	Intolerant, easily frustrated
Stressed and worried; fearful	In confused and indecisive ways	Become paralyzed (and fail to follow a plan)	Anxious
Overconfident, powerful, arrogant	"I'm the exception to the rule. I've got it made. I'll show them. I'll be the center of attention."	Play counselor, impress others with my accomplishments, be generous to a fault	Grandiose
Guilty over never doing enough and driven to do more	Nothing is ever right. "I must make up for past mistakes."	Cut myself off from others	Perfectionistic
Fearful of the future; regretful of the past	If only . . . (fantasizing excessively)	Live according to "should" and not needs	Trapped in a "there and then" mind-set/ way of life
Conflicted internally	"No one knows but me."	Run from help; express destructive feelings; rebel	Defiant

When I start *feeling* . . .	I begin *thinking* . . .	What I *do* is . . .	I *become* . . .
Bored; lonely	"I don't belong… I don't need anyone… I can do it myself… No one cares."	Withdraw; reject help	Isolated; disconnected

Which situations in the chart do you most readily identify with?

_____

_____

Which feelings are most common? Which thoughts are a regular part of your mind-set?

_____

_____

What connection do you see between what we think and feel and what we do?

_____

_____

_____

Go back through the chart and see if you can explain how the elements in each row (thoughts, emotions) can logically lead to overeating.

Look at the last column—which of those words or phrases typically describe you? What do you want to do about that? What words would you prefer others used to describe your personality/character?

_____

_____

A prayer of Jeremiah the prophet: "O LORD, if you heal me, I will be truly healed; if you save me, I will be truly saved. My praises are for you alone!" (Jeremiah 17:14 NLT)

Phases of Relapse

Because relapse is a gradual process building over time, you should be aware of the phases of relapse as well. This lesson can help.

LOOKING AT YOUR *LIFE*

Describe what dynamics are going on in each of the following scenarios.

- You're at the beach. The sand, the water, and the weather—it's all glorious. You get on a floating raft in the warm aquamarine waves out in front of your hotel. You are so relaxed that you doze off. When you awake thirty-five minutes later, you realize that your hotel moved! It's five hundred yards down the beach!

  _____

  _____

- You normally run a tight ship at home—everything spotless and in order and highly organized. Last month, however, was *crazy*. A family medical crisis, a huge musical/drama production at church, kids playing on two sports teams in two different leagues, several quick out-of-town trips, plus you've been nursing a really painful lower back. You wake up one Saturday morning, and notice—for the first time in weeks—how dirty and messy your home is. It looks almost like a frat house!

  _____

  _____

- Six months ago you were extremely passionate about your faith. You had something of a spiritual awakening and couldn't get enough of God. You devoured the Bible and looked forward to small group meetings like a kid looks forward to Christmas. Now, for some reason, you feel blah, ho-hum, disinterested. The Bible seems dry and irrelevant.

_____

_____

_____

The second law of thermodynamics basically says that things tend toward disorder. What examples have you experienced in your own life? If this law is true, what is the solution? How can we avoid losing the gains we've made?

_____

_____

_____

"We must pay more careful attention, therefore, to what we have heard, so that we do not drift away" (Hebrews 2:1).

LEARNING A NEW WAY OF *LIFE*

We must be proactive in watching for relapse. It's easy to drift along. The story of David's adultery with Bathsheba is a case study in how we can gradually end up in places where we don't want to be.

Read 2 Samuel 11, and note the foolish choices David made along the way.

_____

_____

_____

Demas was a Christian brother mentioned in some of Paul's epistles. The final mention of him is rather solemn: "Demas, because he loved this world, has deserted me and has gone to Thessalonica" (2 Timothy 4:10).

What do you suppose happened? What might have been in Thessalonica that caused Demas to chuck everything?

_____

_____

_____

Why do you suppose God included this cautionary tale in His Word?

_____

_____

_____

King Solomon had some huge advantages. He had a godly father, whom the Bible describes as a man after God's own heart (Acts 13:22); he was given an infusion of supernatural wisdom (1 Kings 3:5–15) and the promise of God's presence and protection if he remained faithful to God (1 Kings 9).

Read 1 Kings 11. What happened?

_____

_____

_____

What's the lesson for us?

_____

_____

_____

LOSING IT FOR *LIFE*

Review the stages of relapse below, and see how much you know about what to do to ward off each danger.

- **Complacency**

What is it?

_____

What causes it?

_____

What does it look like in your life?

_____

How can you combat it?

_____

- **Confusion**

What is it?

_____

What causes it?

_____

What does it look like in your life?

_____

How can you combat it?

_____

- **Compromise**

What is it?

_____

What causes it?

_____

What does it look like in your life?

_____

How can you combat it?

_____

- **Catastrophe**

What is it?

_____

What causes it?

_____

What does it look like in your life?

_____

How can you combat it?

_____

— DAY 4 —
Protection from Relapse

In order to prevent relapse, you need to establish a system of protection. That is the focus of this workbook lesson.

LOOKING AT YOUR *LIFE*

"Do not withhold your mercy from me, Lord; may your love and faithfulness always protect me" (Psalm 40:11).

Which of the following kinds of daily protection do you have or do you use?

- ☐ computer virus protection software
- ☐ Internet filters
- ☐ smoke alarms
- ☐ water purification system
- ☐ burglar alarm system
- ☐ vehicle antitheft device
- ☐ sunscreen with high SPF
- ☐ child safety latches on your cabinets
- ☐ safety deposit box
- ☐ surge protectors on sensitive electronics

What kind of protections—emotionally, spiritually, or physically—do you have in place to help you avoid a relapse?

_____

_____

_____

We're nearing the end of this *LIFL* workbook, so let's assess a few things.

What specific, identifiable changes have you made since beginning this new adventure? List at least ten.

_____

_____

_____

_____

_____

What's proving more difficult for you—cutting out certain eating habits or adding exercise routines?

_____

_____

_____

What has been the single most helpful insight you've gained? You're biggest "aha!" revelation?

_____

_____

_____

LEARNING A NEW WAY OF *LIFE*

Remember the Old Testament story of Caleb? Caleb and Joshua boldly (but unsuccessfully) urged the Israelites to trust God and conquer their enemies inhabiting the Promised Land. Because of the people's stubbornness and lack of faith, Caleb spent almost half of his life trudging through a desert wasteland.

"May the Lord direct your hearts into God's love and Christ's perseverance" (2 Thess. 3:5).

Then God gave His people a second opportunity to conquer Canaan. Caleb could have said, "Look, I've done enough already. I fought hard and tried my best once before. And look where it got me. Quite frankly, I'm tired. Why struggle day after day? No thanks. I think I'll kick back and live off the memory of that one shining moment when I really went for it." But he didn't. Instead, here's what happened:

Now the people of Judah approached Joshua at Gilgal, and Caleb son of Jephunneh the Kenizzite said to him, "You know what the LORD said to

Moses the man of God at Kadesh Barnea about you and me. I was forty years old when Moses the servant of the LORD sent me from Kadesh Barnea to explore the land. And I brought him back a report according to my convictions, but my fellow Israelites who went up with me made the hearts of the people melt with fear. I, however, followed the LORD my God wholeheartedly. So on that day Moses swore to me, 'The land on which your feet have walked will be your inheritance and that of your children forever, because you have followed the LORD my God wholeheartedly.'

"Now then, just as the LORD promised, he has kept me alive for forty-five years since the time he said this to Moses, while Israel moved about in the desert. So here I am today, eighty-five years old! I am still as strong today as the day Moses sent me out; I'm just as vigorous to go out to battle now as I was then. Now give me this hill country that the LORD promised me that day. You yourself heard then that the Anakites were there and their cities were large and fortified, but, the LORD helping me, I will drive them out just as he said." (Joshua 14:6–12)

Put yourself in Caleb's sandals. How would you have responded?

_____

_____

_____

_____

Avoid "if only" thinking. It is not compatible with surrender; instead, it reflects an attitude of discontent.

What qualities did Caleb have that you admire?

_____

_____

_____

_____

How does a person develop these virtues?

_____

_____

_____

LOSING IT FOR *LIFE*

In chapter 11 of the *LIFL* book is a list of a number of protections we can build into our lives to avoid relapse. Let's review them and think about them in more detail.

The authors write, "Exercise and physical activity are essential to a healthy lifestyle and must be a part of your regular, daily routine." How is your plan/program to get your body moving coming along? What types of activity have you settled on as most suited for you?

_____

_____

_____

_____

Do you think you've made the switch from viewing your changes in eating as a temporary diet to a whole new way of life? Why or why not?

_____

_____

How can rest and relaxation protect against relapse? What are your favorite replenishing activities?

_____

_____

_____

A huge premise of the LIFL plan is that lasting external change requires a solid internal foundation. What specific steps have you taken to help you develop and maintain a steady, healthy relationship with God? What spiritual disciplines have you incorporated into your regular lifestyle?

_____

_____

_____

What's the wisdom in living one day at a time (Matthew 6:34)?

_____

_____

_____

We've talked about it at length, but how does accountability provide a safety net? List your sources of accountability.

_____

_____

_____

— DAY 5 —
Preserving Our Gains and Moving On

Congratulations! You've done it. You've made it to the end of this workbook. Of course, that doesn't mean the work is done. Losing it for life is a lifestyle, not a short-term project or experiment. But the good news is that you now are armed with information you didn't have a short time ago.

With God's help, you've begun implementing new strategies and plans that really do have the potential to enable you to live in freedom and joy. Let's spend this last section celebrating and remembering a few crucial details.

LOOKING AT YOUR *LIFE*

The word *mediocre* comes from two Latin words, *media*, meaning "in the middle of," and *ocris*, meaning "mountain." Literally then, to be mediocre is to be "midway up the mountain." Perhaps the picture is of a mountain climber who starts out with grand ambitions and big dreams, but who then gets weary during the arduous ascent. Stopping on a ledge to catch his breath, the climber stops focusing on where he still wants to go. Instead, he looks back down at how far he has come and begins to become self-satisfied, complacent. As a result, rather than pressing on for the summit, he settles in. He has become *mediocre.*

With God, it's possible to lose it for life and keep it off. To Him be the glory!

Thinking back, what are some areas where you've been tempted to become mediocre and settle, saying, "Well, it isn't what I originally hoped for, but I guess it's good enough"?

_____

_____

_____

_____

Define *excellence.* How does it require an ever-increasing commitment to make progress?

_____

_____

_____

_____

What part of this program that you have studied and implemented encourages you the most right now?

_____

_____

_____

_____

"But thanks be to God! He gives us the victory through our Lord Jesus Christ" (1 Corinthians 15:57).

LEARNING A NEW WAY OF *LIFE*

The apostle Paul's letter to the Colossian Christians begins with a glorious tribute to Jesus Christ. Notice how He is described:

> The Son is the image of the invisible God, the firstborn over all creation. For in him all things were created: things in heaven and on earth, visible and invisible, whether thrones or powers or rulers or authorities; all things have been created through him and for him. He is before all things, and in him all things hold together. And he is the head of the body, the church; he is the beginning and the firstborn from among the dead, so that in everything he might have the supremacy. For God was pleased to have all his fullness dwell in him, and through him to reconcile to himself all things, whether things on earth or things in heaven, by making peace through his blood, shed on the cross. (Colossians 1:15–20)

> But thanks be to God! He gives us the victory through our Lord Jesus Christ. (1 Corinthians 15:57)

What does it mean that . . .

in Jesus, "all things hold together"?

_____

Jesus has supremacy in everything?

_____

What are the implications of these divine declarations for your life?

_____

Revelation 21 and 22 picture the world to come. Take a few minutes to read these short, concluding chapters of the Bible. What strikes you about this peek into the future? What can we look forward to? How does seeing what is ahead give us hope and renewed motivation now?

_____
_____
_____

What does it tell you about the heart of our God that He is in the process of making everything new (Revelation 21:5)?

_____
_____
_____

LOSING IT FOR *LIFE*

God wants us to succeed in this journey. Here's a list of questions you can use right now (and every morning before you launch out into the day), to help you remember the basics.

- Today—right now—am I surrendered to God? Even if I don't understand everything that is happening, is the attitude of my heart, "Not my will, but Thy will be done"? If not, what's keeping me from this?
- Today—right now—am I engaged and involved deeply with other Christians? Even when I feel like pulling away? Today—

Dear Lord, grant me the serenity to accept things I cannot change, the courage to change the things I can, and the wisdom to know the difference. Amen.

right now—am I participating in healthy community? If not, what's keeping me from this?

- Today—right now—am I giving trusted friends the right to hold me accountable and ask me hard questions in love? If not, what's keeping me from this?

- Today—right now—am I being honest, real, and authentic? Have I renounced a lifestyle of pretending to be what I'm not? If not, what's keeping me from this?

- Today—right now—am I working on renewing my mind— replacing old distorted and unhealthy thinking with God's truth (as revealed in His Word)? How so? What's my plan for today? If not, what's keeping me from this?

- Today—right now—am I maintaining clear boundaries to keep me from returning to sick, sinful behaviors? If not, what's keeping me from this?

- Today—right now—am I committed to forgiving others quickly; that is, keeping short accounts? If not, what's keeping me from this?

- Today—right now—am I being patient with myself when I slip, remembering God's grace and the truth that my journey is a marathon, not a sprint? (Note to self: one misstep or even twenty wrong steps will not wipe me out.) If not, what's keeping me from this?

So don't lose a minute in building on what you've been given, complementing your basic faith with good character, spiritual understanding, alert discipline, passionate patience, reverent wonder, warm friendliness, and generous love, each dimension fitting into and developing the others. With these qualities active and growing in your lives, no grass will grow under your feet, no day will pass without its reward as you mature in your experience of our Master Jesus. Without these qualities you can't see what's right before you, oblivious that your old sinful life has been wiped off the books. (2 Peter 1:5–9 MSG)

For Use in a Group Setting

Each participant should have a *Lose It for Life* book and workbook. Because the workbook follows the eleven book chapters, it will work best in an eleven-week format. The workbook has five lessons (days) for each chapter of the book. Each week, discuss the first lesson (Day 1) for each chapter with your group. Then make sure that everyone finishes the next four days of lessons during the week.

Preparation

To prepare for each week, participants should read the appropriate chapter in the book and then work through the corresponding lessons in the workbook, being sure to answer all the questions. You, as the group leader, should do the same.

Openers

You may want to begin each session with an interesting opener to introduce the topic and initiate discussion. These activities should be light and easy to do. When used well, openers can be very effective. As you think through your own creative openers, here are some sample ideas:

- To begin the Week 1 session, distribute magazines and have group members find ads for diet plans or articles about losing weight. Then ask, "What are the most popular diet plans these days? Which ones have you've tried over the course of your life?"

- Week 2, show the "Red Pill" clip from *The Matrix* DVD.
- Week 3, have the group design a new "breakthrough" diet that focuses on the guidelines you give. For example, break into pairs and have them create a diet centered around the colors orange and yellow; a leftovers only diet; a timed diet (everything must be consumed within a certain time limit), and so forth. Use your imagination. Everyone will enjoy some good laughs as they hear the diet reported. And this will lead naturally into the topic.

After the first week, you may want to precede the opener with a brief time of personal reporting/reviewing. Ask members how they did during the week, and be sure to affirm those who completed their assignments.

Discussion

You'll notice that some of the questions in the *LIFL* workbook are more personal than others. To avoid embarrassing anyone and keep the discussion moving, choose the more neutral questions to highlight in the group sessions. (Note: the "Losing It for Life" section of each lesson focuses on personal application.) Eventually, you will be able to get more personal, especially in Week 10, where we discuss holding each other accountable. You may even want to have group members divide into accountability partners. *(Note: it's important to foster an environment of confidentiality within the group as they share experiences.)*

Wrap-Up

The end of the lesson is the time to encourage members to continue doing the lessons and to follow through on their assignments. You may also want to end with a time of prayer, so members can pray with and for each other.

A Personal Note
from Steve Arterburn

God loves you as you are—please know and believe this truth. But He also wants you to find the weight that is right for you and maintain that weight. Truly, everything and anything is possible for your future. If you surrender your life to God, humble yourself to get the assistance you need, and willingly make the changes you need to make, you will lose the weight and be free of it for life.

Don't be discouraged. If you struggle and wonder why, understand that the journey is difficult! All of us who struggle with overeating share your pain. The reality is that you can stumble back and you can stumble forward . . . just don't ever give up. Thousands of people have successfully traveled this road. This can be your story, too, but you must do whatever it takes to win this battle.

God is for you. Dr. Linda and I are for you. The healing online community at LoseItForLife.com is for you. So come, begin this journey, and look toward the freedom we have experienced that can also be yours. And if I can help you in any way, e-mail me: SArterburn@newlife.com.

Steve

If you are interested in attending a Lose It for Life Institute, call 1-800-NEW-LIFE or visit our websites at NewLife.com or LoseItForLife.com.

APPENDICES

APPENDIX A
Food Journal

Name:				
Date:				
When I ate	Where I ate	What I ate	How much I ate	Was I hungry?

APPENDIX B
Physical Versus Emotional Hunger Chart

When reviewing what you have eaten, it is important to be honest with yourself in order to find out whether it was physical hunger or an emotional feeling that triggered you to eat. Ask yourself the following three questions:

1. Was I experiencing physical or emotional hunger?
2. Before I ate, how did I feel?
3. After I ate, how did I feel?

Physical or emotional hunger?	Before I ate, I felt:	After I ate, I felt:

APPENDIX C
Glycemic Food Index[1]

BAKERY PRODUCTS	GI
Sponge cake	66
Pound cake	77
Danish	84
Muffin	88
Flan	93
Angel food cake	95
Croissant	96
Doughnut	108
Waffle	109

BREADS	GI
Oat bran bread	68
Mixed grain bread	69
Pumpernickel bread	71
White pita	82
Cheese pizza	86
Hamburger bun	87
Rye flour bread	92
Semolina bread	92
Oat kernel bread	93
Whole wheat bread	99
Melba toast	100
White bread	101
Plain bagel	103
Kaiser rolls	104
Bread stuffing	106
Gluten-free wheat bread	129
French baguette	136

BREAKFAST CEREALS	GI
Rice bran	27
Kellogg's All-Bran®	60
Oatmeal, non-instant	70
Special K®	77
Honey Smacks®	78
Oat bran	78
Kellogg's Mueslix®	80
Kellogg's Mini-Wheats® (unfrosted)	81
Multi-Bran Chex®	83
Kellogg's Just Right®	84

	GI
Life®	94
Grape-Nuts®	96
Post Shredded Wheat®	99
Cream of Wheat®	100
Golden Grahams®	102
Puffed wheat	105
Cheerios®	106
Corn bran	107
Total®	109
Rice Krispies®	117
Corn Chex®	118
Cornflakes	119
Crispix®	124
Rice Chex®	127

CEREAL GRAINS	GI
Pearled barley	36
Rye	48
Wheat kernels	59
Rice, instant	65
Bulgur	68
Rice, parboiled	68
Cracked barley	72
Wheat, quick cooking	77
Buckwheat	78
Brown rice	79
Wild rice	81
White rice	83
Couscous	93
Rolled barley	94
Mahatma Premium rice	94
Taco shells	97
Cornmeal	98
Millet	101
Tapioca, boiled with milk	115

COOKIES	GI
Oatmeal cookies	79
Shortbread	91
Arrowroot	95
Graham crackers	106

	GI
Vanilla Wafers®	110
Biscotti	113

CRACKERS	GI
Breton® wheat crackers	96
Stoned wheat thins	96
Rice cakes	110

DAIRY FOODS	GI
Lowfat yogurt, artificially sweetened	20
Chocolate milk, artificially sweetened	34
Whole milk	39
Soy milk	43
Fat-free milk	46
Low-fat yogurt, fruit flavored	47
Low-fat ice cream	71
Ice cream	87

FRUIT AND FRUIT PRODUCTS	GI
Cherries	32
Grapefruit	36
Peach	40
Dried apricots	43
Fresh apricots	43
Canned peaches	43
Orange	47
Pear	47
Plum	55
Apple	56
Apple juice	57
Grapes	62
Canned pears	63
Raisins	64
Pineapple juice	66
Grapefruit juice	69
Fruit cocktail	79
Kiwifruit	83

Mango	86
Banana	89
Canned apricots, in syrup	91
Pineapple	94
Watermelon	103

LEGUMES	GI
Soybeans, boiled	23
Red lentils, boiled	36
Kidney beans, boiled	42
Green lentils, boiled	42
Butter beans, boiled	44
Yellow split peas, boiled	45
Baby lima beans, frozen	46
Chickpeas	47
Navy beans, boiled	54
Pinto beans	55
Black-eyed peas	59
Canned chickpeas	60
Canned pinto beans	64
Canned baked beans	69
Canned kidney beans	74
Canned green lentils	74
Fava beans	113

PASTA	GI
Protein enriched spaghetti	38
Fettuccine	46
Vermicelli	50
Whole-grain spaghetti	53
Meat-filled ravioli	56
White spaghetti	59
Capellini	64
Macaroni	64
Linguine	65
Cheese tortellini	71
Durum spaghetti	78
Macaroni and cheese	92
Gnocchi	95
Brown rice pasta	113

ROOT VEGETABLES	GI
Sweet potato	63
Carrots, cooked	70
Yam	73
White potato, boiled	83
White potato, steamed	93
White potato, mashed	100
New potato	101
Rutabaga	103
Potato, boiled, mashed	104

French fries	107
Potatoes, instant	114
Potato, microwaved	117
Parsnips	139
Potato, baked	158

SNACK FOOD AND CANDY	GI
Peanuts	21
Mars M&Ms® (peanut)	46
Mars Snickers® Bar	57
Mars Twix® Cookie Bars (caramel)	62
Chocolate bar, 1.5 oz	70
Jams and marmalades	70
Potato chips	77
Popcorn	79
Mars Kudos® Whole Grain Bars	87
Mars® Bar	91
Mars Skittles®	98
Life Savers®	100
Corn chips	105
Jelly beans	114
Pretzels	116
Dates	146

SOUPS	GI
Canned tomato soup	54
Canned lentil soup	63
Split pea soup	86
Black bean soup	92
Canned green pea soup	94

SUGARS	GI
Fructose	32
Lactose	65
Honey	83
High-fructose corn syrup	89
Sucrose	92
Glucose	137
Maltodextrin	150
Maltose	150

VEGETABLES	GI
Artichoke	<20
Argali	<20
Asparagus	<20
Broccoli	<20
Brussels sprouts	<20
Cabbage, all varieties	<20
Cauliflower	<20

Celery	<20
Cucumbers	<20
Escarole	<20
Eggplant	<20
Beet	<20
Chard	<20
Collard	<20
Kale	<20
Mustard greens	<20
Spinach	<20
Turnip	<20
Lettuce, all varieties	<20
Mushrooms, all varieties	<20
Okra	<20
Peppers, all varieties	<20
Green beans	<20
Snow peas	<20
Spaghetti squash	<20
Young summer squash	<20
Watercress	<20
Wax beans	<20
Zucchini	<20
Tomatoes	23
Dried peas	32
Green peas	68
Sweet corn	78
Pumpkin	107

[1]Glycemic Index numbers are provided by the World Health Organization.

APPENDIX D
Two Weight-Loss Plans

For both plans, consult the following chart to plan meals; it's important to eat the number of servings listed for each food group. By eating the specified number, you will reduce carbohydrates but still get the proper amounts of food from other food groups to maintain a healthy weight-loss plan.

Food Group	1,500–1,800 Daily Calories			1,800–2,200 Daily Calories		
	Servings	Calories	Carbs (g)	Servings	Calories	Carbs (g)
Protein	9	495	0	14	890	0
Fats	6	270	0	8	360	0
Nuts	1	200	4	1	200	4
Vegetables	5	125	25	5	125	25
Starches	4	320	60	4	320	60
Fruits	2	120	30	2	120	30
Dairy	0.5	45	6	0.5	45	6
TOTAL		1,575	125		2,060	125

This plan is tailored to fit your calorie and carbohydrate needs while helping you lose about one to two pounds per week. Before you know it, you'll be losing the weight and loving your new low-carb lifestyle! Choose your desired number of daily calories and limit eating to the foods listed while observing the serving sizes listed in the appropriate column. All calorie levels are approximate. The following five-day meal plan allows 125 grams of carbs per day.

THE SMART LOW-CARB WEIGHT-LOSS PLAN MENU

Recipes included on pages 492–501

MONDAY	Calorie Level 1,500–1,800	Calorie Level 1,800–2,200
Breakfast		
Fried Eggs in Vinegar*	1 serving	1 serving
Fat-free milk	1/2 cup	1/2 cup
Apple juice	1/2 cup	1/2 cup
Whole wheat bread	1 slice	1 slice
Butter spray, non-fat	1 tsp.	1 tsp.
Snack		
Nectarine, pear, or apple	1	1
Lunch		
Grilled chicken tenders	4 oz.	5 oz.
brushed w/ Italian dressing	1 tsp.	1 tbsp.
Red leaf lettuce	1 cup	1 cup
Carrot, shredded	1/4 cup	1/4 cup
Cucumber, sliced	1/2 cup	1/2 cup
Italian dressing	2 tsp.	2 tbsp.
Snack		
Walnuts	1 oz.	1 oz.
Dinner		
London broil	4 oz.	5 oz.
Spanish-Style Green Beans*	1 serving	1 serving
Couscous	1/2 cup	1/2 cup
Snack		
Orange-Walnut Biscotti*	2	2
Total Calories	**1,640**	**1,880**
Total Carbs	**125**	**125**

TUESDAY	Calorie Level 1,500–1,800	Calorie Level 1,800–2,200
Breakfast		
Cherry Cream of Rye Cereal*	1 serving	1 serving
Fat-free milk	1/2 cup	1/2 cup
Turkey sausage	1 oz.	1 oz.
Snack		
Apple	1	1
Lunch		
Tuna	3 oz.	4 oz.
Celery, chopped	1/4 cup	1/4 cup
Onion, chopped	1/4 cup	1/4 cup
Mayonnaise, reduced-fat	2 tbsp.	1/4 cup
Green olives	10 small	10 small
Green leaf lettuce, torn	1 cup	1 cup
Whole wheat bread	1 slice	1 slice
Snack		
Pecans	1 oz.	1 oz.
Dinner		
Pork Chops Baked w/Cabbage and Cream*	1 serving	1 serving
Steamed butternut squash	1/2 cup	1/2 cup
Snack		
Pumpernickel bread	1 slice	1 slice
Swiss cheese, reduced-fat	1 oz.	1 oz.
Butter spray, non-fat	1 tsp.	2 tsp.
Total Calories	**1,670**	**1,960**
Total Carbs	**127**	**127**

WEDNESDAY	Calorie Level 1,500–1,800	Calorie Level 1,800–2,200
Breakfast		
Scrambled egg	1	2
Orange juice	1/2 cup	1/2 cup
Rye toast	1 slice	1 slice
Butter spray, nonfat	1 tsp.	2 tsp.
Fat-free milk	1/2 cup	1/2 cup
Snack		
Kiwi	1	1
Lunch		
Salad of lentils, cooked	1/2 cup	1/2 cup
Turkey breast, cooked and cubed	3 oz.	4 oz.
Carrots, sliced	1/2 cup	1/2 cup
Peppers, chopped	1/2 cup	1/2 cup
Peas, cooked	1/4 cup	1/4 cup
Olive oil	2 tsp.	1 tbsp.
Cheddar cheese, low-fat	1/2 oz.	1/2 oz.
Snack		
Brazil nuts	1 oz.	1 oz.
Dinner		
Stir-Fried Chicken and Broccoli*	1 serving (4 oz. chicken)	1 serving (5 oz. chicken)
Snack		
Pecan Muffins*	1	1
Butter	1 tsp.	2 tsp.
Total Calories	**1,590**	**1,890**
Total Carbs	**123**	**123**

THURSDAY	Calorie Level 1,500–1,800	Calorie Level 1,800–2,200
Breakfast		
Pecan Muffins*	1	1
Cottage cheese, low-fat	2 tbsp.	6 tbsp.
Peach	1	1
Fat-free milk	1/2 cup	1/2 cup
Snack		
Grapefruit	1/2	1/2
Lunch		
Sandwich of two rice cakes		
topped w/ sardines or salmon,		
boneless, skinless	4 oz.	5 oz.
Cream cheese, low-fat	2 tbsp.	2 tbsp.
Tomato	2 slices	2 slices
Zucchini, sticks	1/2 cup	1/2 cup
Snack		
Almonds	1 oz.	1 oz.
Dinner		
Lamb chop topped	4 oz.	5 oz.
w/ garlic powder	1/8 tsp.	1/8 tsp.
Mint leaves	2 tsp.	1 tbsp.
Barley, cooked	1/2 cup	1/2 cup
Stewed tomatoes	1 cup	1 cup
Green beans,	1/2 cup	1/2 cup
sautéed in olive oil	2 tsp.	3 tsp.
Snack		
Whole wheat bread	1 slice	1 slice
Butter spray, nonfat	1 tsp.	2 tsp.
Chicken, sliced	1 oz.	2 oz.
Total Calories	**1,700**	**1,950**
Total Carbs	**122**	**122**

FRIDAY	Calorie Level 1,500–1,800	Calorie Level 1,800–2,200
Breakfast		
Sweet potato, cooked and topped	1/2 cup	1/2 cup
with walnut oil or canola oil	1/2 tsp.	1 tsp.
Walnuts, chopped	1 oz.	1 oz.
Coconut, shredded	1 tbsp.	2 tbsp.
Pineapple, crushed	1/4 cup	1/4 cup
Chicken breast, cooked	—	2 oz.
Fat-free milk	1/2 cup	1/2 cup
Lunch		
Salad of spinach	2 cups	2 cups
Chickpeas	1/2 cup	1/2 cup
Egg, hard-cooked	1	2
Artichoke hearts	1/2 cup	1/2 cup
Olive oil	2 tsp.	3 tsp.
Lemon juice	1 tbsp.	1 tbsp.
Whole wheat pita	1/2	1/2
Snack		
Monterey Jack cheese, low-fat	2 oz.	2 oz.
Dinner		
Breaded Baked Cod*	1 serving	1 serving
Red cabbage, sautéed	1/2 cup	1/2 cup
in sesame oil	1 tsp.	2 tsp.
Yellow squash, steamed	1/2 cup	1/2 cup
Butter spray, non-fat	1 tsp.	1 tsp.
Cantaloupe Sorbet*	1 serving	1 serving
Snack		
Popcorn, air-popped	3 cups	3 cups
Butter spray, non-fat	1 tsp.	2 tsp.
Monterey Jack cheese, reduced fat	2 oz.	2 oz.
Total Calories	**1,640**	**1,980**
Total Carbs	**124**	**124**

THE SMART LOW-CARB WEIGHT-LOSS PLAN RECIPES

Breaded Baked Cod with Tartar Sauce

Cantaloupe Sorbet

Cherry Cream of Rye Cereal

Fried Eggs with Vinegar

Orange-Walnut Biscotti

Pecan Muffins

Pork Chops with Cabbage and Cream

Spanish-Style Green Beans

Stir-Fried Chicken with Broccoli

Breaded Baked Cod with Tartar Sauce

Ingredients:

TARTAR SAUCE

1/2   cup reduced-fat mayonnaise or Lemonaise Lite

11/2 tbsp. lemon juice

1   tbsp. finely chopped dill or sweet pickles

2   tsp. mustard

2   tsp. capers, drained and chopped

2   tsp. chopped parsley (optional)

FISH

2   slices whole wheat bread

2   eggs or 1/2 cup EggBeaters

1   tbsp. water

11/4 lbs. cod or scrod fillet, cut into 1" pieces

1/2   tsp. salt (or salt substitute for a lower-sodium choice)

1/4   tsp. ground black pepper

Serves: 4
Calories Per Serving: 268
Preparation Time: 30 minutes
Difficulty: Easy

Cooking Instructions:

1. To make the tartar sauce: In a small bowl, combine the mayonnaise, lemon juice, dill, mustard, capers, and parsley. Cover and refrigerate.
2. To make the fish: Preheat the oven to 400°F. Coat a baking sheet with cooking spray.
3. Place the bread in a food processor, and process into fine crumbs. Place in a shallow bowl. In another bowl, beat the eggs and water together. Season the fish with the salt and pepper.
4. Dip the fish into the egg mixture and then into the bread crumbs. Place fish on the prepared baking sheet. Generously coat the breaded fish with cooking spray.
5. Bake until fish pieces are opaque inside, about 10 minutes. Serve with the tartar sauce.

Per Serving Nutrition:

Fat:	10 g
Saturated fat:	2 g
Cholesterol:	174 mg
Carbs:	14 g
Protein:	30 g
Fiber:	1 g
Sodium:	734 mg*

* Using a salt substitute will lower the total sodium.

Tips:

- If you buy your fish fresh, use within two days. Keep fish in its market wrapper in the refrigerator.
- Eating fish regularly offers many health benefits: omega-3 fatty acids are believed to offer protection against heart disease, depression, and irregular menstrual cycles.

Cantaloupe Sorbet

Ingredients:

4	frozen cantaloupes, slightly thawed
1	frozen banana, sliced
1/4	cup Splenda
1	tbsp. lime juice
2	tsp. grated lime peel
1/8 –1/4	tsp. ground cinnamon

Serves: 6
Calories Per Serving: 61
Preparation Time: 4–5 hours
Difficulty: Easy

Cooking Instructions:

1. In a food processor, combine the cantaloupe, banana, Splenda, lime juice, lime peel, and cinnamon. Process until smooth.

2. Scrape into a shallow metal pan. Cover and freeze for 4 hours or overnight. Using a knife, break the mixture into chunks. Process briefly in a food processor to a smooth consistency before serving.

Per Serving Nutrition:

Fat:	0 g
Saturated Fat:	0 g
Cholesterol:	0 mg
Carbs:	15 g
Protein:	1 g
Fiber:	2 g
Sodium:	11 mg

Tips:

- Cantaloupe is a powerful source of beta-carotene.
- Cantaloupe not only offers protection against cancer but can help keep your skin lovely!
- To pick the juiciest, sweetest cantaloupe at the store, look for a melon that is heavy and without obvious injuries. The fragrance should be strong and sweet.
- Savory or lightly sweetened sorbets are customarily served either as a palate refresher between courses or as dessert.

Cherry Cream of Rye Cereal

Ingredients:

- 1 1/4 cup water
- 1 1/4 cup apple cider
- 1/4 tsp. salt or salt substitute
- 1 cup cream of rye cereal
- 1 tbsp. low-sugar or no-sugar-added cherry fruit spread
- 1/8 tsp. ground nutmeg
- 1/8 tsp. ground cardamom
- 1 1/2 tbsp. chopped hazelnuts (optional)

Serves: 4
Calories Per Serving: 208
Preparation Time: 10 minutes
Difficulty: Easy

Cooking Instructions:

1. Combine the water, cider, and salt in a saucepan and bring to a boil over medium heat. Stir in the cereal and reduce heat to low. Cook, uncovered, until thick, stirring occasionally, 3-5 minutes. Remove from heat and stir in the fruit spread.
2. Spoon into bowls and sprinkle with nutmeg, cardamom, and hazelnuts. Serve hot.

Per Serving Nutrition:

Fat:	1 g
Saturated Fat:	0 g
Cholesterol:	0 mg
Carbs:	45 g
Protein:	4 g
Fiber:	6 g
Sodium:	168 mg

Fried Eggs with Vinegar

Ingredients:

2	tbsp. butter or nonfat butter spray
8	large eggs or 2 cups EggBeaters
1	tsp. salt or salt substitute
1/4	tsp. ground black pepper
1/8	tsp. dried marjoram or basil
4	tsp. red wine vinegar
1	tsp. chopped parsley (optional)

Serves: 4
Calories Per Serving: 206
Preparation Time: 10 minutes
Difficulty: Easy

Cooking Instructions:

1. Melt 1 tablespoon of butter in a large nonstick skillet over medium-low heat. Add the eggs, and sprinkle with the salt, pepper, and marjoram (work in batches if necessary). Cover and cook until the whites are set and yolks are almost set, 3 to 5 minutes. (For steam-basted eggs, add 1 tsp. of water to the pan and cover with a lid.)
2. Remove eggs to plates. Place the skillet over low heat and add the remaining 1 tablespoon of butter. Cook until the butter turns light brown, 1 to 2 minutes. Add the vinegar. Pour the vinegar mixture over the eggs. Sprinkle with parsley. Serve hot.

Per Serving Nutrition:

Fat:	16 g
Saturated Fat:	7 g
Cholesterol:	440 mg
Carbs:	1 g
Protein:	13 g
Fiber:	0 g
Sodium:	764 mg

Orange-Walnut Biscotti

Ingredients:

- 2/3 cup walnuts
- 1/4 cup sugar
- 11/4 cup whole-grain pastry flour
- 1/4 cup cornmeal
- 1 tsp. baking powder
- 1/4 tsp. salt or salt substitute
- 1/4 cup butter, softened or nonfat butter spray
- 1/4 cup Splenda
- 2 large eggs or 1/2 cup EggBeaters
- 2 tsp. grated orange peel
- 1/2 tsp. orange extract

Serves: 24
Calories Per Serving: 76
Preparation Time: 11/2 hours
Difficulty: Easy

Cooking Instructions:

1. In a food processor, combine the walnuts and 2 tablespoons of the sugar. Process just until walnuts are coarsely ground. Transfer to a large bowl and add the flour, cornmeal, baking powder, and salt. Stir until combined.

2. In a large bowl, and using an electric mixer, beat the butter, Splenda, and remaining 2 tablespoons of sugar until light and fluffy. Beat in the eggs, orange peel, and orange extract. Gradually beat in the flour mixture until dough is smooth and thick. Divide the dough into two equal-sized discs. Refrigerate for 30 minutes or until dough is firm.

3. Preheat the oven to 350°F. Coat a baking sheet with cooking spray.

4. Shape each disc into a 12" log. Place both logs on the prepared baking sheet. Bake for 25 to 30 minutes, or until golden brown. Remove the logs to wire racks to cool.

5. Cut each log on a slight diagonal into $1/2$"-thick slices. Place the slices, cut side down, on the baking sheet and bake for 5 minutes. Turn the slices over, and bake for 5 minutes longer, or until dry. Remove biscotti to wire racks to cool.

Per Serving Nutrition:

Fat:	5 g
Saturated fat:	2 g
Cholesterol:	23 mg
Carbs:	8 g
Protein:	2 g
Fiber:	1 g
Sodium:	68 mg

Tips:

- Walnuts are a good source of alpha-linolenic acid, which can reduce your risk of heart attack and stroke.

Pecan Muffins

Ingredients:

$11/2$ cups whole grain pastry flour

$1/4$ cup soy flour

$21/2$ tsp. baking powder

$1/2$ tsp. salt or salt substitute

$1/2$ tsp. ground nutmeg

$1/2$ cup toasted pecans, chopped

$1/2$ cup vegetable oil

$1/2$ cup low-sugar or no-sugar-added apricot or peach fruit spread

2 large eggs or $1/2$ cup EggBeaters, lightly beaten

$11/2$ tsp. vanilla extract

$1/8$ tsp. liquid stevia* or Splenda

Serves: 12
Calories Per Serving:
  One muffin, 218
Preparation Time: 25 Minutes
Difficulty: Easy

Available in most health-food stores

Cooking Instructions:

1. Place a rack in the middle position in the oven. Preheat the oven to 375°F. Coat a 12-cup muffin pan with cooking spray or line with paper cups.
2. In a large bowl, whisk together the pastry flour, soy flour, baking powder, salt, nutmeg, and pecans.

3. In a small bowl, combine the oil, fruit spread, eggs, vanilla extract, and stevia. Add to the flour mixture, stirring just until the dry ingredients are moistened.

4. Spoon into the prepared muffin cups until three-quarters full. Bake 12–14 minutes or until a toothpick inserted in the center of a muffin comes out clean. Serve warm.

Per Serving Nutrition:

Fat:	12 g
Saturated Fat:	1 g
Cholesterol:	35 mg
Carbs:	20 g
Protein:	4 g
Fiber:	3 g
Sodium:	193 mg

Tips:

- Whole-wheat pastry flour is available at most health-food stores.
- Whole grains reduce your risk of heart disease, cancer, and other chronic illnesses. Always choose whole-grain breads and pasta over any made from refined white flour.

Pork Chops Baked with Cabbage and Cream

Ingredients:

1	small head (1½ lbs.) green cabbage, cored and finely shredded
4	boneless pork chops (6 oz. each), each 3/4" thick
1/2	tsp. salt or salt substitute
1/4	tsp. ground black pepper
2	tsp. olive oil
1/2	cup half-and-half
1	tsp. caraway seeds
1/2	tsp. sweet Hungarian paprika
1	tsp. dried marjoram or thyme
1/2	cup (2 oz.) shredded low-fat Swiss cheese

Serves: 4
Calories Per Serving: 463
Preparation Time: 50 minutes
Difficulty: Average

Cooking Instructions:

1. Preheat the oven to 350°F.

2. Bring a large pot of salted water to a boil over high heat. Add the cabbage and cook until soft, 4–5 minutes. Drain in a colander and allow to dry on paper towels.

3. Season meat with 1/4 teaspoon of the salt and pepper. Heat the oil in a large ovenproof skillet over high heat. Add meat and cook just until browned, 1–2 minutes. Remove to a plate.

4. Discard any fat in the skillet and heat the skillet over low heat. Stir in the cabbage, half-and-half, caraway seeds, paprika, marjoram, and the remaining $1/4$ teaspoon of salt. Cook and stir until heated through, about 5 minutes. Remove from heat and place chops on a plate. Place cabbage in skillet and arrange the pork over the cabbage, adding any juices accumulated on the plate. Sprinkle with the cheese. Bake until a meat thermometer registers 160°F for medium-well, about 25 minutes.

Per Serving Nutrition:

Fat:	20 g
Saturated Fat:	9 g
Cholesterol:	165 mg
Carbs:	12 g
Protein:	53 g
Fiber:	4 g
Sodium:	460 mg

Tips:

- Vegetables like cabbage help reduce your risk of heart disease, cancer, and stroke
- Cabbage is also high in calcium, which protects bone density.

Spanish-Style Green Beans

Ingredients:

1	lb. green beans, trimmed and cut into 2" lengths
3	tbsp. olive oil
1	onion, chopped
1	small green bell pepper, chopped
1	tomato (4 oz.), peeled, seeded, and coarsely chopped
2	cloves garlic, minced
1/4	tsp. salt or salt substitute
1/8	tsp. ground black pepper
2–3	tbsp. coarsely chopped, pitted kalamata olives
2	tsp. drained capers (optional)

Serves: 4
Calories Per Serving: 162
Preparation Time: 30 minutes
Difficulty: Easy

Cooking Instructions:

1. Combine the beans, oil, onion, bell pepper, tomato, garlic, salt, and black pepper in a saucepan over medium heat. Cook, stirring, until the vegetables start to sizzle, 2–3 minutes.

2. Reduce the heat to low, cover, and cook, stirring occasionally, until the beans are very tender but not falling apart, 20–25 minutes. Stir in olives and capers and heat for 1 minute. Serve warm, at room temperature, or chilled.

Per Serving Nutrition:

Fat:	12 g
Saturated Fat:	2 g
Cholesterol:	0 mg
Carbs:	13 g
Protein:	2 g
Fiber:	6 g
Sodium:	230 mg

Tips:

- Eating more vegetables helps you feel full and satisfied longer.
- Fiber-rich foods, such as green beans, help lower cholesterol levels.

Stir-Fried Chicken and Broccoli

Ingredients:

1/2	cup chicken broth
3	tbsp. Chinese oyster sauce
2	tbsp. orange juice
1	tbsp. plus 11/2 tsp. low-sodium soy sauce
2	cloves garlic, minced
2	tsp. fresh ginger, minced
1	tsp. sesame oil
1/4	tsp. hot-pepper sauce (optional)
1	tbsp. cornstarch
1	tbsp. plus 11/2 tsp. cold water
3	tbsp. vegetable oil
1	lb. boneless, skinless chicken breasts, cut into thin strips
1	large bunch (2 lbs.) broccoli, cut into small florets
5	scallions, sliced
	sesame seeds (optional)

Serves: 4
Calories Per Serving: 321
Preparation Time: 20 minutes
Difficulty: Easy

Cooking Instructions:

1. In a small bowl, combine the broth, oyster sauce, orange juice, soy sauce, garlic, ginger, sesame oil, and hot-pepper sauce.
2. In a cup, dissolve the cornstarch in the cold water.
3. Heat the oil in a large wok or skillet over high heat until the oil just starts to smoke. Add the chicken and cook, stirring constantly, until it is no longer pink on the surface, about 30 seconds. Add the broccoli and cook, stirring constantly, until it turns bright green and the chicken is half-cooked, about 2 minutes.
4. Pour in the broth mixture and cook for 2 minutes, stirring frequently.
5. Stir in the scallions and cornstarch mixture. Cook and stir until the sauce comes to a boil and thickens, and the chicken is cooked through, about 1 minute.
6. Sprinkle with the sesame seeds.

Per Serving Nutrition:

Fat:	14 g
Saturated Fat:	1 g
Cholesterol:	66 mg
Carbs:	18 g
Protein:	34 g
Fiber:	8 g
Sodium:	692 mg

Tips:

- Avoid buying broccoli with yellow tips. If it isn't fresh, it won't taste as good.
- Eating broccoli and other cruciferous vegetables regularly will help lower your risk of cancer.

THE WALKER'S WEIGHT-LOSS PLAN

To lose weight, your goal is to burn more calories a day than you eat. Remember these six essential factors:

1. CONTROL YOUR CALORIES. If you exercise three days a week or less and do only minimal daily activity, a good daily calorie level is 1,350. You could lose up to two pounds per week at this level. If you exercise four days a week by walking, jogging, or doing in-home cardio exercise, you could increase your calorie level to 1,600 each day and still lose up to two pounds per week.

2. INCREASE YOUR FIBER INTAKE. Choose high-fiber foods over low-fiber foods. Each gram of fiber eaten can cancel out nine calories from your daily caloric intake! Try high-fiber multigrain breakfast cereals, barley, whole-wheat bread, and fruits such as pears and raspberries. Eat four servings a week of legumes such as beans, peas, and lentils. Some ideas for how to get lentils into your diet include bean or lentil salad, vegetable chili, low-fat refried beans, baked beans, and bean burritos.

3. REPLACE HIGH-FAT FOODS WITH CHOICES THAT ARE LOWER IN FAT. Read all food labels and try to stay within the range of no more than 25 percent of your calories coming from fat. Good choices include: avocados, olives, peanut butter, and nuts. Try olive and canola oil for cooking, in your salad dressings, or on your bread. Favor unsalted nuts over chips or other snack foods.

4. EAT AT LEAST ONE FIBER-RICH FRUIT OR VEGETABLE EACH DAY. The choices are many! Carrots, sweet potatoes, squash, tomatoes, cantaloupes, apricots, oranges, grapefruit, papayas, red peppers, or broccoli.

5. ELIMINATE OR REDUCE SUGAR. Remember that too much sugar turns to fat!

6. REDUCE SALT. According to the USDA, too much sodium can elevate blood pressure and lead to stroke. Too much salt can also cause water retention. Avoid canned or pre-packaged foods in favor of the frozen or fresh variety. Read all food labels to make sure the sodium content is within reasonable limits. If you're trying to lose weight, you should have no more than 2,000 mg of sodium per day. Salt is literally in everything, so be careful when eating out and ask your waiter or waitress to "hold the salt" on your order.

THE WALKER'S WEIGHT-LOSS PLAN MENU

Recipes included on pages 508–11

MONDAY

Breakfast

1/2   grapefruit

1   slice whole wheat toast

1   tbsp. low-sugar or no-sugar-added fruit spread

Midmorning Snack

3/4   cup Concord grape juice

1   cup oatmeal

1   cup fat-free milk

Lunch

1   cup black bean soup

1   wedge cornbread

1   cup spinach salad topped with 1/2 cup orange sections

Midafternoon Snack

1   oz. reduced-fat cheddar cheese

2   tbsp. walnuts

1   apple

Dinner

1   cup cooked whole wheat pasta shells tossed with 1 tbsp. olive oil and 2 cloves garlic

1   cup broccoli

1/2   cup red bell pepper slices

Evening Snack

1   cup reduced-sodium tomato juice

4   whole wheat crackers

Nutrition Information:

Calories:	1506
Fat:	45 g
Saturated Fat:	10 g
Fiber:	23 g
Sodium:	2168 mg

Tips:

- To find whole wheat bread, check the ingredients list; the first ingredient should be "whole wheat flour."
- Concord grape juice has almost five times the antioxidant power of orange juice.
- Today's improved reduced-fat cheeses taste as good as the real thing.
- Eating mini-meals (at breakfast, midmorning snack, lunch, midafternoon snack, dinner, and evening snack) may help prevent weight gain.
- Chop garlic, then let it "rest" for 15 minutes before cooking so that healing phytochemicals have a chance to develop.
- Processed tomato products are concentrated sources of lycopene, a likely prostate cancer fighter.

TUESDAY

Breakfast

- 1/2 whole wheat English muffin
- 1 tsp. trans-free margarine or non-fat butter spray
- 1 poached or hard-cooked egg or 1/2 cup EggBeaters
- 1 pear

Midmorning Snack

- 1/2 cup low-fat vanilla yogurt
- 1/2 cup low-fat granola

Lunch

- 2 slices whole wheat bread with 2 oz. reduced-fat mozzarella cheese and 1 roasted bell pepper (packed in water) or fresh basil leaves

Midafternoon Snack

- 1/4 cup hummus
- 1/2 cup cucumber slices

Dinner

- 3 oz. poached salmon
- 1 cup brown rice
- 1/2 cup no-salt-added stewed tomatoes
- 1 cup steamed kale

Evening Snack

- 1/2 cup calcium-fortified orange juice
- 1 banana

Nutrition Information:

Calories: 1506
Fat: 38 g
Saturated fat: 10 g
Fiber: 21 g
Sodium: 1337 mg

Tips:

- Check ingredients lists; look for margarine without the words "partially hydrogenated."
- Mix your yogurt and granola the night before and freeze. By the time you get ready to eat your snack at work, it should be defrosted.
- Choosing fruits and vegetables with vivid colors helps you zero in on the nutrient powerhouses.
- The Italian section of the ethnic food aisle has ready-to-eat jarred red bell peppers. If you're concerned with sodium levels, and the sodium is high on the pre-prepared items, stick with fresh vegetables.
- Look for calcium-fortified red grapefruit juice too.
- Poaching is very healthy and quite easy. Bring water (enough to cover the fish), a bay leaf, a lemon slice, and a little salt or salt substitute to a boil in a skillet. Lower to a simmer; then place the fish in the liquid. Cook gently for about 8 minutes or until cooked through.

WEDNESDAY

Breakfast

- 3/4   cup hot whole wheat cereal
- 1/2   cup frozen blueberries, thawed
- 1   cup fat-free milk

Midmorning Snack

- 1   slice toasted whole wheat raisin bread
- 1   tbsp. natural or low-fat peanut butter

Lunch

- 1   small bean burrito
- 8   grape tomatoes, halved and tossed with 2 oz. crumbled reduced-fat feta cheese

Midafternoon Snack

- 1 serving Papaya Power Shake*

Dinner

- 2   oz. roasted chicken breast
- 1   cup mashed butternut squash
- 1   cup brussels sprouts
- 1/2   cup corn kernels mixed with 1/4 cup cooked barley and 2 tsp. canola oil

Evening Snack

- 1   extra large baked apple with 2 tsp. honey or brown sugar

Nutrition Information:

Calories: 1529
Fat: 45 g
Saturated Fat: 15 g
Fiber: 30 g
Sodium: 2609 mg

Tips:

- Blueberries are the top source of antioxidants among all fruits and vegetables.
- Choose natural peanut butter to avoid trans-fatty acids.
- Healthy microwavable burritos are available in the frozen food case.

THURSDAY

Breakfast

- 1/2 toasted whole wheat bagel topped with 1/4 cup reduced-fat ricotta cheese
- 3 finely chopped prunes

Midmorning Snack

- 1 cup low-fat plain yogurt with 1/2 sliced banana and 1 tbsp. chopped walnuts

Lunch

Pasta salad made with:

- 1 cup cooked whole wheat rotini or pasta spirals
- 1/2 cup broccoli
- 1/2 cup yellow bell pepper
- 1/2 tomato, chopped
- 1 tbsp. olive oil
- 1 tsp. vinegar

Midafternoon Snack

- 2 rye crispbread sheets
- 2 tbsp. light cream cheese
- 1/2 cup frozen strawberries, thawed

Dinner

- 1 serving Carrot Soup with Lime and Chiles*
- 6 large shrimp broiled with 1 tbsp.of low-sodium teriyaki sauce
- 1 cup cooked whole wheat couscous
- 1/2 cup green peas

Evening Snack

- 1/2 cup pear slices tossed with 1/2 oz. blue cheese or brie

Nutrition Information:

Calories:	1586
Fat:	46 g
Saturated fat:	15 g
Fiber:	28 g
Sodium:	1803 mg

Tips:

- For an extra flavor boost, try lemon- or orange-flavored prunes.
- Lightly toasting walnuts in a small skillet for a few minutes really brings out the flavor.
- If you are cooking for just one or two, it makes sense to grab vegetables from the supermarket salad bar.
- Look for brands with 4–5 grams of fiber per two-cracker serving, such as WASA Fiber Rye Crispbread and Natural Rye crisp crackers.

FRIDAY

Breakfast

- 1 cup fat-free milk
- 1 Raisin Bran Muffin*
- 1/2 cup grapes

Midmorning Snack

- 1 slice toasted cracked-wheat bread topped with
  1/2 mashed banana
- 1 tangerine

Lunch

- 1 cup tabbouleh
- 1 raw carrot
- 1 whole wheat pita round

Midafternoon Snack

- 1 cup reduced-sodium tomato soup made with
  1/3 cup fat-free milk
- 8 rye crisp rounds

Dinner

- 1 serving Spicy Lentils*
- 1/2 cup brown rice
- 1 cup steamed spinach mixed with
  1/2 cup diced canned tomatoes

Evening Snack

- 1 brown rice cake
- 1/2 oz. reduced-fat cheddar cheese

Nutritional Information:

Calories: 1523
Fat: 22 g
Saturated fat: 3.8 g
Fiber: 26 g
Sodium: 2869 mg

Tips:

- Make a batch of tabbouleh from a mix (available in the rice aisle), but substitute lemon juice for some oil.
- Rice cakes have exploded with flavors in the past few years, so take your pick.
- In the winter, canned tomatoes have far more flavor than fresh.
- The instant versions of bean soup that require only boiling water are great! But watch the sodium levels!

THE WALKER'S WEIGHT-LOSS PLAN MENU RECIPES

Carrot Soup with Lime and Chiles

Papaya Power Shake

Raisin Bran Muffins

Spicy Lentils

Carrot Soup with Lime and Chiles

Ingredients:

1	tbsp. olive or canola oil
1	large onion, finely chopped
2	large cloves garlic, chopped*
1/2	lb. peeled, ready-to-eat baby carrots
1/2	cup uncooked instant brown rice
2	cans (14.5 oz. each) fat-free, reduced-sodium chicken broth
1	cup water
1/2	tsp. salt or salt substitute
1	tbsp. chopped green chilies
	juice of 1 lime (about 2 tbsp.)

Serves: 4
Calories Per Serving: 130
Preparation Time: 35 minutes
Difficulty: Easy

* *1 tbsp. prepared chopped garlic can be substituted*

Cooking Instructions:

1. Heat the oil in a large nonstick saucepan over medium heat. Add the onion and sauté for 3 minutes. Add the garlic and sauté 1 minute longer.
2. Add the carrots, rice, broth, water, and salt to the saucepan. Bring to a boil; then reduce the heat to medium low. Simmer, partially covered, for 20 minutes, or until the carrots are tender. Stir in the chilies and lime juice.
3. Puree the soup in a food processor or blender. The best method is to place half of the solids in the food processor and add just enough of the broth to liquefy the carrots and rice. Add the rest of the solids; then stir the puree back into the remaining broth.

4. Reheat if necessary. Serve warm. If desired, garnish with chopped fresh cilantro, thinly sliced scallions, a dollop of plain yogurt, and additional chopped chili peppers.

Per Serving Nutrition:

Fat:	4 g
Saturated Fat:	0.5 g
Cholesterol:	0 mg
Carbs:	21 g
Protein:	5 g
Fiber:	3 g
Sodium:	717 mg*

*Using a salt substitute will lower the total sodium.

Papaya Power Shake

Ingredients:

1	papaya, peeled, seeded, and cut up
1	cup low-fat plain yogurt
1/2	banana
1/2	cup no-sugar-added pineapple chunks
1/2	tsp. dried mint
4	ice cubes, slightly crushed

Serves: 4
Calories Per Serving: 88
Preparation Time: 5 minutes
Difficulty: Easy

Cooking Instructions:

1. Combine all ingredients in a blender and process until smooth.

Per Serving Nutrition:

Fat:	1 g
Saturated Fat	1 g
Cholesterol:	4 mg
Carbs:	17 g
Protein:	4 g
Fiber:	2 g
Sodium:	44 mg

Tip:

- This shake also works well with canned mango spears, which are available in the produce aisle of most supermarkets.

Raisin Bran Muffins

Ingredients:

1   cup low-fat buttermilk

3/4   cup bud-style bran cereal (such as Bran Buds, 100% Bran, or Fiber One)

1/2   cup golden raisins

1/2   cup shredded carrots

1   egg or 1/4 cup EggBeaters

1/3   cup honey

1/4   cup canola oil

1   tsp. vanilla extract

1   cup whole wheat flour

1   tsp. baking soda

1   tsp. ground cinnamon

1   tbsp. honey-crunch wheat germ (optional)

> Serves: 12 muffins
> Calories per Serving: 164
> Preparation Time: 45 minutes
> Difficulty: Easy

Cooking Instructions:

1. Preheat the oven to 425°F. Line a 12-cup muffin pan with paper liners; coat the papers with cooking spray.
2. In a medium bowl, combine the buttermilk, cereal, raisins, carrots, egg, honey, oil, and vanilla extract. Let it stand for 15 minutes.
3. In a large bowl, combine the flour, baking soda, and cinnamon. Make a well in the center and add the buttermilk mixture all at once. Stir just enough to moisten the flour.
4. Divide the batter evenly among the muffin cups. Sprinkle the tops with wheat germ. Bake for 15–20 minutes, or until a toothpick inserted in the center comes out clean.

Per Serving Nutrition:

Fat:	6 g
Saturated Fat:	1 g
Cholesterol:	18 mg
Carbs:	28 g
Protein:	4 g
Fiber:	3 g
Sodium:	131 mg

Tips:

- If you can't find high-fiber/low-sugar oat bran muffins, these are a great substitute.
- Make a double batch of these for fast breakfast treats.

Spicy Lentils

Ingredients:

1	tbsp. canola oil
1	cup onion, finely chopped
2	tsp. ground ginger
1	tsp. ground cumin
1	cup dried red or brown lentils
3	cups water
3/4	tsp. salt or salt substitute
2	tbsp. fresh cilantro, finely chopped
1	tbsp. lemon juice

Serves: 4
Calories Per Serving: 167
Preparation Time: 35 minutes
Difficulty: Easy

Cooking Instructions:

1. Heat the oil in a medium saucepan. Add the onion and sauté, stirring often, for 5 minutes or until tender. Stir in the ginger and cumin and sauté 30 seconds longer.
2. Add the lentils, water, and salt. Heat to a boil. Reduce the heat to low and simmer, partially covered, for 15 minutes.
3. If the lentils are tender, uncover and gently boil until most of the liquid evaporates. If the lentils are too hard, continue to cook, partially covered, ten minutes longer or until lentils are tender.*
4. Remove lentils from heat and stir in cilantro and lemon juice. Serve warm. Serve this soupy, stew-like dish in a shallow bowl over brown rice.

* Cooking time for lentils can vary from 15 minutes to as long as 1 hour, depending on the type and age of the lentils. Red lentils (which turn yellow when cooked) cook very quickly because they are split, and after 15 to 20 minutes, they soften to a puree. Brown lentils hold their shape better but can take longer to cook.

Per Serving Nutrition:

Fat:	4 g
Saturated Fat:	0 g
Cholesterol:	0 mg
Carbs:	25 g
Protein:	10 g
Fiber:	6 g
Sodium:	406 mg

Physical Exercises

THE TEN-MINUTE WORKOUT

Tone up and trim down! Set aside a few minutes several times a day for these great exercises and you'll shed those excess pounds! Remember: keep your routine short and simple. Have weights handy and do any combination of these simple exercises at structured or random times. Over time you will notice better muscle tone and increased strength.

Lean muscle has very little fat and burns more calories than underdeveloped muscle. Keeping your muscles lean requires physical resistance that can be achieved by lifting light weights several minutes daily. If you have your doctor's permission, you can follow this simple workout.

1. BICEPS. You need three-pound, four-pound, or five-pound hand weights, or equivalent weights using water or sand-filled plastic bottles. A half-gallon container filled with water weighs about four and a half pounds. A sand-filled plastic half-gallon container weighs seven and a half pounds. Double these weight amounts for a gallon size. You do not have to fill the containers completely; approximate and determine a comfortable weight.

Keeping your arms down at your sides, hold one weight in each hand against each thigh. Slowly lift your arms parallel to the floor or ground. Slowly return your arms to the original position. Repeat gradually five to ten times.

Hold weights next to your thighs (starting position). Bend your arms up and then continue the motion to lift weights over your head. Repeat slowly five to ten times.

2. TRICEPS. Hold weights next to your thighs. Slowly raise both forearms so they are parallel to the floor or ground and make a 90-degree angle. Slowly lower weights to the starting position. Return to the 90-degree angle and repeat movement five to ten times. Hold weights with your arms extended downward. Slowly shrug your shoulders (lifting weights with shoulder muscles). Repeat five to ten times.

3. LEGS. Hold weights against thighs. Slowly squat; then rise. (Do not squat to a position that is uncomfortable.) Repeat five to ten times. Using weights, bend your arms up and hold weights against your chest. Slowly slide one leg forward as far as you comfortably can while keeping the other leg stationary; then return your leg to the starting position. Repeat movement with other leg. Repeat five to ten times per leg.

4. ARM CURL. Hold weights and extend arms downward at sides with palms facing forward. Alternately curl weights in each arm upward while keeping elbows at the same level each time. Slowly repeat five to ten times per each arm.

5. ANKLE WEIGHTS. Strap a light ankle weight on each leg, and do leg lifts standing or sitting; move legs to the side one at a time while standing, or together when sitting. Slowly repeat movements five to ten times. Do not overdo this exercise!

THE IN-HOME CARDIO ROUTINE

If you prefer to exercise at home or need to stay indoors because of bad weather, try this in-home cardio routine. Set aside twenty to thirty minutes. It's okay if you're not able to go the full thirty-minute session at first. Remember, any movement is better than none!

Begin at a level you can maintain. Then slowly add a few minutes to each session. Do each of the moves for two to three minutes, alternating options throughout. Rotate your schedule between doing this routine two days a week and walking the other two days. This rotation schedule will provide variety as well as alternate the workout for your muscles.

Eight options

MARCHING OR RUNNING IN PLACE. This is great as a warm-up before your routine starts. Be sure to work your whole body by pumping your arms and getting your knees nice and high.

CROSSOVERS. Stand and place your hands behind your head. Lift your left knee up to your right elbow and then lower it again. Do the same with the other side of your body. Repeat for two to three minutes. (You'll find this also works on your waistline!)

KICKS. Stand and bring your fists to the level of your chest (as if you are blocking an imaginary opponent). Raise your left knee to your waist and then kick your lower leg forward to extend your leg. Tighten your abs as you kick in the air. Lower and repeat with the other leg. Repeat for two to three minutes, continuing to switch legs. (This move is called a front kick in kickboxing.)

PUNCHES. Bend your knees slightly and punch forward with your right arm (imagine you're boxing). Release and repeat with your left arm. Do this exercise for two to three minutes. (You'll find this routine great for toning your arms.)

JUMP ROPE. Skipping rope is great for the whole body. To bring in variety, try jogging or skipping like a boxer as you jump. Continue for two to three minutes.

JUMP SQUATS. Stand with your feet together and arms at your sides. Then squat as if you are going to sit in a chair. Keep your abs pulled in and your torso straight. Jump up into the air, land, and repeat. Slightly bend your knees as you land to minimize the impact. Continue for two to three minutes. (You may find this exercise challenging, but do the best you can. You'll find it's great for your rear end!)

WAIST TWISTS. Imagine you're skiing down a hill. Place your feet together and lightly jump and pivot your knees and toes to the right. Lift your right elbow out to the right (at shoulder height) and extend your left arm out to the left at the same time. Repeat the move in the opposite direction without lowering your arms. Continue for two to three minutes.

JACK-IN-THE-BOX. Squat as though you're sitting in a chair, keeping your feet together. Then jump up and spread your hands and feet out so you make an X with your arms and legs (like a jumping jack). Repeat for two to three minutes. (You'll find this exercise great for your inner and outer thighs!)

PRACTICE RELAXATION

Relaxation is a great substitute for overeating. The problem is many of us don't know how to relax. We become fidgety and bored and end up reaching for food. When a highly stressful period hits (at work, for instance), put a time limit on the amount of time you will give to thinking about it. To relax in spite of the stress, build into your day moments of distraction and practice relaxation exercises.

Deep Muscle Relaxation

There are a number of easy relaxation exercises you can do to de-stress without using food. If you carry stress in your physical body, deep muscle relaxation may be for you. It's easy to do. Just clench your fist, hold it tense, and then relax it. Do this again and then move on to another muscle in your body. In deep muscle relaxation, you are taking each muscle group, tensing it, and then releasing it. This exercise teaches you the difference between tension and relaxation. Practice deep muscle relaxation up to thirty minutes a day if you carry a lot of tension in your body. You can practice in the morning when you wake up and start your day refreshed, or you can practice in the evening before bedtime to calm yourself down. The more you practice, the easier it will become for you to relax.

Deep Breathing

Another easy technique is deep breathing. Slowly inhale and breathe deeply from your abdomen—now you are deep breathing. When we get tense, we tend to take short, shallow breaths from our chest. But deep breathing is slow and originates in the abdomen. When you feel stressed and want to eat, take a few deep breaths and relax your body. Do this several times a day if need be. The great thing about deep breathing is you can do it anywhere—in traffic, at work, in the house, or even in the park.

LOSE WEIGHT IN JUST THIRTY DAYS˙

Walking is easy, cheap, convenient, and not likely to result in injury. Rebecca Gorrell, director of fitness and movement therapy at Canyon Ranch in Tucson, Arizona, helped develop three walking workouts guaranteed to have you dropping pounds in just thirty days.

The higher the intensity of your walk, the more calories you'll burn. But how do you know at what intensity you're working? An easy, low-tech method to use is the Borg Scale for Rate of Perceived Exertion (RPE). No arithmetic or heart-rate monitors are needed.

To use it, monitor your body and consider how hard you are working. Is your breathing heavy? Are you sweating? Do your muscles feel warm? Are they burning? Now, rate how you feel.

˙ All walking plans are adapted from www.LoseItForLife.com.

Borg Scale for Rate of Perceived Exertion (RPE)	
6 7 8	Very, very light (lounging on the couch)
9 10	Very light (puttering around the house)
11 12	Fairly light (strolling leisurely)
13 14	Somewhat hard (normal walking)
15 16	Hard (walking as if in a hurry)
17 18	Very hard (jogging/running)
19 20	Very, very hard (sprinting)

Borg RPE scale, © Gunnar Borg, 1970, 1985, 1994, 1998.

Week #	Time	Length	Plateau-Busting Plan	RPE*
Week 1	35 min.	5 days	Warm-up (5 min.)	10–11
			Normal walk (5 min.)	13
			Speed up (5 min.)	15
			Recovery (10 min.)	13
			Speed up (5 min.)	15
			Cool-down (5 min.)	0–11
Week 2	35 min.	5 days	Warm-up (5 min.)	10–11
			Normal walk (5 min.)	13
			Speed up (5 min.)	16
			Recovery (10 min.)	13
			Speed up (5 min.)	16
			Cool-down (5 min.)	10–11
Week 3	45 min.	5 days	Warm-up (5 min.)	10–11
			Normal walk (5 min.)	13
			Speed up (5 min.)	16
			Recovery (8 min.)	13
			Speed up (5 min.)	16
			Recovery (7 min.)	13
			Speed up (5 min.)	16
			Cool-down (5 min.)	10–11
Week 4	45 min.	5 days	Warm-up (5 min.)	10–11
			Speed up (5 min.)	16
			Recovery (5 min.)	13
			Speed up (5 min.)	16
			Recovery (5 min.)	13
			Speed up (5 min.)	16
			Recovery (5 min.)	13
			Speed up (5 min.)	16
			Cool-down (5 min.)	10–11

*RPE is Rate of Perceived Exertion

Plan #1: The Plateau-Busting Plan

Have you stopped losing weight even though you regularly walk? Perhaps you've reached a plateau. Try adding intervals to your program or increase your pace. Set new goals to achieve increased weight loss.

Plan #2: The Muscle-Toning Circuit Plan

Shape your muscles when you walk! This plan is for you if you want firmer muscles, need some variety, and have been walking regularly. Try the different techniques in the muscle-toning circuit to firm up your muscles (toning exercises follow chart).

Week #	Time	Length	Muscle-Toning Circuit Plan (See below for exercise descriptions.)	RPE*
Week 1	30 min.	5 days	2 min. each segment	13–15
Week 2	40 min.	5 days	3 min. each segment	13–15
Week 3	50 min.	5 days	4 min. each segment	13–15
Week 4	60 min.	5 days	5 min. each segment	13–15

*RPE is Rate of Perceived Exertion

EXERCISE DESCRIPTIONS

1. HILLS OR STAIR CLIMBING firms up the fronts and backs of your calves and thighs.

2. RACE WALKING shapes your abdomen and upper back muscles. You race walk by taking shorter, quicker steps. Use your arms for more power, keeping them bent at 85- to 90-degree angles.

3. THE BUTT SQUEEZE tones the gluteus muscles. Use your normal walking form, but as you press off the toes of your back leg, squeeze your buttocks firmly. Be careful not to tense your lower back.

4. BACKWARD WALKING strengthens the back and abdomen. Do your walk backward. Tuck your belly in and put your hands on your hips. You'll find your abs and back doing all the work. For safety, try this only on a level track or path.

Plan #3: The Incline Walking Plan

Take your walking exercise to the next level and burn up to 50 percent more calories in the process by raising the incline on the treadmill in your home or gym. Follow this routine every other day, and you will want to rest your muscles between these workouts.

STEP ONE: Before adding your first hill, start out with a five-minute slow walk. Use a brisk pace for ten minutes.

STEP TWO: Begin with five minutes of level walking. Add five minutes of walking hills. Try to maintain the same speed whether walking level or at an incline. At first, you may only be able to walk a 1 percent incline. A great goal is a 5 percent incline. Please don't do more than a 7 percent incline—steeper inclines will put too much strain on your back, hips, and ankles.

STEP THREE: Alternate the level walking and the incline walking, going as long as you can. Of course, the longer you go, the better the workout! Cool down for five more minutes.

STEP FOUR: Stretch for at least ten minutes when you are done, focusing on the muscles in your lower body, back, and shoulders.

Dysfunctional Thought Record[3]

Date	Situation	Emotion / Intensity	Automatic Thought	Rational Response / Intensity	Outcome

3 Beck, A.T., Rush, A.J., Shaw, B.F., & Emory, G. *Cognitive Therapy of Depression*. New York: Guilford. 1979.

The Healthy 100s
Diet and Weight-Loss Plan

By

Stephen Arterburn, M.Ed.

INTRODUCTION

Most of us who struggle with losing weight and keeping it off realize that the only way to lose weight is to burn off more calories than we take in. We go through all sorts of gyrations to make that possible, but they all either help us burn more calories than we take in or they don't. Over the long haul, most of them don't. Most of them only benefit us temporarily, if you call short-term progress then disappointment a benefit. But here is the irrefutable truth about weight-loss attempts and plans. If what goes in equals what burns up, weight stays the same. And of course if more calories go in than are burned up, fat arrives and hangs around. If this is true, then it seems that all of us weight warriors would be quite proficient at calorie counting. It should be second nature to us or almost like a second language. But if you are like me, you only know the calorie count of fewer than twenty foods unless the count is stated boldly on the bag or bottle.

It makes sense that the more we know about calorie content of a lot of foods, the better decisions we can make about selection and portion size. We need a way to learn the calorie content of most of the food we eat. (Just a warning: nothing I present here reverses the law that the best-tasting stuff usually contains the most calories.) Additionally we need to know many different exercises to burn off calories, and we need to know how long we have to exercise to burn off the amount we need to burn. And to add to our knowledge, we need to know how many calories are burned off from participating in various activities such as mowing a lawn, washing a dog, or painting a house. If we know how to easily make these calculations, we can modulate our activity to overcome our calorie intake. The more we know, the more likely it is we will be effective in our efforts to lose weight and keep it off.

For years, people have written, e-mailed, tweeted, and Facebooked their desire for Lose It for Life to have a specific diet and weight-loss plan. We have always been for anything that works. Now we are for this specific plan because, like the rest of the material in the book, this is something that can be done for the rest of your life. And if you can't do it for the rest of your life, why do it at all?

You may be stuck in your weight loss or stuck in your head and starting to gain again. You may have tried so many things to get back on track that you don't remember what the track is or where and how you got off it. So I have tried to provide a way for you to learn a plan that is easy to remember and hard to forget.

There is an old saying we have all heard: "A picture is worth a thousand words." I think pictures might be worth getting a thousand or more calories out of your diet. Here is how the concept works. If I ask you to memorize all the various calorie content numbers of one hundred foods, it would be very difficult to remember all of those numbers if they have no pattern or flow to help in the memory process. But there is a way to remember calorie content, and you will find it easy to accomplish.

If I told you that most doughnuts have around 300 calories, you might remember that the next time you had one; but over time that number would most likely fade. But if the only thing you were ever concerned with were 100-calorie portions, you would only have to memorize one number: the number 100. Everything we do in this plan revolves around 100-calorie portions of food. But here is the good news. You might forget that a whole doughnut has about 300 calories, but if I show you a picture of one-third of a doughnut, that picture will stick in your head (if you are able to stick things there). We don't tend to forget pictures. So I have provided you with some pictures of some 100-calorie portions of food. (There is an expanded list in my book *The Healthy 100s*.)

If we can look a few times at the portions, we are likely to remember them for much longer than we can remember a number. Similarly if I ask you to memorize a list of calorie-burn numbers associated with exercises and activities, you would have a hard time keeping those in the current memory bank. You would have to learn calories plus duration plus intensity. But if the only number you have to remember, in addition to 100, is the time, it will be twice as easy to grasp how much to do each exercise to accomplish your goal. So I have also provided a list of exercises that each burn off 100 calories at a time.

Once again, the key here is that I have made the calculations simple by only presenting what 100 calories looks like. I have provided pictures of 100 foods in 100-calorie portions. If you study these pictures, I think you will agree that a picture is worth a thousand calories.

I want to see you grow on the inside while you shrink on the outside. I hope this appendix makes it all easier and more effective for a lifetime. If this helps you, please let me know at SArterburn@newlife.com.

THE 100-CALORIE FOOD

Following this section are the foods in their most one hundredly form. Take a look. Take a few looks. Then determine to memorize what these portions look like. If you don't memorize them, memorize the ones you eat the most. It might be best to imagine a dinner table set for ten—or, if you are really bright (or just have an effectively working memory) you might imagine a dinner table set for twenty. Imagine a different 100-calorie portion on each plate. You might even want to put the foods on the table in alphabetical order. Give it a try. Once you have one table set and served, pick a different style of table and silverware and china, and set and serve another table of 100-calorie portions. Then set another and another until you have learned as many of the 100-calorie portions as possible. All I ask is that you try this method before you discount it. I think you are going to be surprised at how easy it is to recall those portions around the table.

100-CALORIE PORTION INDEX

Plate: 8" side plate   Spoon: 1 Tbsp.   Glass: 12 oz.   Ramekin: 5 oz

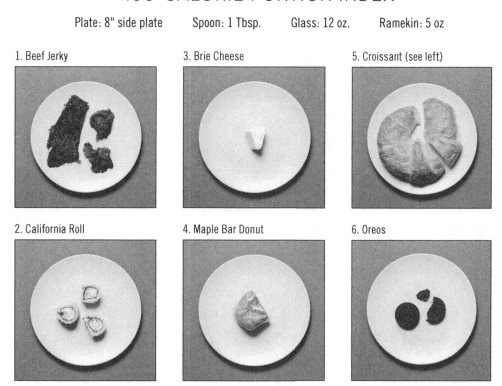

1. Beef Jerky   3. Brie Cheese   5. Croissant (see left)

2. California Roll   4. Maple Bar Donut   6. Oreos

7. Frozen Waffle

11. Roasted Butternut Squash

15. Meatballs in Tomato Sauce

8. Potato Chips

12. Mac 'n' Cheese

16. Sweet Potato Fries

9. Marinated Tofu

13. Chips and Salsa

17. Breaded Chicken Tender

10. Apple Slices

14. Veggie Patty

18. Popcorn Shrimp

19. Orange Slices

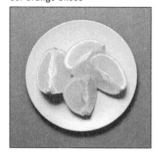

23. Baby Carrots

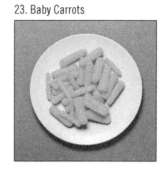

27. Greek Salad

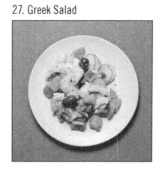

20. Avocado (see left)

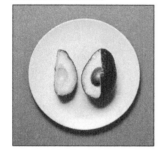

24. Blueberry Muffin (see top)

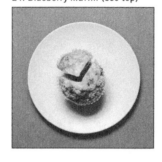

28. Cheese Ravioli

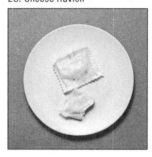

21. Corn Cob

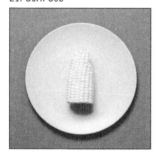

25. Deli Turkey Meat

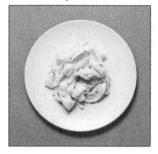

29. Cracker + Cheddar

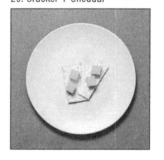

22. Bean and Cheese Burrito (right)

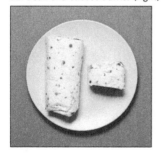

26. Salami

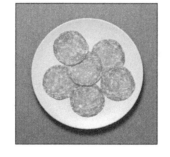

30. Peanut Butter and Jelly Sandwich

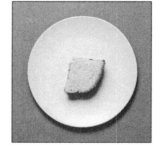

31. Roasted Chicken Breast, no skin

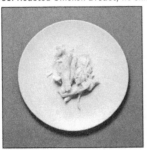

35. Coleslaw

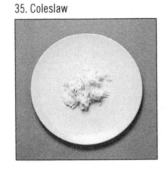

39. Vegetarian Lasagna

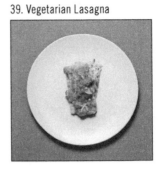

32. Roasted Chicken Breast, with skin

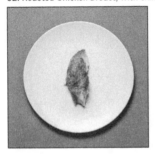

36. Hot Dog (see top)

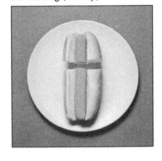

40. Steamed Broccoli

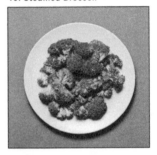

33. Chicken Breakfast Sausage

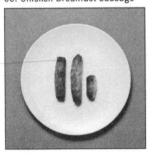

37. Cheese Crackers

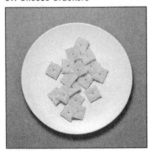

41. Bacon

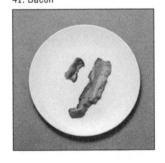

34. Edamame Beans

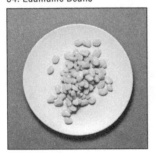

38. Caesar Salad

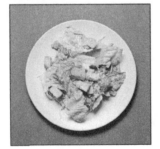

42. BBQ Chicken Pizza

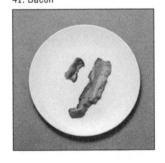

43. Scrambled Egg Whites

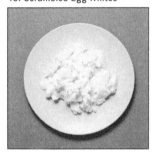

47. Salmon Filet

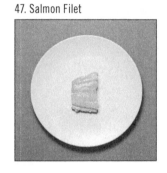

51. Trail Mix

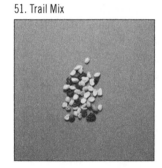

44. Hard-Boiled Egg

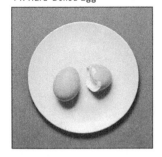

48. Marinated Flank Steak

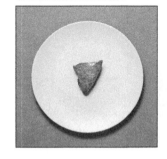

52. Peanut M&Ms

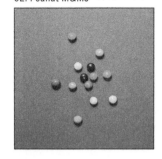

45. Chicken Patty

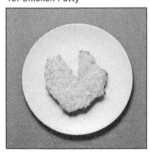

49. Dill Pickles

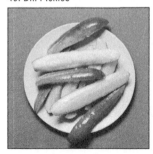

53. Banana

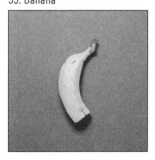

46. Canned Tuna, in water

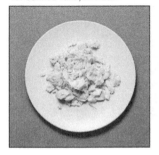

50. Whole Grain Bread

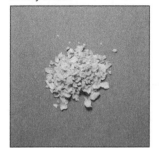

54. Dry Cereal

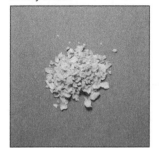

55. Spaghetti Noodles

59. Roasted Peanuts

63. Microwave Popcorn

56. Wheat Crackers

60. English Muffin

64. Red Grapes

57. Gummy Bears

61. Boiled Baby Potatoes

65. Chocolate Covered Pretzels

58. Pretzel Rods

62. Blueberries

66. Chocolate Chips

67. Snickers Bar (top)

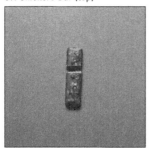

68. Oatmeal Raisin Cookie

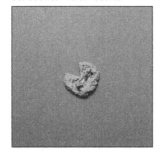

69. Low Moisture String Cheese

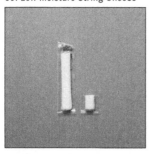

70. Granola Bar (top)

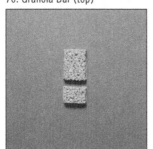

71. Small, Fresh Mango

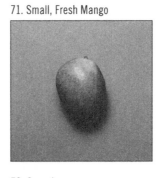

72. Granola

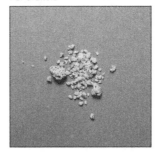

73. White Rice, Uncooked

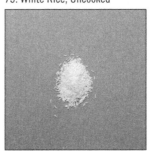

74. Butter

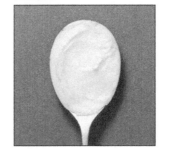

75. Canola Oil

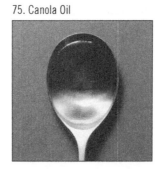

76. Peanut Butter

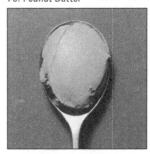

77. Ranch Dressing

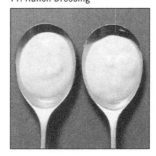

78. Honey

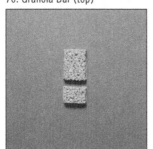

79. Low-fat Chocolate Milk

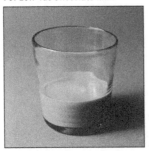

83. Light Beer

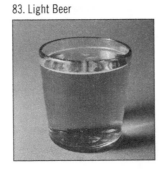

87. Chocolate Pudding

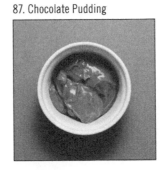

80. Coca-Cola

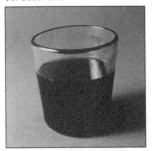

84. Low-fat Milk

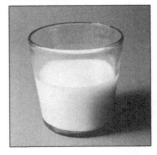

88. Beef Chili

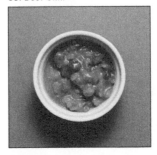

81. Orange Juice

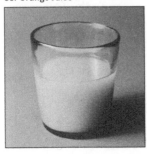

85. Unsweetened Soymilk

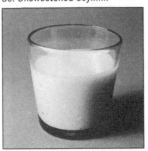

89. Baked Beans

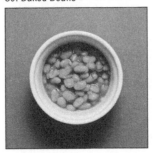

82. Sports Drink

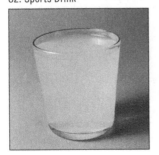

86. White Wine

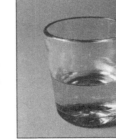

90. Lentils, Cooked

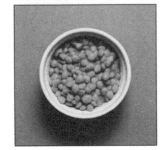

91. Teriyaki

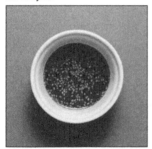

95. Cookies 'n' Cream Ice Cream

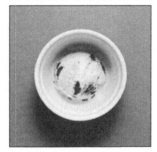

98. Blueberry Jam

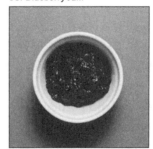

92. BBQ Sauce

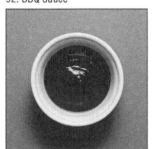

96. Hummus

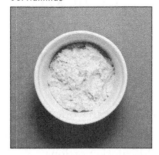

99. Brown Sugar

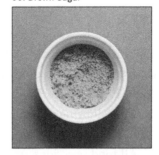

93. Low-fat Yogurt

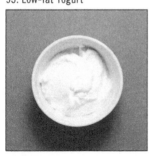

97. Steel-Cut Oats

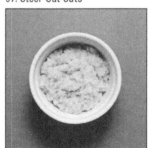

100. Ketchup

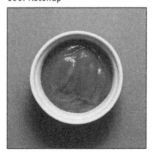

94. Black Bean Soup

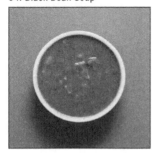

SHOPPING

In addition to these handy pictures, there is good news at the supermarket. There is a trend in the grocery store to help you with your Healthy 100s project. Everything from chips to nuts is prepackaged in 100-calorie portions. These are particularly prevalent in the snack sections of the store. They make it easy to stock the cabinets with goodies you love in a portion size you can use. I especially love the popcorn bags in 100-calorie portions. (But watch the salt content.)

THE PLAN

There is no rocket science here. If you eat in 100-calorie portions and you are on a 1,200-calorie diet, you make twelve 100 calorie selections a day in the area of food, while you can choose unlimited portions of water. Seem too sparse? Then try the 1,800, 2,400, or the 3,600 version.

The following example of how this can work with a 2,400-calorie diet (even though it is so ridiculously simple, I probably don't really need to spell it out.)

All food selections are in 100-calorie portions.

Breakfast

2/3 cup plain low-fat yogurt
2 cups of raspberries
1 hard-boiled egg
1 slice toast with 1 tsp. of jam

Morning Snack

1 small banana
20 roasted peanuts
1 cup of orange juice

Lunch

2.5 oz skinless chicken breast
45 steamed edamame beans
4 slices of pineapple
1 8-oz cup of 1% milk

Afternoon Snack

1/2 cantaloupe

2 tsp. peanut butter and one half apple

2 cups reduced-sugar cranberry cocktail

Dinner

1 small baked sweet potato

11/2 cups steamed chopped broccoli

3 oz. baked cod

4.5 oz glass of wine or 8 oz. Gatorade

1 slice of bread with 1 tsp. jam

2 Oreos or 100-calorie Oreo crisp pack

Bedtime Snack

25 seedless frozen grapes

1 cup non-fat yogurt

1 cup strawberries mixed into yogurt

A few observations about this 2,400-calorie food plan: first of all, you are eating every two to three hours, so you don't have to fill up at any one meal or snacktime, thinking you have to make it last for five hours until you get to eat or drink again. You will feel great about the blood sugar stability that comes from eating moderate amounts six times a day versus large amounts three times a day.

Secondly, there is a lot of food to be consumed in a day on this 2,400-calorie, 100-calorie portion diet. You stick to portion control at 100 and it is surprising how many things you get to eat in a day. You literally could do this for the rest of your life. And most people are going to lose weight on a 2,400-calorie diet if they are doing the right amount of exercise.

THE 100-CALORIE EXERCISES

Here are the activities that can burn 100 calories.

1. Brisk walk—15 minutes
2. Vacuum—25 minutes
3. Gardening—20 minutes

4. Doing housework—25 minutes
5. Ironing—25 minutes
6. Playing volleyball—12 minutes
7. Dancing—20 minutes
8. Running in place—12 minutes
9. Biking—20 minutes
10. Golfing—30 minutes
11. Swimming—15 minutes
12. Aerobics—10 minutes
13. Mowing—25 minutes
14. Painting—20 minutes
15. Weight Training—15 minutes
16. Playing Frisbee—30 minutes
17. Running a mile—12 minutes
18. Jumping rope—10 minutes
19. Climbing stairs—20 minutes
20. Window shopping—40 minutes

The bottom line is that if you can exercise for thirty minutes with any kind of intensity, you will most likely burn off 300 calories for the day.

The reality of the exercise burn and food consumption equation is that most people cannot exercise enough to lose a substantial amount of weight. To remove 1,200 calories from your body is much easier accomplished by not eating those calories in the first place rather than by trying to exercise that many calories off. So it is the combination of portion control and moderate exercise that seems to benefit the most people for the longest time.

A Final Note

There is a phrase that will keep you from losing and keeping weight off. That phrase is: "All I have to do is . . ." I have listened to overweight people utter that phrase as if it were a mantra. Part of the problem is that they don't ever do whatever they think is all that they have to do. Weight loss is not easy. It takes more than just an eating and exercise plan. It requires doing the work internally and relationally so that the loss is supported. So take this food and exercise plan only alongside the rest of the truths in the other sections of the book.

Notes

Getting Started

1. Nanci Hellmich, "Obesity in America Is Worse Than Ever," *USA Today*, October 9, 2002.
2. Mayo Clinic Women's Health Source. *Causes of Obesity* 6, no. 4 (April 2002).
3. Ibid.

Chapter 1: What Do You Have to Lose?

1. Nanci Hellmich, "Obesity in America Is Worse Than Ever," *USA Today*, October 9, 2002.
2. J. H. Crowther, E. M. Wolf, and N. Sherwood, "Epidemiology of Bulimia Nervosa," in M. Crowther, et al., eds., *The Etiology of Bulimia Nervosa: The Individual and Familial Context* (Washington, D.C.: Taylor & Francis, 1992), 1–26.
3. S. Arterburn and D. Stoop, *Seven Keys to Spiritual Renewal* (Wheaton, IL: Tyndale House Publishers, 1998).
4. Hellmich, "Obesity in America."

Chapter 2: Take the Red Pill

1. Fyodor Dostoevsky, *The Brothers Karamazov* (New York: Macmillan, 1922).
2. Tara Parker-Pope, "The Diet That Works: What Science Tells Us About Weight Loss," *Wall Street Journal*, April 22, 2003.
3. Ibid.
4. "Happy All the Time," words and music by A. B. Simpson. © 1990 New Spring, a division of Brentwood-Benson Music Publishing (ASCAP).
5. Dostoevsky, *The Brothers Karamazov*.

6. Parker-Pope, "The Diet That Works."

7. Ibid.

8. Simpson, "Happy All the Time."

Chapter 3: Lose Dieting (for Life!)

1. Adapted from Doreen Virtue, *Constant Craving A-Z* (Carlsbad, CA: Hay House, 1999), http://www.utexas.edu/student/cmhc/outreach/8traits.html.

2. Beth Moore, *Jesus, The One and Only* (Nashville: B&H Publishing, 2002), 211.

3. Ibid.

Chapter 4: The Doctor Is "In"

1. Mayo Clinic Women's Health Source, *Causes of Obesity* 6, no. 4 (April 2002).

2. http://instruct1.cit.cornell.edu/courses/ns421/BMR.html.

3. Ibid.

4. Patrick J. Bird, "Ask the Experts: Why Does Fat Deposit on the Thighs and Hips of Women and Around the Stomachs of Men?" Scientific American.com, http://www.scientificamerican.com/article.cfm?id=why-does-fat-deposit-on-t.

5. Ibid.

6. Denise Mann, "Stress May Cause Fat Around the Midsection in Lean Women," September 22, 2000, http://my.webmd.com/content/article/28/1728_ 61643 .htm?lastselectedguid={5FE84E90-BC77-4056A91C-9531713CA348}.

7. Lee Bowman, "Sleep Loss a Factor in Holiday Weight Gain," *Orange County Register*, December 25, 2002.

8. Robert K. Su, MD, posted in the Virginia Pain Clinic, Portsmouth, Virginia, 1985. Used with permission.

9. National Institute of Diabetes and Digestive and Kidney Diseases, "Do You Know the Health Risks of Being Overweight?" http://win.niddk.nih.gov/publications/health _risks.htm.

10. Ibid.

11. Ibid.

12. Ibid.

13. Ibid.

14. Ibid.

15. Ibid.

16. Ibid.

17. From the Metropolitan Life Insurance Company. See www.halls.md/ideal-weight/met .htm for the pros and cons of these charts.

18. Mayo Clinic Women's Health Source, *Causes of Obesity*.

19. http://instruct1.cit.cornell.edu/courses/ns421/BMR.html.

20. Ibid.

21. Bird, "Why Does Fat Deposit?"
22. Mann, "Stress May Cause Fat."
23. Su, Virginia Pain Clinic posting.
24. National Institute of Diabetes and Digestive and Kidney Diseases, "Do You Know?"
25. Ibid.
26. Ibid.
27. Ibid.
28. Ibid.
29. Ibid.

Chapter 5: Nutrition Transformed

1. Nancy Stedman, "The Hunger-Proof Diet," *Reader's Digest*, January 1999, 96.
2. Charles Platkin, "If You Want to Lose Weight, You Need More Than a Miracle Food," *The Honolulu Advisor*, Shape Up, November 27, 2002.
3. Lisa Davis, "Holy Cow, Look What Makes You Thin," *Reader's Digest*, July 2002, 107–11.
4. "'Oreos Too Dangerous for Our Kids,' Suit Says," *Orange County Register*, May 13, 2003.
5. Samantha Heller, "The Hidden Killer," *Men's Health*, September 2003, 116–18.
6. Jeffrey Kluger, "Fessing Up to Fats," *Time*, July 21, 2003.
7. Heller, "The Hidden Killer."
8. *The Society for Neuroscience*, "Brain Briefings: Sugar Addiction," October 2003, http://web.sfn.org/content/Publications/BrainBriefings/sugar.html.
9. Angela Pirisi, "A Real Sugar High?" *Psychology Today*, January 1, 2003, http://www.psychologytoday.com/articles/200301/real-sugar-high.
10. Carol Sorgen, "Snack Attack: Coping with Cravings," October 14, 2002, http://my.webmd.com/content/article/51/40783.htm?z=2731_00000_0000_ep_01.
11. M. B. Engler, *Journal of the American College of Nutrition* 23 (June 2004). News release, University of California, San Francisco, June 2004.
12. Felicity Stone, "Health Tip: Breakfast Benefits," *Forbes.com*, http://www.forbes.com/health/feeds/hscout/2004/05/20/hscout518894.html.
13. Tara Parker-Pope, "The Diet That Works: What Science Tells Us About Weight Loss," *Wall Street Journal*, April 22, 2003.
14. Nanci Hellmich, "'Clean Your Plate' Tradition Coming Back to Bite Us," *USA Today*, September 24, 2003.
15. *Men's Health*, Nutritional Briefs, May 2003, 50.
16. Parker-Pope, "The Diet That Works."
17. B. Wansink, "The Influence of Assortment Structure on Perceived Variety and Consumption Quantities," *Journal of Consumer Research* (March 2004).
18. ABC Online Home, News in Science, "Chocolate Cake Addiction: It's Real," April 24, 2004, http://www.abc.net.au/science/news/stories/s1091988.htm.

19. Nanci Hellmich, "10 Ways to Make It a Habit to Eat Less, Eat Better and Exercise More," *USA Today*, January 6, 2004.

20. Pirisi, "A Real Sugar High?"

21. *The Society for Neuroscience.* "Brain Briefings: Sugar Addiction."

22. Platkin, "If You Want to Lose Weight."

23. Davis, "Holy Cow."

24. "Oreos Too Dangerous."

25. Heller, "The Hidden Killer."

26. *Men's Health*, Nutritional Briefs.

Chapter 6: *Move It* and *Lose It*

1. Tara Parker-Pope, "The Diet That Works: What Science Tells Us About Weight Loss," *Wall Street Journal*, April 22, 2003.

2. Christopher Vaughan, "VA Study Points to Higher Fitness Levels as Predictor of Longer Life," *Stanford Report*, March 20, 2002, http://news.stanford.edu/news/2002/march20/HEART.html

3. J. M. Jakicic, et. al., "Prescribing Exercise in Multiple Short Bouts Versus One Continuous Bout: Effects on Adherence, Cardio Respiratory Fitness, and Weight Loss in Overweight Women," *International Journal of Obesity and Related Metabolic Disorders* (1995), 19, 893–901.

4. "How Much Exercise Is Enough?" http://www.mayoclinic.com/invoke.cfm?objectid=02ACDB54-6F65-438B-9E7613BC252B0842.

5. "Fitness Fundamentals," developed by the President's Council on Physical Fitness and Sports, http://www.hoptechno.com/book11.htm.

6. Nanci Hellmich, "Walking Off 'Secret Flab,'" *USA Today*, January 15, 2003.

7. Medline Plus, "Muscle Atrophy," http://www.nlm.nih.gov/medlineplus/ency/article/003188.htm.

8. "Exercise Fuels the Brain's Stress Buffers," APA online, Psychology in Daily Life, http://helping.apa.org/daily/neurala.html.

9. "Bulk Up Your Brain," REV, 19, March and April 2004, www.cnn.com/health.

10. J. Wilmore, "Exercise, Obesity and Weight Control," http://www.fitness.gov/activity/activity7/obesity/obesity.html.

11. The American Council on Exercise. "Fit Facts: Can Exercise Reduce Your Risk of Catching a Cold?" http://www.acefitness.org/fitfacts/fitfacts_ display.cfm?itemid=79.

12. "Aerobic Exercise: Why and How?" Mayoclinic.com, special to CNN.com Health Library, April 1, 2003, http://www.cnn.com/ HEALTH/library/EP/00002.html.

13. Quiz taken from www.LoseItForLife.com.

14. Atlantic Health Science Corporation, "My Heart, I Take Care of It," http://www.ahsc.health.nb.ca/hearthealth/highriskactivities.shtml.

15. "Fitness Fundamentals," developed by the President's Council on Physical Fitness and Sports.

16. Information taken from www.LoseItForLife.com.

17. Vicki Pierson, "Starting an Exercise Program," http://www.primusweb.com /fitnesspartner/library/activity/startexercise.htm.

18. Michael Stefano, "When It Comes to Exercise, Less Is More," http://www.seekwellness .com/fitness/less_is_more.htm.

19. "Walking, a Step in the Right Direction." NIH Publication No. 01-4155 (March 2001), http://www.niddk.nih.gov/health/nutrit/walking/walkingbro/walking.htm#okaywalk.

20. Wendy Bumgardner, "What Is Planter Fasciitis and Heel Spur?" http://walking.about .com/cs/heelpain/f/heelpain.htm.

21. "Fitness Fundamentals," developed by the President's Council on Physical Fitness and Sports.

22. J. Wilmore, "Exercise, Obesity and Weight Control."

Chapter 7: Coming Out (of the Eating Closet)

1. Carin Gorrell, "Sarah Ferguson, The Duchess Weighs In," *Psychology Today*, January/ February 2002, 35.

2. Based on questions adapted from Linda Mintle, *Breaking Free from Compulsive Overeating* (Lake Mary, FL: Charisma House, 2002).

Chapter 8: Changing the Viewing

1. Dr. Linda Mintle, Story adapted from *A Daughter's Journey Home* (Nashville, TN: Integrity, 2004).

2. A. T. Beck, et. al., *Cognitive Therapy of Depression* (New York: Guilford, 1979).

Chapter 10: Community—The Connection Cornerstone

1. R. Stuart, "Do Intimate Partners Help or Hinder Weight Loss?" *Psychology Today*, January/February 2002.

2. Ibid.

3. Ibid., 43.

CPSIA information can be obtained at www.ICGtesting.com
Printed in the USA
LVOW03s0740200814

399820LV00001B/1/P